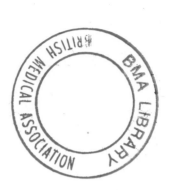
Clinical Radiology

for medical students
and health practitioners

second edition

William S C HARE

Professor Emeritus
The Department of Radiology
The University of Melbourne

b

Blackwell
Science
Asia

Distributors

Blackwell Science Asia Pty Ltd
54 University Street
Carlton, Victoria 3053, Australia

Orders: Tel: 03 9347 0300
         Fax: 03 9349 3016
         Email: info@blacksci-asia.com.au
         www.blackwell-science-asia.com

North America
Blackwell Science, Inc.
Commerce Place, 350 Main Street
Malden, MA 02148-5018

Orders: Tel: 617 388 8250
                 800 759 6102
         Fax: 617 388 8255

Canada
Copp Clark Professional
200 Adelaide Street, West, 3rd Floor
Toronto, Ontario M5H 1W7

Orders: Tel: 416 597 1616
                 800 815 9417
         Fax: 416 597 1616

United Kingdom
Marston Book Services Ltd
PO Box 87
Oxford OX2 0DT

Orders: Tel: 01865 791155
         Fax: 01865 791927
         Telex: 837515

©1999 by
Blackwell Science Asia Pty Ltd

Editorial Offices:

54 University Street, Carlton
Victoria 3053, Australia

Osney Mead, Oxford OX2 OEL
25 John Street, London WC1N 2BL

23 Ainslie Place, Edinburgh EH3 6AJ

350 Main Street, Malden
MA 02148-5018, USA

Other Editorial Offices:

Blackwell Wissenschafts-Verlag GmbH
Kuerfürstendamm 57
10707 Berlin, Germany

Zehetnergasse 6
1140 Wien, Austria

Production Editor: Brett Lockwood

Design & Typesetting: John Bedovian,
The University of Melbourne Design & Print Centre

Printed in Australia

Cataloguing-in-Publication Data

Hare, W. S. C. (William Samuel Calhoun).
Clinical radiology for medical students and health practitioners.

2nd ed.
Includes index
ISBN 0 86793 007 1

1. Radiology, Medical. 2. Diagnosis, Radioscopic.
I. Title.

616.0757

The aim of this book is to encourage the logical use of radiology tailored to the clinical status of individual patients. Long before Roentgen's epoch-making discovery, clinical medicine was well-established, based on history-taking, physical examination, and a sound knowledge of pathology. Used appropriately, radiology can assist greatly in elucidating clinical problems with, in most instances, minimal inconvenience to the patient.

And whilst it is true that for many patients radiology has provided an earlier and more specific diagnosis, a more confident prognosis, and a sound basis for therapy, it is evident that not infrequently radiology is used inappropriately, adding unnecessarily to the radiation burden of the community and escalating costs of medical services. Since the first edition of this text eight years ago, the centenary of Roentgen's discovery of x-rays has come and gone and the flow of significant radiological advances has continued on. Developments in computed tomography, ultrasound, and particularly magnetic resonance imaging, have replaced a number of more invasive diagnostic techniques which required hospitalization. Such sectional imaging techniques are expensive and not readily available in some areas, so throughout this book a balanced view of diagnostic protocols is presented.

This book does not describe radiological procedures in any detail. It is helpful for all health practitioners to know what is involved for patients who undergo radiological examinations, but this is best gained by visits to radiology departments. It is not recommended that the book be read cover to cover. Chapter One deals with general principles and should be read early in one's clinical experience. Other chapters should be referred to in respect to particular problems which arise during clinical practice. For those seeking more detailed information a key reference book is quoted at the end of most chapters. This edition has been expanded to include relevant material in paediatric, obstetric and gynaecological radiology and orthopaedics and the number of illustrations has been greatly increased. It is certainly not a radiographic atlas and visits to the film libraries of radiology departments are recommended to gain more familiarity in interpretation.

In the preparation of this text my thanks are due to Mr John Bedovian, Design and Print Centre, The University of Melbourne; and to Mrs Claire Beriman, librarian, for her typing skills, and Mr Ian Hood, technical officer, who prepared many illustrations, both of the Department of Radiology, The University of Melbourne. In addition, I thank the following for help in providing radiographs: Drs Christine Acton, Tony Apanis, Nathan Better, Frank Burke, Michael Ditchfield, Joseph Ferrucci, Stacey Goergen, Meier Lichtenstein, Alan McKenzie and Michael Scott, and particularly my radiological colleagues in the University department.

W. S. C. Hare
Melbourne, February 1999

Chapter 14   Musculo-Skeletal System

Chapter 15   Joints

Index

1.1 What Do We Mean by Diagnosis?

Patients present to their doctor for various reasons. Many, perhaps the majority, present because they feel unwell, others because they discover a physical abnormality, and another group for routine 'checkups' or the monitoring of normal functions such as pregnancy. They all seek reassurance and relief and expect prompt attention.

The **management** of patients includes **diagnosis**, an appreciation of **prognosis**, and the prescription and monitoring of appropriate **treatment**.

Diagnosis is the doctor's concept of the nature of the pathological process causing the patient's illness. It is important to dwell a moment and consider the meaning of diagnosis in some detail. After all, diagnosis is what this book is all about and muddled thinking concerning this phase of patient management has significant implications.

Diagnosis is a word derived from the Greek and literally means 'distinguishing between'. It is commonly held that a diagnosis has not been made unless a specific pathological process has been identified precisely. In medicine there are at least two flaws in this attitude. First, whereas it is easy to determine precisely that a flat tyre is due to a puncture, in many illnesses the true cause remains obscure. Even at autopsy, the pathologist, recognized generally as the final arbiter, is often left in a quandary. Secondly, the patient's condition frequently requires treatment before the series of tests leading to a specific diagnosis can

be completed. It is better, I believe, to consider diagnosis as a dynamic process, open to review throughout the period of patient management, but serving as the basis for planning treatment. This viewpoint is crucial in understanding the role of diagnostic imaging procedures and we can now consider how it applies in practice.

A detailed history and thorough clinical examination form the basis of diagnosis. As a result the doctor is in a position to list a number of diagnostic possibilities. Frequently the list may be long and on other occasions short, but, in medicine, it is virtually never possible clinically to arrive at a totally exclusive specific diagnosis. Even with traumatic fracture of the shaft of a long bone in a young person there is a remote possibility of pathological fracture. As well as listing possibilities the doctor arranges them in order of probability. The most probable pathology is designated as the **'provisional diagnosis'**. With the increasing use of computers in medicine, systems for weighting these probabilities quantitatively have been proposed. It is at this stage of management, following history taking and clinical examination that important decisions must be made. Not only should the course of treatment be considered, but also the question of whether further diagnostic information is required. The decision to investigate a patient further is a most important one, not only for the patient's welfare, but also because of the economic implications of overusing diagnostic services. Nowadays an extensive range of tests is available, and many of them are expensive.

The reasons for further investigation following history and clinical examination can be listed. Practitioners are encouraged to analyse the motive for further investigation in their patients and the influence the results have on patient management. Alas, all too frequently, diagnostic investigations are requested without due consideration, and do not contribute to management.

1. Investigations to clarify the diagnosis

When faced with a number of significant diagnostic probabilities investigation may help to refine the list, increasing certain probabilities and diminishing, and perhaps excluding, others. For example, in an elderly alcoholic patient who has lost weight, but has no other physical findings, the probabilities might well include cirrhosis and some form of neoplasia. If a chest radiograph shows widespread small spherical lung opacities consistent with metastases, the probability of advanced neoplasia is increased to the point of virtually excluding other possibilities and no further investigation may be required. In practice the extent to which a diagnostic test alters the order of probabilities at the time of clinical provisional diagnosis is a measure of its diagnostic value.

2. To confirm the provisional diagnosis

If there is a very high probability, after clinical examination, that a patient's condition is due to a particular pathological condition, then the need to perform diagnostic investigations to confirm this opinion can be seriously questioned. For example, if a patient presents extremely ill and a provisional diagnosis of pulmonary oedema secondary to cardiac failure is made with a high degree of confidence, it is of little if any value in management to request a chest x-ray, particularly if that examination leads to further physical disturbance

and delay in treatment. Later on, in particular cases, further investigation may be indicated.

3. Investigation to obtain detailed information concerning a particular diagnosis

This is frequently a prelude to surgery. For example, a patient presents with painless haematuria with no clues in the history or physical examination to suggest the possible pathology. If intravenous urography reveals a space-occupying lesion in the kidney and ultrasound shows the mass to be solid, the investigation has clarified the diagnosis and renal cell carcinoma emerges as the highly probable provisional diagnosis. In such a case computed tomography is justified to obtain more detail prior to surgery, including demonstration of the inferior vena cava and renal vein, and a chest radiograph to determine the extent of spread.

4. Diagnostic tests to monitor the progress of disease and the results of treatment

Although valuable in this regard, it is important that such investigations should be requested with due respect to the natural history of the disease process. The economic implications of too frequent investigations for this purpose are considerable and many such tests performed for this reason do not contribute to patient management. As an example one could cite the too frequent use of chest x-rays to follow the clearing of lobar pneumonia.

5. Investigations to detect evidence of disease at a sta before clinical manifestation

This is the philosophy behind various screening programs and is based on the concept that detecting abnormalities at an early stage may benefit the individual. A sceptic has been known to comment 'a normal person is one who has not been adequately investigated!'.

In summary, diagnosis is the process of establishing a concept of the underlying cause of disease. Based on the history and clinical examination a provisional diagnosis, i.e. the most likely cause, is made and serves as the basis for initial treatment, but it is provisional on the way the illness develops and the results of diagnostic investigations which might be sought. Thus, diagnosis is a dynamic process throughout an illness and remains under review. Special investigations may be required to narrow down the number of diagnostic possibilities, a process often referred to as **differential diagnosis**, and radiology plays a major role.

Making a provisional diagnosis is very much a matter of experience. Remember, common diseases occur most commonly and it is only the tyro who hears hoofbeats and calls 'zebra'!

1.2 Diagnostic Imaging Investigations

The object of diagnostic imaging is to demonstrate pathological processes beyond the scope of the clinical bedside examination. Since 1895, when Roentgen discovered x-rays, many developments have occurred to increase the sensitivity and specificity of diagnostic imaging. Nowadays, the clinician is faced with a wide choice of tests and it is important that the most appropriate investigation is requested in a given clinical situation. Experience is important in deciding this and increasingly clinicians are seeing the value of early consultation with the radiologist in planning protocols for complex diagnostic problems.

Nowadays diagnostic images may be produced using x-rays, radionuclides, ultrasound, or magnetic resonance, and the various techniques employing these modalities will be described. Within each radiation category, the various methods will be presented in order of increasing sophistication and this follows roughly the order in which they became available historically. And, because of the increasing complexity of equipment necessary, the more recent methods are the more expensive.

X-ray imaging
Plain radiography
The use of an x-ray beam with a film/screen/cassette recording device to produce two-dimensional static images of various parts of the body is basic to most diagnostic imaging studies.

Although providing much information it is important to realize that plain radiography has limited ability to differentiate between tissues. The absorption of x-rays is directly proportional to the physical thickness and the density (specific gravity) of the tissue traversed but, more importantly, is proportional to the fourth power of the atomic number of the elements in the beam. Thus, the following densities, in increasing order of absorption, can be recognized:

- Air.
- Fat.
- Soft tissues (including body fluids).
- Calcifications.
- Teeth.

Air

Air causes the least absorption of x-rays because of its low density and the low atomic numbers of the elements concerned, namely carbon, hydrogen, oxygen, nitrogen. As a result, air appears black on the film and acts as a naturally occurring contrast medium in the lungs and gut where it is an aid to diagnosis. Air is readily detected when in abnormal situations.

Fat

Fat is almost as dark as air on plain films and is easily confused with it. Very occasionally fat within certain lesions, such as a dermoid cyst or lipoma, can give the clue to the diagnosis. It is the small amount of fat surrounding organs and in muscle planes which allows plain radiography to demonstrate the outlines of many soft tissue structures, particularly in the abdomen.

Soft tissues

On plain radiography all soft tissue structures, including collections of body liquids, appear about the same grey density. Slight variations occur according to the bulk of soft tissue in the path of the x-ray beam but for practical purposes organs such as the heart, liver, spleen and kidneys are equally and moderately opaque. The outlines of these structures are seen because of the adjacent low density of air or a small layer of fat. Abnormal fluid collections such as cysts or effusions also appear of soft tissue density. An advantage of the newer imaging modalities (see below) is to differentiate between these various soft tissue densities in the body.

Calcifications

The presence of calcium, with a relatively high atomic number, causes considerable absorption of x-rays resulting in a whiter area on the radiograph. The site and pattern of calcification can be helpful in diagnosis, e.g. gall stones; calcified liver hydatid.

Teeth

The densest tissues in the body are the teeth and this high density and shape allows identification. Occasionally this is helpful in identifying dental elements as foreign bodies within the respiratory passages or sometimes within a dermoid cyst.

Plain radiographs are two-dimensional images of three-dimensional objects. From experience, radiologists, in many instances, are able to assess the depth of structures in radiographs but it is conventional to obtain a second view at right angles to develop the three-dimensional concept, e.g. a postero-anterior and lateral film of the chest.

Tomography

Tomography is a technique which provides a radiograph at a particular level within the body, which may be selected. It provides an image free from overlying, and underlying, opacities and assists in clarifying uncertainties in conventional radiographs. The tomogram, or laminagram as it is sometimes called, is obtained by moving the x-ray tube and the cassette about an adjustable fulcrum during exposure, resulting in blurring of all objects except those in the particular plane of interest. Computed tomography (CT) and ultrasound (US) have largely replaced this method.

Fluoroscopy

The modern fluoroscope consists of an image intensifier tube coupled to a television chain. Movement within the body can be studied with it and recordings made using videotape, a cine camera, or a series of static films.

Contrast radiography

The limitations of plain radiography and fluoroscopy were realized early in the history of radiology. The introduction of contrast media to broaden the scope of imaging gave rise to many fascinating stories. A number of the media owe their introduction to accidental events and astute observations.

There are two major categories of contrast media.

Positive contrast media

These substances are denser than soft tissues and contain materials, usually iodine or barium, with a relatively high atomic number. They appear whiter than soft tissue on plain radiography.

Negative contrast media

These substances are less dense than soft tissues and appear darker on the radiograph. Almost always the negative contrast used is air or carbon dioxide.

The wide range of contrast examinations now available can be placed in the following categories.

1. Injection of contrast medium into natural body orifices

Contrast medium has been introduced into literally all of the human orifices. Whilst in some instances this is a simple matter, e.g. ingestion of barium, in others it is complex, e.g. the pancreatic duct by endoscopy.

2. Injection of contrast medium into sinuses and fistulae

Valuable information may be obtained by retrograde filling of such abnormal communications.

3. Injection of contrast medium into body cavities or ducts

Where no external orifice exists diagnostic information can be obtained by using a needle to introduce the positive or negative contrast medium. Examples include lumbar puncture to perform myelography, i.e. outlining the subarachnoid space with contrast medium, or percutaneous needle puncture of the renal pelvis to outline the ureter, a technique called antegrade pyelography.

4. Injection of contrast medium into blood vessels

Because of the universal nature of the vascular system the development of contrast media which can be injected safely into the blood vessels was a major advance and opened the whole field of angiography. However, a number of problems required solution before satisfactory images were obtained. Rapid dilution meant that filming had to be made precisely at the time of injection of the contrast bolus. Needling, or catheterization of vessels was necessary to deliver the contrast medium to the region of interest. Also, the movement of the blood and the blood vessels required very short exposure times to avoid blurring. These problems have been solved and today high quality rapid serial angiography or cineangiography in all parts of the body is now available.

Digital subtraction angiography (see 'digital radiography' below) has brought further benefits.

5. Contrast medium excretion studies

The intravenous injection of certain water soluble contrast media leads to dense outlining of the urinary tract, i.e. the intravenous urogram. The oral ingestion of certain iodine compounds absorbed from the small bowel and conjugated in the liver, as is bilirubin, results in dense outlining of the gall bladder bile, i.e. the oral cholecystogram.

Computed tomography (CT)

In the last two decades machines have been developed utilizing a computer to analyse the x-ray beam after it has passed through the patient. These techniques make it possible to differentiate subtle soft tissue density differences. They provide information with relatively little discomfort for the patient compared with the invasive and sometimes risky alternatives previously employed.

In CT the computer is used to produce cross-sectional images of the body. A narrow beam of x-rays passes through the body and the emerging energy activates detectors which translate the data received into digital form for computing. The CT section is produced by rotating the x-ray tube and detectors in circular fashion around the body so that data is collected from multiple exit points on the arc. The computation of this vast amount of mathematical information takes only seconds to derive a quantitative point by point density assessment within the slice scanned. When these density values are displayed as shades of grey, with dense structures shown as white and less dense as black, a body section resembling a radiograph is produced. However, the sensitivity is far greater than radiography so that it is possible to differentiate white and grey matter within the brain. Furthermore, CT provides a quantitative density measurement in terms of Hounsfield units (HU) named after the inventor of CT. A 'region of interest' can be selected on the displayed CT image, even as small as a single pixel, and the density recorded. Approximate ranges are as follows:

Fat	< - 75 HU.
Body fluids	< 25 HU.
Soft tissues	25–90 HU.
Calcification	> 90 HU.

Because the two-dimensional sections are thin, it is necessary to make multiple contiguous sections to develop a three-dimensional concept of the anatomy. CT scanners can only section transversely, i.e. axially, but this deficiency is overcome by computer manipulation of the data so as to reconstruct images in the sagittal and coronal planes. More recently, **helical CT** scanners have become available in which the ring of detectors and the x-ray tube move in a spiral or helical fashion so that the data from a volume of tissue can be collected very rapidly, compared with the original technique of obtaining contiguous slices. Helical CT allows the computer to produce reconstructed images in any plane, and using a 3D program the data can be displayed on a monitor, allowing rotation, so that the region can be viewed from all angles. The latest software applications to helical CT data have resulted in **virtual endoscopy,** in which the radiological data is viewed on the monitor as though through the endoscope. The bronchial tree and large intestine (Plate 1.1 in colour plates section) have already been studied in this way.

CT, particularly helical CT, may be used to show vascular anatomy. CT sections are made after the intravenous injection of a large contrast medium bolus. Referred to as **dynamic CT** or **computed tomography angiography** (CTA), the method is replacing conventional catheter angiography in certain clinical situations, e.g. pulmonary embolism and aortic dissection.

Digital radiography

Computerisation of x-ray images has many benefits and the trend is gradually towards the recording of images, not on film, but on x-ray-sensitive detectors which provide the data on which the computer reconstructs the image. The computer is a convenient means of storing images and transmitting them, and if required, a series of minified images can be recorded from the computer onto a single sheet of film as in CT.

Apart from the high initial cost of equipment, the method allows a considerable saving in film costs. A particular application of great benefit financially has been the introduction of **digital subtraction angiography** (DSA). In this technique the video signal from the television camera of standard image intensifier fluorographic equipment is converted to a digital signal and the TV image is stored in the computer. Just prior to injecting contrast medium into the blood vessel, TV images of the region are stored and then followed by the series of contrast-containing images. The digital function of the computer allows subtraction of the data obtained prior to contrast injection from the contrast images so that, when played back to the video monitor, the images show only the blood vessels of interest with minimal background which is subtracted out. In addition the computer can be programmed to enhance the contrast image within the blood vessel so that a smaller volume of contrast medium can be injected by the radiologist reducing further any discomfort to the patient. Again there is a considerable saving in film costs.

Risks of x-ray imaging

X-rays are a form of ionising radiation which have biological effects which, for practical purposes, can be divided into carcinogenic effects in somatic structures, and genetic effects on reproductive cells. In this regard, medical radiation, mainly imaging, contributes only about 20% to the population dose, the major contribution coming from the natural background. Although the risks of carcinogenesis from diagnostic imaging are low and studies of exposed populations have not revealed any direct evidence of genetic damage, it is important to keep radiation doses as low as reasonably achievable in order to minimize these risks, particularly as it is assumed that the radiation burden is cumulative throughout life. Certain tissues are more sensitive to x-rays, particularly thyroid and breast and particular care is taken to protect those regions. Similarly, the gonads and the developing foetus require special attention. For women in the reproductive age group, special measures are required to avoid irradiating an unsuspected early pregnancy. The crucial period is now recognized as about the sixth week of pregnancy when active organogenesis is taking place. **When planning pelvic or abdominal radiography in this age group, it is important to perform it in the first or second week following menstruation.**

Radionuclide imaging

Radionuclides, which emit gamma rays that are more penetrating than x-rays can be administered intravenously or occasionally by ingestion or injection into body cavities, and their position in the body demonstrated using a gamma scintillation camera. Radionuclides can be used to label particular molecules selected to target an organ of interest, e.g. the use of sulphur colloid labelling to achieve selective uptake by the reticulo-endothelial system. Although a range of radionuclides is available for specific purposes, the development of technetium 99m as a scanning agent has been a major advance. This radionuclide can be prepared in the laboratory when required from its molybdenum parent quite readily so that storage and transport problems are overcome. Also, it has a short half-life of about six hours so that disposal is not a particular hazard. This radionuclide can also be labelled without difficulty. Static images, such as in a bone scan, can be obtained or a series of dynamic scans can be performed with radionuclides which allows the function of an organ to be assessed, e.g. glomerular filtration rate. A further advantage is that radionuclide imaging is relatively non-invasive, i.e. does not require vascular catheterization. Because radionuclide images demonstrate only the position of the radioactive material, very little information is provided concerning the surrounding normal tissue

anatomy. Also, as with plain radiography, using a single gamma camera, the images are two-dimensional, and with large organs such as the liver, it is necessary to obtain two emission images at right angles to assist localization of abnormalities.

Single Photon Emission Computed Tomography (SPECT)

Recently, more detail of focal lesions has been obtained using a technique similar to x-ray CT, employing an arc of detectors.

Positron Emission Tomography (PET)

This technique uses very short-lived radionuclides, produced in a cyclotron, to study metabolic processes in various sites, particularly the brain and heart (Plate 1.2 in colour plates section).

Risks of radionuclide imaging

Although the biological effects are similar to x-radiation, the dosage to patient and personnel is quite different in quality, being determined by the half-life of the radionuclide employed, whereas with x-radiation, the dosage is determined by the finite length of the short exposure. Furthermore, the intravenous route results in a total body exposure until the labelled molecule reaches its target. For these reasons, the preparation, selection of dosage, handling and disposal of radionuclides requires particular attention.

Ultrasound imaging (US)

Ultrasound is a compression wave similar to audible sound but of higher frequency. The ultrasound transducer, which is placed on the skin surface using a fluid coupling medium, emits very short ultrasound pulses which are generated by the vibration of the small ceramic tile at its tip. For most of the time between pulses the transducer acts as a detector of the returning echoes which are digitized and used by the computer to reconstruct the image. Echoes are produced at interfaces between tissues differing in their ultrasonic conduction properties. Thus, homogeneous structures such as cyst fluid produce minimal echoes whilst fat, due to lobulation and septa, is highly echogenic. To produce a sectional image, the transducer is moved across the body surface. The image, produced by the narrow beam of ultrasound, is two-dimensional, if we disregard the finite but narrow width of the beam. Thus, as with CT and SPECT, it is necessary, using US, to make a series of contiguous sections to build up a three-dimensional concept. However, US has the advantage that sections can be made both transversely and longitudinally, compared with CT which can only produce transverse images. From the data in the computer, selected images are photographed onto film for reporting. When viewing ultrasound images the convention is that transverse body sections are viewed as from the foot end of the patient and longitudinal images are viewed with the head end to the viewer's left. Another important advantage of US is that the computer provides continuous real-time images so that movement within the tissues in the ultrasound beam can be viewed on the monitor and can be recorded on videotape.

Transluminal US

Probes and catheters have been developed for use in various body cavities and through orifices. Transoesophageal US is useful in diagnosing dissecting thoracic aortic aneurysm, transgastric US for detailed pancreatic imaging, transvaginal US for pelvic organs, and transrectal US for prostatic imaging. The close proximity of adjacent tissues to the transducer allows for greater detail than the transabdominal pathway.

Vascular US

US allows the measurement of velocity of flow in blood vessels dependent on the **Doppler effect**. The change in the frequency of sound when a railway train passes by is well known and this change in frequency is dependent on velocity.

Thus, US is able to display not only the anatomical dimensions of vascular structures, but also the flow characteristics. Flow data can be recorded in various ways. **Duplex Doppler** displays the anatomical US image with the sampling site and, separately, the flow graph for that site (Fig. 10.13). **Colour Flow Doppler** (CFD), in which the flow is colour-coded, displays flow superimposed on the anatomical image (Plate 4.8 in colour plates section). **Power Doppler**, a new technique, provides colour-coded flow data, superimposed on the anatomical image, based on the total energy of flow, rather than just kinetic energy as in CFD; it is proving to be valuable in certain regions, e.g. kidney (Plates 1.3 and 4.9 in colour plates section). A further addition to vascular US is the availability of **US contrast media**. Tiny encased gas bubbles injected intravenously pass through the lungs and appear hyperechoic in the vessels being studied (Plate 1.4 in colour plates section).

Risks of US imaging

US is non-ionizing in its effect and, although US can be used to damage tissues, at the energies employed in diagnostic imaging it seems free of harmful effects. In obstetrics, foetal activity increases during US examination and it is prudent that the number of examinations during pregnancy should be restricted to providing clinically significant information.

Magnetic Resonance Imaging (MRI)

This rapidly expanding newer diagnostic modality employs a strong magnetic field and radio waves. The technique images hydrogen protons, which are universally spread throughout the body. The quality of the images depends on the distribution and density of hydrogen protons and the nature of the molecules in the vicinity. It also depends on whether the hydrogen protons are static or moving, as in blood. The patient lies within a very strong magnetic field which brings the hydrogen protons into alignment, which is disturbed when a pulse of radio waves is introduced. After the pulse, as the protons realign, signals are returned to the circular array of detectors and the images are reconstructed by computer. Soft tissue differentiation in the MRI scans produced is exquisite in certain tissues, particularly the brain, but tissues low in hydrogen content, e.g. bone, do not produce a significant signal and appear black. To enhance the quality of MRI and particularly to display pathological tissue, paramagnetic intravenous contrast materials, such as **gadolinium**, are available. More recently **magnetic resonance angiography (MRA)** has been developed and has the potential to replace many conventional angiographic examinations. MRA is non-invasive, requiring only an intravenous injection of gadolinium, and the vascular images can be displayed with background subtraction as in DSA. The latest MRI development has reduced the acquisition time to a point where breathing is not a problem and abdominal imaging is a reality. As a result tubular systems such as biliary and pancreatic ducts can be displayed. **MR cholangio-pancreatography (MRCP)**, requiring no contrast medium, is already replacing ERCP in some centres. Further developments will see the development of functional MRI in which metabolic changes in certain tissues will be detectable.

Risks of MRI

The powerful magnetic fields employed may attract metallic objects, imposing a strict routine in performing MRI to exclude that possibility. Patients with metallic and electronic implants such as heart pacemakers, bionic ears, or brain aneurysm clips, recently applied, are generally excluded. The short duration within the high magnetic field and the use of radio waves at this stage appear to be harmless, as does the use of gadolinium contrast medium.

Historical review of imaging

From this galaxy of available diagnostic imaging tests, you will perceive an evolutionary trend during the past century since the discovery of x-rays. The major deficiency of plain radiography, fluoroscopy, and plain film tomography, was the inability to differentiate between the soft tissues of the body. The development of contrast media helped to overcome this problem to some extent. Contrast studies of the gut, the biliary system, and the urinary tract could be performed with little inconvenience to the patient. Other contrast studies, particularly angiography, were more invasive, often requiring hospitalization and were performed with significant risk and discomfort to the patient. Radionuclide studies heralded the ability of radiologists to demonstrate directly differences in the nature of soft tissues and this has now reached a high level of sophistication with the introduction of US, CT and MRI. DSA improved the quality of conventional angiography but nowadays non-invasive techniques of imaging the blood vessels are available including Doppler ultrasound, helical CT scanning following intravenous contrast injection, and more recently MRA. As a result of these developments, diagnostic imaging has become less invasive with reduced risk and less discomfort for the patient. Hospitalization is no longer required and, although these new technologies are expensive, they have the potential for reducing the costs, not only in hospital bed time, but in resources, e.g. film and contrast medium.

1.3 Interventional Radiology

Because radiologists develop a spatial orientation to the anatomy displayed on TV monitors and have developed skills in catheterization and manipulation of instruments under x-ray control, a logical extension has been towards radiologists treating an ever-widening range of conditions, once diagnosed. These interventional techniques include the biopsy of tissue, drainage of fluid collections or obstructed duct systems. Stenotic lesions can be dilated using balloons and if necessary to maintain patency, stents of various kinds may be inserted. Embolotherapy is used to occlude bleeding points or close vascular malformations or aneurysms in certain sites. Calculi and foreign bodies may also be removed in some patients. The trend towards interventional radiology has many benefits. General anaesthesia and hospitalization are rarely required and the absence of a skin wound minimizes the convalescent period.

1.4 The Diagnostic Imaging Department

In many instances when further diagnostic information is required during clinical management you will call on the radiology department. The resources of these departments are extensive in terms of equipment and personnel and it is important that you learn to utilize these departments wisely. Many aspects of radiology will be learnt from department visits but certain generalities in respect to the specialty should be appreciated.

Radiology is a referral specialty

Radiologists function as true consultants in that they only accept patients referred from clinicians. This is an important consideration at this time, when the financial implications of self-referral are under scrutiny.

The objective nature of the information obtained

In radiology, the objective evidence on which the radiologist's report is based remains available for further analysis. The film can be viewed and the conclusions reviewed and criticized. The films of previous studies often assist greatly in diagnosis and departments expend considerable effort in maintaining film files for this purpose.

The radiological data stands on its own

The radiologist describes the abnormalities seen in the diagnostic imaging examination recorded in the films. Based on these findings and the information provided, the radiologist provides a conclusion as to the most likely diagnosis. In this regard, his opinion on diagnosis is independent of others. It is important to provide clinical notes for the radiologist. Clinical information is necessary to plan the examination and in drawing conclusions. In reaching a conclusion the radiologist weighs up the probabilities based on the objective data available in the images obtained and assesses them in respect to the clinical picture. It is important that the objectivity of diagnostic imaging be retained. It is a valid criticism of many forms of endoscopy, for example, that the diagnosis is purely subjective and no photographic image is provided.

Radiologist – patient relationship

Radiologists generally do not pass on their findings to the patient but communicate directly to the clinician by way of the report, and in addition, verbally when indicated. For the most part the radiologist adopts a 'low-key' role in patient dealings particularly in respect to non-invasive, non-contrast studies. To this end, the provision of adequate clinical notes is important when referring patients to the radiologist. When this information is not available the radiologist is then obliged to establish the clinical picture by interviewing the patient directly. With invasive techniques carrying a significant risk, and particularly in the field of interventional radiology where radiological methods are employed in treatment, it is mandatory that the radiologist explain the potential hazards to the patient and obtain consent. As much as possible it is important that the referring clinician should gain the confidence of the patient, explaining the possible risks. Too frequently patients are referred to radiology with no idea of what the investigation might involve.

The radiologist as a consultant

We have seen that radiologists function as consultants in that they accept only referred patients and issue their opinion in the form of the radiological report. With the increasing range of diagnostic investigations available radiologists are encouraged to expand their consultant role to assist in the planning of appropriate investigations in complex cases. Considerable savings in patient discomfort and finance may result if early in management the clinician and radiologist confer on the question of diagnostic probabilities in a particular case and develop a protocol aimed at a speedy resolution of the problem.

1.5 Interpreting Diagnostic Images

The undergraduate medical course is not designed to produce a diagnostic imaging expert. Nevertheless, interested students can develop these skills to above-average levels through their own efforts by way of leisure time spent in the radiology film library. All students should become competent in recognizing the commonly encountered abnormalities seen in x-ray films.

To assist in interpretation the following approach may prove helpful.

1. Know the normal

Some experience of this will have been gained during tutorials in radiographic anatomy. Every opportunity of analyzing normal diagnostic images should be taken as it is only against a background of understanding the normal that you will be able to detect abnormalities.

2. Spot the abnormalities

Develop a system for studying the images obtained from the various diagnostic investigations. Go over the images, systematically covering the entire field. Do not preset your mind by reading the clinical information. However, when you have studied the images without the clinical knowledge, then read the notes and review the images again with this information in mind. The single most important function in studying diagnostic images is to detect the abnormalities.

3. Determine the anatomical situation of each abnormality

Students have a tendency to 'naturally assume'. Confronted with a rounded opacity in a PA chest film the student may assume that it is within the lung, completely disregarding the possibility of it being on the chest wall or in any tissues along the line of the x-ray beam. It is most important to consider both views at right angles wherever possible when dealing with plain radiography. Admittedly, radiologists do take short cuts. A cluster of opacities typical of gall stones, if seen on an antero-posterior film in the upper right quadrant of the abdomen, will be interpreted by most as being gall stones even though the lateral is not obtained. This is a matter of experience and perhaps a reflection of medicine being an art rather than a science. It is a valuable exercise for students to go through the logic of determining the anatomical site of each abnormality they see in diagnostic images.

4. Study the radiopathology of each lesion

Having detected an abnormality and determined as best one can the anatomical site, the lesion itself should be carefully analyzed. Basic pathological features such as size and shape are important parameters and the presence of calcification and its pattern can provide important clues to aetiology.

5. Consider the diagnostic possibilities from the data obtained

Having studied the images carefully it is time to collate the evidence obtained from the investigation. It is important that all abnormalities have been detected, their anatomical site determined and their pathological features, as shown by the imaging technique, carefully analyzed. A list of diagnostic probabilities can be drawn up and it is important to realize that this list, based purely on the findings, is independent of the list developed by the clinician at the time of the clinical examination.

6. Relate the findings to the clinical data

This is the stage at which the availability of comprehensive clinical information can allow you to refine the radiological list of probabilities. Also, you will be able to assess the impact of the imaging test on the provisional diagnosis made clinically.

7. Which additional tests are indicated to further clarify the diagnosis

Consideration should be given to the most appropriate test to be performed, if any, in the interests of patient management. If further differentiation between conditions is crucial to management then this is an important further step to take. Should the line of treatment be clear from tests already performed, irrespective of the precise diagnosis, then the wisdom of proceeding further for a more specific diagnosis is open to question.

1.6 Medico-Legal Considerations

Litigation, particularly in affluent countries, is becoming more prevalent, and claims of negligence in respect to radiology share in the increase. In general, these claims are negated if it can be shown that practitioners have performed to prevailing standards and the best of their ability. For primary care practitioners who refer patients to radiologists, the following comments include some of the problems which may arise in which the referring doctor may be vulnerable.

1. An imaging test is no substitute for adequate history-taking and clinical examination of the patient.

2. Selecting the type of diagnostic examination is the responsibility of the primary care practitioner. For example, in a patient with melaena, a request for a barium enema might be appropriate to exclude a right-sided colon cancer, and it is not the role of the radiologist to point out that a barium meal or endoscopy might be the more likely to demonstrate the primary cause for the bleeding. Likewise, if oral cholecystography is requested, it is not the role of the radiologist to indicate that ultrasound is generally more informative. Also it is the role of the referring practitioner to realize that a painful knee in a child may result from hip disease and request x-rays accordingly.

3. The referring practitioner is advised to always read carefully and appreciate the details of the radiologist's report. It is the referring doctor's perogative to disagree with the report and to discuss the matter, but it would be considered negligent to totally disregard it. Mismanagement resulting from failure to read an x-ray report has led to litigation.

4. Primary care practitioners should be guided predominantly by the clinical situation and not blindly accept radiology reports. Radiologists, like others, are fallible and miss diagnoses on occasions. For example, posterior dislocation of the shoulder is not infrequently misdiagnosed and a negative shoulder report should not be accepted if clinical suspicion continues.

5. When requesting a radiological examination, the primary care practitioner has a role in describing to the patient briefly what will be involved and obtaining consent. For more complex examinations carrying a significant risk, and particularly angiography and interventional procedures, this is a shared responsibility with the radiologist, but it is important that the patient be informed by the referring practitioner.

6. Referring practitioners have a responsibility when requesting abdominal and pelvic radiological examinations on women of reproductive age to advise them that the examination should be performed, if not an emergency, in the first half of the menstrual cycle.

Reference

Eisenberg, R. L., *Radiology: An Illustrated History*, Mosby, 1992.

2.1 Paranasal Sinuses, Pharynx and Larynx

Paranasal sinuses

In recent years the role of radiology has changed with the advent of endoscopic sinus surgery and a better understanding of paranasal sinus physiology. Normally the epithelium is coated with a 'mucus blanket' and the ciliary movement directs the stream of mucus in each sinus towards the natural ostium. About two litres per day of secretion is produced by the sinonasal mucosa. The frontal, ethmoidal and sphenoidal sinuses drain into the space between the middle and inferior turbinates, an area referred to as the **ostiomeatal complex**. Sinusitis is now considered, in most cases, secondary to obstruction arising in the ostiomeatal complex and is potentially reversible if the nasal obstruction is cleared. Plain radiography is no longer indicated for clinical sinusitis and CT is the primary investigation. A limited CT study with coronal sections (Fig. 2.1) is obtained to demonstrate the details of the ostiomeatal complex and for guidance in endoscopic surgery.

Although plain radiography may show evidence of tumour (Fig. 2.2) CT is the definitive investigation for neoplasms in this region, of which 60% arise in the maxillary antra and 30% in the nasal cavity. MRI may provide more detail if the tumour involves the cranial cavity.

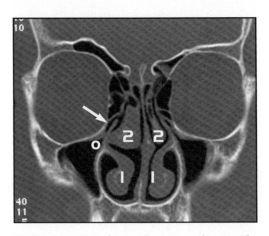

Fig. 2.1 Coronal CT showing the ostiomeatal region. The ostium (o) of the maxillary antrum leads to the infundibulum (arrow) which enters the middle meatus. The inferior (1) and middle (2) turbinates are well shown.

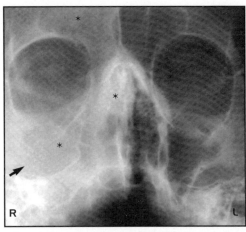

Fig. 2.2 Carcinoma of the right maxillary antrum. Compared with the left side note the destroyed right lateral antral wall (arrow) and the opacity of the right frontal and ethmoidal sinuses and antrum (asterisks) indicating extension of the tumour into the nasal cavity obstructing sinus drainage.

Pharynx and larynx

Nasopharyngeal carcinoma is common in Asiatics and CT is indicated to demonstrate the extent of the lesion and spread. Juvenile angiofibroma (Fig. 2.3) is an unusual benign tumour which may be quite large, extending into surrounding tissues. It is extremely vascular, occurring in adolescent males and tending to regress with sexual maturity. Arising in the nasopharynx, bleeding is often the first symptom. The extent of the tumour is clearly shown by CT, MRI or angiography and preoperative transcatheter embolisation avoids excessive haemorrhage.

Carcinoma involving the vocal cords (Fig. 2.4), usually squamous, presents clinically early on and CT is used to define the extent. Carcinomas extrinsic to the vocal cords and in the hypopharynx may present late with palpable lymph nodes the first sign. Contrast-enhanced CT is indicated to demonstrate the extent of the primary and abnormal nodes.

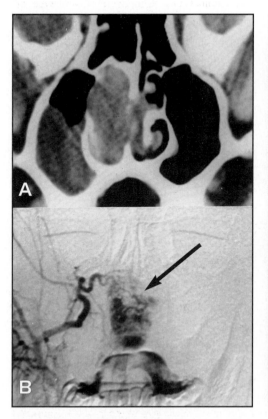

Fig. 2.3 Juvenile angiofibroma in a 16 year old male. (A) A soft tissue mass expands the right nasal cavity in this coronal CT section. The opacity in the floor of the right maxillary antrum is an incidental mucosal retention cyst. (B) A selective external carotid digital subtraction angiogram shows the mass (arrow) to be very vascular. The tumour was embolised prior to surgery.

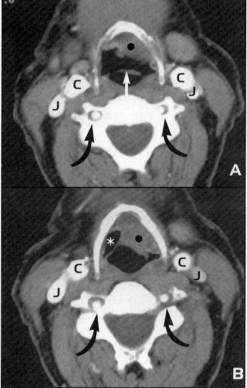

Fig. 2.4 Laryngeal carcinoma (●) involving the left pyriform fossa and extending superiorly. The two contrast-enhanced CT sections, (A) 1 cm higher than (B), show the soft tissue mass posterior to the hyoid bone. The epiglottis (top arrow) is seen in (A) and the patent right pyriform fossa (*) compares with the occluded fossa on the left. The carotid arteries (C) and jugular veins (J) and the vertebral arteries (curved arrows) have enhanced strongly with contrast.

2.2 Plain Chest Radiography

The plain chest radiograph is an extremely valuable diagnostic investigation, due largely to the widespread uniform distribution of air in the lungs which acts as a natural negative contrast medium. Soft tissue abnormalities are contrasted against this background of air. For this reason the plain chest radiograph provides a much greater range of information than plain radiography of other parts of the body. Almost certainly, it will continue to be the first imaging investigation for diagnostic problems in the thorax. The test is relatively inexpensive and the radiation dose, particularly to the gonads, is very low in adults.

The two standard views obtained are the **postero-anterior** view with the patient's anterior chest wall against the cassette and a **lateral** view with the side of suspected pathology adjacent to the cassette. The prime reason for performing a postero-anterior view rather than antero-posterior is not to avoid cardiac enlargement, because that problem does not arise when the film is made at the standard distance of two metres. The main reason is to allow the patient to be postured so that the scapulae will be projected clear of the upper lung fields. Students should develop a system for studying the chest film to include the sub-diaphragmatic region, the cardio-mediastinal contour, the shoulder girdle and thoracic cage, the tissues in the neck and a detailed study of the lungs. It is important to be familiar with the positions of the interlobar fissures and the normal distribution of pulmonary vascular opacities. Remember that air-filled bronchial shadows do not extend significantly beyond the hila.

Pulmonary and pleural opacities revealed in the plain chest film can usually be placed into one of a number of categories. For each type of radiological abnormality there is a list of possible causes. The list of probabilities is then correlated with the clinical information to arrive at a provisional diagnosis. Further diagnostic tests may be required to confirm the diagnosis and to establish the correct course of treatment. Students should become familiar with these commonly encountered abnormalities.

2.3 Single Mass in the Lung

With PA and lateral chest films there is usually no difficulty in determining that such a mass is within lung tissue and not in overlying structures such as the breast. With marginal opacities close to chest wall, diaphragm or mediastinum, it may be difficult to be sure and CT may be of help. Sometimes a loculated interlobar pleural effusion may simulate an intra-pulmonary mass.

A rounded isolated soft tissue density mass seen in the lungs on plain radiography (Fig. 2.5) may be due to:

* Primary bronchogenic carcinoma.
* Unruptured hydatid cyst.
* Granuloma (particularly tuberculoma).
* Solitary metastasis.
* Unruptured lung abscess.
* Hamartoma.

Usually the appearance of the homogenous soft tissue mass gives no clue as to the aetiology. Sometimes calcium is present in tuberculoma and hamartoma, and this may help in differentiation. The clinical information might narrow the number of possibilities. Bronchogenic carcinoma accounts for most solitary lung lumps. It is rare below the age of 40 years and does not calcify. **Pancoast's tumour** is a bronchogenic carcinoma

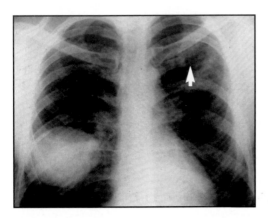

Fig. 2.5 Single rounded soft tissue mass in lower right lung field. Diagnosis: Hydatid cyst. Appearance is non-specific, but note surgical resection of left 5th rib posteriorly from previous cyst removal (arrow).

in the lung apex which is exophytic, invading the neck tissues, and may cause Horner's syndrome. Prior to rupture a hydatid cyst is homogenous and in contrast to liver hydatids calcification is rarely seen. A tuberculoma may be suggested by the presence of other calcified foci within the lungs or calcification in the mass. This is not always the case but with any pulmonary opacity the possibility of tuberculosis should be paramount because of the availability of effective treatment and the public health implications. The previous history may favour solitary metastasis, e.g. if the patient has had melanoma resected. Lung abscesses may be residual following pneumonia or may be pyaemic in origin. Hamartomas are generally small, not more than about 2cm in size, and there may be calcification within the mass.

Further imaging tests

In the past thoracotomy was frequently required because of the difficulty in obtaining a specific diagnosis of an isolated round mass. With newer techniques this is required only occasionally. CT differentiates the solid masses from those containing fluid, such as hydatid cyst, lung abscess, or even interlobar effusion (Fig. 2.6). For solid nodules, percutaneous fine needle biopsy under radiological control is now used widely to confirm a diagnosis of carcinoma, particularly

when bronchoscopy with biopsy has been unrewarding. However, this technique requires needling of the chest and a small pneumothorax frequently occurs. A number of special techniques have been developed to differentiate between benign and malignant pulmonary nodules. Thin section CT through the nodule allows the tissue densities to be measured and after contrast medium, if the tissue enhances by more than 20 HU (Hounsfield units), it is almost certainly malignant. CT also allows assessment of the

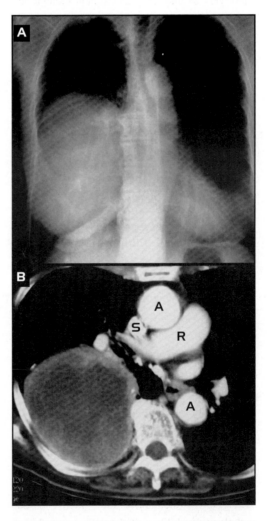

Fig. 2.6 (A) Large single rounded mass in lower right lung field. (B) CT shows the mass to be solid with lower density centrally due to necrosis. Diagnosis: Bronchogenic carcinoma. A = Aorta. S = Superior vena cava. R = Right pulmonary artery.

remaining lung fields to detect further nodules, e.g. metastases, and provides information concerning the mediastinal lymph nodes (see section 2.10). If bronchogenic carcinoma is suspected, CT is extended to include the adrenals, which are a common site for metastases from lung.

Currently, if a pulmonary nodule is detected on plain radiography, detailed CT is required and if the nodule is solid, and does not contain calcium, and particularly if it enhances strongly with contrast material, percutaneous needle biopsy is indicated for tissue diagnosis.

2.4 Multiple Rounded Masses in the Lungs

These lesions may be seen on plain radiography or the multiplicity of lesions may be revealed by CT in a patient thought to have a solitary mass on plain films. This finding alters significantly the aetiological possibilities compared with a solitary mass.
• Multiple metastases.
• Multiple unruptured hydatid cysts.
• Multiple pyaemic abscesses.
• Multiple granulomata, e.g. rheumatoid nodules.

The overwhelming majority of patients with this finding have multiple neoplastic metastases. Hydatid cysts when multiple tend to be moderately large and relatively few in number. Multiple pyaemic abscesses may be seen as a result of intravenous drug administration by addicts. Granulomata very occasionally may cause confusion with metastatic disease and this possibility should be considered, particularly in rheumatoid patients.

2.5 Lobar and Segmental Consolidation

Consolidation of lung tissue occurs when alveoli fill with fluid or soft tissue and produces an homogenous area of opacity on the radiograph (Fig. 2.7). When consolidation is confined to a lobe or anatomical segment, and the area is not collapsed, there are very few causes to consider.
• Pneumonic consolidation.
• Pulmonary infarction.
• Infiltrating processes e.g. alveolar cell carcinoma or lymphoma.

Lobar pneumonic consolidation is usually diagnosed without difficulty clinically, and radiography documents the extent of the pathology. In children, it should be remembered, lower lobe pneumonia may present with

abdominal symptoms and upper lobe consolidation may mimic a nervous system abnormality, e.g. meningitis. The alveolar exudate of pneumonia commences as a focus within a lobe and spreads throughout the lobe by way of the pores of Cohn. The first sign on the chest film is an ill-defined area of mottled opacity which becomes confluent and homogeneous as the process progresses. It is not uncommon for an entire lobe to become uniformly opaque.

There are two important radiological signs of pulmonary alveolar consolidation:
1. *The air bronchogram.*
2. *The silhouette sign.*

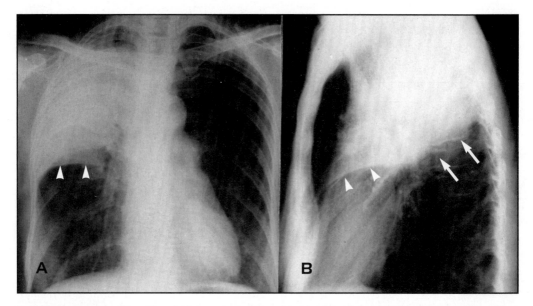

Fig. 2.7 Postero-anterior (A) and lateral (B) showing pneumonic consolidation involving most of the right upper lobe without volume loss. The horizontal (arrowheads) and the upper extent of the oblique (arrows) fissures make up the lower margins of the opaque lung.

1. The air bronchogram

Normally the bronchial outlines cannot be traced beyond the hila. In pneumonia, as the peribronchial alveoli become filled with exudate, the air in the respiratory passages can be seen by contrast with the consolidated adjacent tissue (Fig. 2.8). The presence of such an air bronchogram is an important sign confirming the intra-alveolar nature of the pulmonary opacity.

2. Silhouette sign

This is important in chest radiology and helps to localise consolidated lung tissue. The air in the lungs normally allows an excellent demonstration of the margins of the mediastinal structures and diaphragm. If immediately adjacent lung tissue becomes consolidated and opaque, the normal silhouette is lost at the point of contact (Figs 2.14, 2.16). Whenever two soft tissue densities within the chest are hard up against each other then the silhouettes of these two structures are lost at the line of contact. However, if there is air-containing lung between the consolidated lung and the other soft tissue structure then their overlapping outlines remain visible. For example,

consolidation of the right middle lobe (Fig. 2.14) will result in loss of the right heart border, but consolidation in the right lower lobe lies well posteriorly and the right heart border will still be seen on the PA chest film.

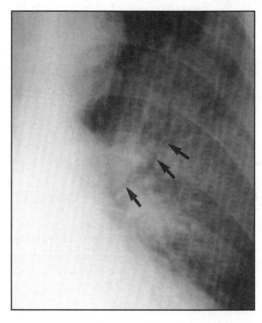

Fig. 2.8 Patchy alveolar consolidation due to pulmonary oedema. Note the air bronchogram (arrows).

A **pulmonary infarct** is generally smaller than the opacity resulting from lobar pneumonia. Infarcts are peripherally situated and broadly based on a pleural surface (Fig. 2.9). In some cases confusion with pneumonia can arise because both conditions share some clinical features, including fever and often haemoptysis. It is important to bear this in mind in atypical cases of pneumonia, as infarction may have resulted from pulmonary embolus. If this is suspected, further investigations may be indicated including radionuclide lung scans and studies of the lower limb veins (see sections 2.13, 3.12).

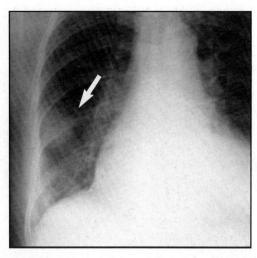

Fig. 2.9 Typical peripheral pulmonary infarct (arrow) abutting the right chest wall with a curved medial margin. Marked cardiomegaly.

Follow-up chest x-rays in pneumonia

Well-established pneumonic consolidation takes at least two weeks to clear completely radiologically, even though there may be a highly satisfactory clinical response. Thus, if treatment is proceeding satisfactorily there is no purpose in re-examining the patient radiologically prior to this time. It is the film made several weeks after the pneumonia which the clinician likes to know is normal consistent with complete resolution. If there is persisting opacity or evidence of collapse in the area, this suggests a complication or underlying pathology. In the older age groups the possibility of bronchial carcinoma is ever present. Persistence of the lung opacity over a long period also brings to mind the possibility that pulmonary infarction was the diagnosis rather than pneumonia. Persisting opacity in the region, particularly if associated with low grade fever in a patient remaining unwell, is consistent with the development of an empyema in the pleural cavity (Fig. 2.24).

2.6 Lung Cavities

A localized rounded lesion in the lung containing air, or air-fluid level when erect, is referred to by radiologists as a **cavity** (Fig. 2.10). It is important to realize that by far the commonest cavity in the lung is the emphysematous bulla. However, bullae have such thin walls that they are not usually seen in chest films unless they become very large. Thus, they are not included in the following list, which includes the vast majority of pulmonary cavities.

• Tuberculosis.
• Necrotic bronchogenic carcinoma.
• Ruptured hydatid cyst.
• Ruptured lung abscess.
• Cavitating infarct.

Bronchogenic carcinoma is the commonest of these nowadays, but tuberculosis is put first because of its public health implications. All of these causes may give rise to cavities which are virtually indistinguishable one from the other. Lesions elsewhere in the lungs, particularly the apices, may favour tuberculosis as a cause. Lung abscesses most commonly occur as a complication of pneumonia, particularly

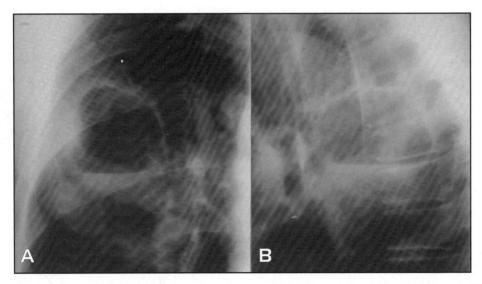

Fig. 2.10 Cavity in right mid-zone with an air-fluid level and thin wall in postero-anterior (A) and lateral (B) erect film. The appearance is non-specific. Diagnosis: Bronchogenic carcinoma.

staphylococcal or klebsiella infection. An extremely peripheral situation of a cavity is consistent with a cavitating infarct. Very occasionally, crumpled membrane can be seen projecting above the surface of the fluid level in a ruptured hydatid cyst giving rise to the so-called **water-lily sign** (Fig. 2.11). It is important to appreciate that the thickness of cavity walls and the degree of irregularity are non-specific. Also, it is very uncommon for pulmonary metastases to cavitate, so they are not included in the list. Occasionally a cavity may be complicated by the presence of a fungus ball or **mycetoma** which is shown to be mobile by a film in a different posture (Fig. 2.12).

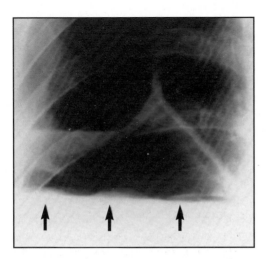

Fig. 2.11 Large ruptured hydatid cyst in right hemithorax. Note the daughter cysts (arrows) projecting above the air-fluid level ('water-lily sign').

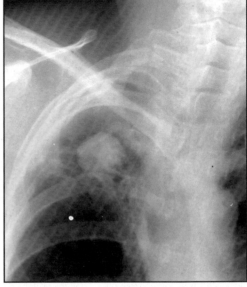

Fig. 2.12 Mycetoma within a residual pleural cavity following right upper lobectomy.

2.7 Lobar Collapse

A collapsed lobe may easily escape detection on the chest film, with serious consequences. Secondary changes within the collapsed lobe, particularly pneumonia, may be a source of trouble and the lesion causing the lobar collapse, e.g. bronchogenic carcinoma, may be significant.

It is important for students to become familiar with the appearance of structures which help to determine the space relationships in the chest. The positions of the oblique and right horizontal fissures are important landmarks. The vascular markings within a lobe become crowded as the lobe shrinks and those in the adjacent lung become more widely spread with over-expansion (**compensatory emphysema**). The central position of the trachea and mediastinum is influenced by alterations in volume of the two lungs. Similarly, the difference in level of the two hemidiaphragms (normally not exceeding 1.5 cm and normally with the right slightly higher than the left) may be increased accordingly. Incidentally, the trachea below the level of the suprasternal notch does not lie in the midline in adults when the aortic arch is placed normally on the left side, but deviates to the right.

Causes of lobar collapse

- Bronchial occlusion (**obstructive collapse**).
- Compression of lung, e.g. pleural fluid or pneumothorax (**compressive collapse**).
- Loss of lung tissue due to necrosis and scarring (**destructive collapse**).

Appearance of collapsed lobes

Two features will help the student understand the appearances seen on chest films when a collapsed lobe is present, particularly due to bronchial obstruction (Fig. 2.13).

1. The peripheral surface of the collapsed lobe remains in contact with the parietal pleura.
2. As air is absorbed from the alveoli the collapsing lobe becomes uniformly opaque and smaller.

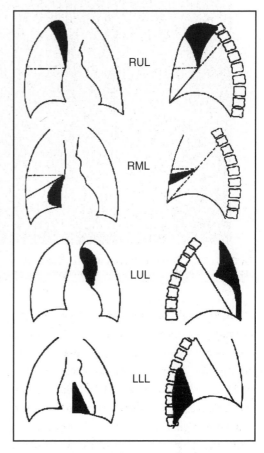

Fig. 2.13 Diagram of PA and lateral views of lobar collapse. Note that the visceral and parietal pleura of the collapsing lobe remain in contact as the lobe rotates to assume its final position.

Note: A segmental bronchus but not a lobar bronchus may be totally blocked without radiological changes because of collateral air flow through the pores of Cohn.

Each of the five lobes needs separate consideration.

Right middle lobe (Fig. 2.14)

The lobe collapses down to a wafer-like opacity without significantly changing its position. In the PA view the silhouette of the right heart border is lost because of the adjacent middle lobe opacity.

Right upper lobe (Fig. 2.15)

The horizontal fissure moves upwards as the lobe reduces in volume. The peripheral visceral and

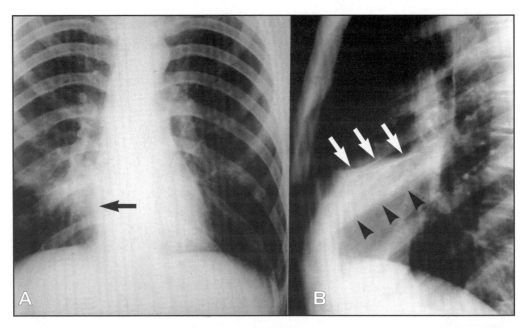

Fig. 2.14 Collapsed right middle lobe. In the PA (A) view the silhouette of the right heart border is lost where it abuts the collapsed and consolidated right middle lobe (arrow). In the lateral view (B) the collapsed lobe is seen as a triangular density overlying the heart. Arrows indicate the horizontal and arrowheads the oblique fissures.

parietal pleura remain in contact as the collapsing lobe swings medially to take up a position beside the superior mediastinum. Confusion may occur with mediastinal pathology, e.g. lymphadenopathy, causing mediastinal widening.

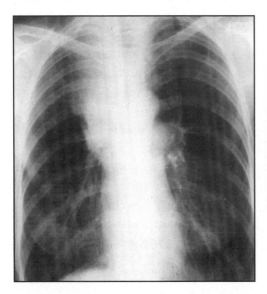

Fig. 2.15 Collapsed right upper lobe. The airless lobe lies adjacent to the superior mediastinum.

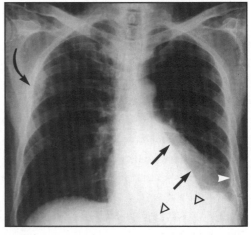

Fig. 2.16 Collapsed left lower lobe due to bronchogenic carcinoma. The edge of the lobe is clearly seen behind the heart (arrows). Bone metastasis (curved arrow) involves the right fifth rib. A small left pleural effusion is present (solid arrowhead). Note loss of the silhouette of the left hemidiaphragm abutting the collapsed lobe (open arrowheads).

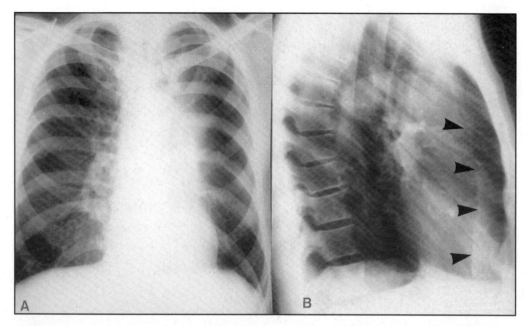

Fig.2.17 Collapsed left upper lobe. Note the loss of silhouette of the left upper heart border and the anteriorly displaced oblique fissure lying vertically behind the sternum (arrowheads).

Right lower lobe

The collapsed lobe moves medially and posteriorly to a paravertebral position. Isolated collapse of the entire lobe is rare. Usually the apical segment is spared because its segmental bronchus arises higher than the basal segments. If the whole lobe collapses the right middle lobe also collapses because the usual lesion responsible is a carcinoma in the bronchus intermedius, i.e. the right main bronchus below the origin of the right upper lobe bronchus.

Left lower lobe (Fig. 2.16)

The lobe collapses to take up a position in the left paravertebral gutter behind the heart. In a properly penetrated chest radiograph the partially collapsed left lower lobe can be seen through the heart shadow. The silhouette of the medial portion of the left hemidiaphragm is lost where it contacts the collapsed lower lobe.

Left upper lobe (Fig. 2.17)

This lobe collapses forwards and medially. In lateral views the oblique fissure can be detected lying well anteriorly. As collapse continues the opaque lobe moves medially to abut on the mediastinum giving an appearance which the unwary may incorrectly interpret as a mediastinal mass.

Collapse of a whole lung (Fig. 2.18)

Complete occlusion of a main bronchus results after some days in an airless and totally collapsed lung. The hemithorax is uniformly opaque and mediastinal structures are displaced towards the side of the lesion. It is this mediastinal displacement which distinguishes the appearance from massive pleural effusion when the mediastinum is displaced away from the opacity.

Causes of obstruction to a tubular structure

Radiology is frequently concerned with demonstrating obstruction to tubular structures within the body. In this book, when considering the aetiology of obstruction to a tube, the abnormalities will be set out in the following manner.

A. Mechanical:

- Within the lumen.
- Within the wall.

- Outside the wall.
- In the organ beyond (where appropriate, e.g. Ca stomach obstructing the oesophagus).

B. Functional:
- Due to muscular dysfunction.

Causes of bronchial obstruction

A. Mechanical:

In the lumen.
- Foreign body (particularly in children).
- Mucous plug (e.g. postoperatively and in asthmatics).

In the wall.
- Bronchogenic carcinoma.
- Tuberculous stricture.

Outside the wall.
- Lymph node masses, direct invasion, e.g. carcinoma of the oesophagus.

B. Functional:
- Bronchospasm.

Although plain radiography demonstrates lobar collapse, CT is indicated to provide more detail of the cause of collapse, and if tumour is present, the state of the adjacent lymph nodes (Fig. 2.27).

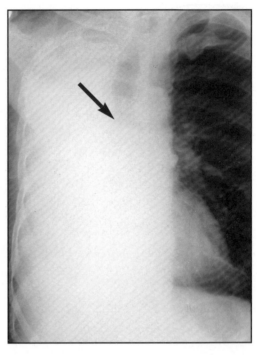

Fig. 2.18 Collapsed right lung. Total loss of the silhouette of the right hemidiaphragm and right side of the mediastinum which is displaced to the right. Diagnosis: Bronchogenic carcinoma of right main bronchus. Note: Absence of air in bronchi distally and air in displaced trachea (arrow).

2.8 Pneumothorax

Spontaneous pneumothorax is quite common in emergency departments. When small, there may be no clinical signs and the diagnosis must be made from the chest film. Students should be able to detect the abnormality.

The radiograph should be made with the patient erect so that the air can move to the apical region. If an AP view is made with the patient supine, a small pleural gas collection can be missed. A small pneumothorax is diagnosed by seeing the lung edge in the apical region lying very slightly medially, and the absence of vascular markings in the air-filled space overlying it (Fig. 2.19). When very small, the diagnosis may

be confirmed by performing a film on expiration. The volume of the hemithorax reduces and the lung edge is displaced further medially by the trapped air and the abnormality becomes more apparent.

With larger pneumothoraces the diagnosis may be made clinically and on the film the lung edge may be seen extending as far down as the diaphragm (Fig. 2.20). Very large pneumothoraces tend to compress the underlying lung to a point where the homogeneously opaque lobes, or lobe, are seen adjacent to the mediastinum. If a ball-valve effect is present in the pleura a **tension pneumothorax** may develop with marked

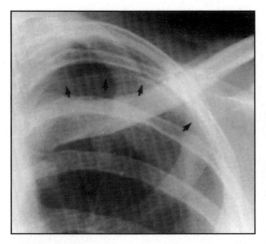

Fig. 2.19 Small left apical pneumothorax. The lung edge (arrows) is clearly seen.

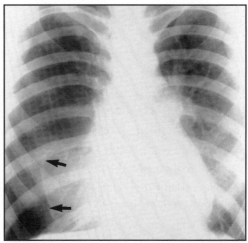

Fig. 2.20 Large right pneumothorax. Note the collapsed lung edge (arrows).

displacement of the mediastinum to the opposite side and a potentially fatal outcome. The diagnosis should always be considered in any case of acute progressive dyspnoea and the clinical features should enable rapid diagnosis, without radiology, and prompt treatment. Chest radiographs of pneumothorax may also show evidence of the cause.

1. Traumatic

Rib fractures may be present consistent with chest wall trauma. Most likely the pneumothorax results from bursting of the lung following sudden compression with a closed glottis, in similar fashion to the bursting of a paper bag when compressed rapidly. The apical region is relatively unsupported and is the usual site of the rupture. This is considered more likely than the lung being lacerated by fractured rib ends.

2. Spontaneous

This is due to rupture of a tiny emphysematous bleb, usually in the apical region, and rarely the bleb or bulla can be seen bulging from the apex into the pneumothorax space if looked for carefully.

3. Iatrogenic

Attempted insertion of a central venous pressure catheter into the subclavian vein may produce a pneumothorax. If, unwittingly, an infusion is given through a misplaced catheter a tension hydropneumothorax may result which is potentially fatal. If doubt exists as to the catheter placement a chest film should be obtained. Pneumothoraces also occasionally follow percutaneous lung biopsy or even brachial plexus block. Air may also be introduced during the drainage of a pleural effusion but careful technique should avoid this unless the underlying lung tissue is unable to expand to fill the available space.

4. Rupture of adjacent air-containing structures

Occasionally rupture of the oesophagus secondary to vomiting results in a pneumothorax, usually left-sided. Such a finding indicates a surgical emergency in these usually elderly patients. Rarely a pulmonary cavity or a gas-containing liver abscess may rupture into the pleural space.

2.9 Pleural Effusion

In the erect chest film the typical appearance (Fig. 2.21) shows the pleural opacity tapering away from below upwards with the major concentration of fluid appearing to lie peripherally in the hemithorax. This is more apparent than real and due to the x-ray beam having to pass through a relatively greater depth of pleural fluid peripherally than in the more central parts of the hemithorax (Fig. 2.22). In the lateral view the accumulations of fluid appear to lie posteriorly and anteriorly for the same reason.

The presence of a small amount of fluid in the pleural space may escape detection clinically and an accumulation of less than about 250 mL will not be seen on a PA chest film made erect, as it is hidden by the diaphragm. However, in the erect position, because the posterior costophrenic sulcus is deeper, fluid accumulates there first under gravity and can be seen in a lateral view. In doubtful cases, the diagnosis can be confirmed by obtaining a lateral decubitus view with the suspicious side of the patient downwards and using a horizontal x-ray beam (Fig. 2.23). The fluid will then be demonstrated lying along the lateral chest wall. This manoeuvre may be helpful in differentiating a small pleural effusion from fibrous adhesions obliterating the costophrenic sulcus.

Loculated effusions

Occasionally, an effusion becomes trapped due to pleural adhesions and this can give rise to a confusing appearance. Fluid trapped in a sub-pulmonic position above the diaphragm (Fig. 2.23) may be confused with elevation of the hemidiaphragm itself. The **lateral decubitus view** will help to solve the problem. Fluid trapped within an interlobar fissure may be confused with an intrapulmonary mass. An empyema following pneumonia (Fig. 2.24) may be seen as a broadly - based dome-shaped opacity bulging into the hemithorax from the chest wall.

Causes of pleural effusion

A pleural effusion may be the first evidence of disease and it is important to consider the large

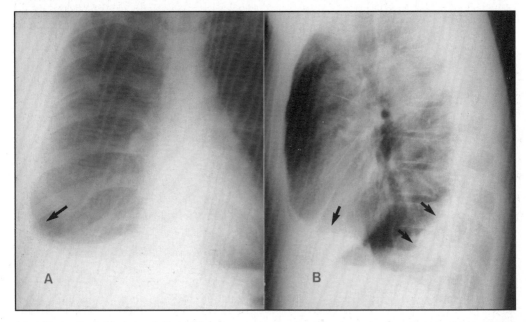

Fig. 2.21 Small right basal pleural effusion filling the costo-phrenic sulcus (arrows) seen best laterally in the PA view (A) and posteriorly and anteriorly in the lateral (B). For explanation see Fig. 2.22.

number of causes for such a collection. In an individual case, the possibilities can be narrowed down by considering whether the collection is unilateral or bilateral and by performing pleural tap to study the nature of the fluid itself.

Bilateral pleural effusions point to a generalized cause such as cardiac failure. The effusions of cardiac failure may differ considerably in size on the two sides, but it is virtually always the right-sided effusion which is the larger. A unilateral effusion points to focal disease related to that hemithorax. Because an effusion is sometimes detected radiologically without any strong clue clinically as to aetiology, it is valuable to consider possibilities on an anatomical basis. Further help

can then be obtained by aspirating the effusion, noting its appearance, and performing cytology and microbiology.

Generalized:
• Cardiac failure.
• Nephrotic syndrome.
• Autoimmune disease e.g. SLE.

Underlying lung:
• Bronchogenic carcinoma.
• Infarct.

Note: Pleural effusions very rarely, if ever, occur in sarcoidosis.

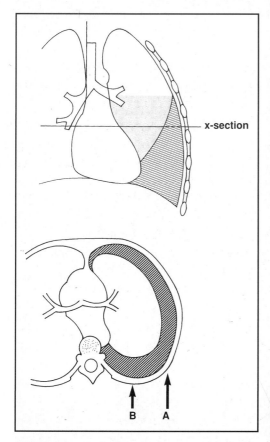

Fig. 2.22 Diagrams of a PA view of a pleural effusion (above) and an axial cross-section (below). Although the effusion envelops the lung uniformly the x-ray beam (B) medially has more air and less fluid to pass through than the lateral beam (A) explaining the characteristic appearances in Fig. 2.21. The same applies to the lateral view.

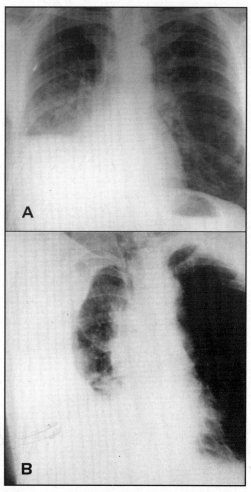

Fig. 2.23 Infrapulmonary effusion. In the PA view (A) the pleural fluid is trapped beneath the lung. The lateral decubitus film (B) confirms the diagnosis using a horizontal beam with the patient lying on the right side.

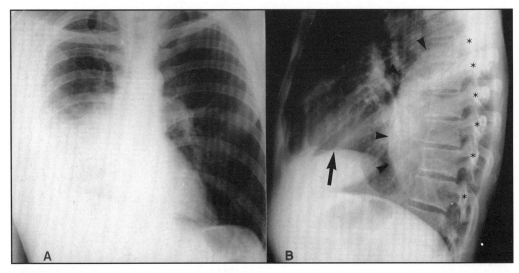

Fig. 2.24 Loculated right-sided empyema. In the right lateral view (B) note the position of the right ribs posteriorly (asterisks), the right hemidiaphragm (arrow) and the anterior margin of the empyema (arrowheads).

Pleura:

- Metastatic carcinoma.
- Tuberculosis.
- Malignant mesothelioma.

Chest wall:

- Trauma.

Mediastinum:

- Traumatic aortic rupture.
- Thoracic duct rupture.

Subdiaphragmatic:

- Acute pancreatitis (usually left-sided).
- Subphrenic abscess.

Nature of the fluid

Transudates, frequently bilateral, are found with generalized causes. The fluid due to bronchogenic carcinoma may be a transudate, an exudate, even purulent, or bloodstained. Bloodstaining indicates pleural involvement, with a worse prognosis, and is the usual finding with metastatic pleural cancer. Although less common nowadays a pleural effusion was a common first presentation of tuberculosis in the past, preceeding the development of an intrapulmonary lesion in many cases. Haemothorax may result from chest wall trauma but a left-sided haemothorax following a decelerating injury should suggest the possibility of traumatic aortic rupture. A chylous, or milky, effusion suggests a thoracic duct lesion, either obstruction or rupture, following trauma, including surgery. A watery white fluid is typical of hydatid cyst fluid but a hydatid rupturing into the pleural space, an uncommon event, usually results in a hydropneumothorax. Subdiaphragmatic causes usually produce an effusion with relatively low protein, sometimes called sympathetic effusion. If the focus extends through the diaphragm then the findings in the fluid will be more specific.

The chest x-ray as a guide to pleural tapping

PA and lateral films show the site of maximum fluid collection and are a good guide to the optimal puncture site so long as the procedure is performed in the erect position. It is important to accurately count the rib spaces. Having decided the point of maximum fluid it is usual to make the needle puncture one space lower.

Ultrasound is also useful in localizing pleural collections in contact with the chest wall and for guiding aspiration. Students should realize that generally ultrasound is useless in the air-containing lungs as the technology is based on the

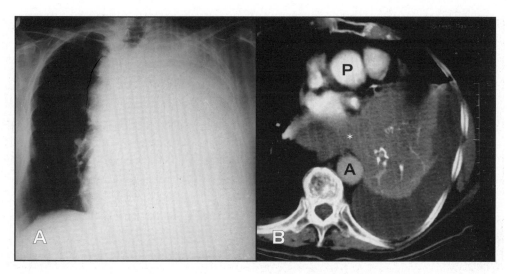

Fig. 2.25 (A) Very large pleural effusion with moderate mediastinal displacement. (B) CT following intravenous contrast injection clearly differentiates the less dense pleural effusion from the collapsed lung containing contrast-filled blood vessels and a soft tissue mass (*) which extends directly into the mediastinum between the pulmonary artery (P) and descending aorta (A). Diagnosis: Bronchogenic carcinoma.

velocity of sound transmission in soft tissues.

The state of the underlying lung

After aspiration, chest radiography is disappointing as a means of determining the state of the underlying lung. CT is recommended prior to aspiration if a pulmonary abnormality is suspected (Fig. 2.25).

2.10 Hilar Lymphadenopathy

Normally, the bronchopulmonary lymph nodes surrounding the bronchi at the hila are not seen on plain radiography. When they enlarge, the hilar opacities increase in size and the lateral margins of the nodes give the hila a lobulated appearance (Fig. 2.26). Because the nodes have air-containing lung separating them very slightly from the adjacent hilar vessels, the vessels can be traced medially through the enlarged hilar opacities. This helps to differentiate lymphadenopathy from dilatation of the vessels themselves when the vascular branches can only be traced back as far as the hilar margins. If hilar enlargement is suspected, CT is indicated, particularly in older age groups when bronchogenic carcinoma may be present (Fig. 2.27).

Causes of hilar lymphadenopathy

- Sarcoidosis.
- Lymphoma.
- Leukaemia (particularly lymphatic).
- Primary tuberculosis (particularly in children).
- Metastatic carcinoma.
- Pneumoconiosis.

Although commonly both hilar and mediastinal nodes enlarge, some diseases, e.g. sarcoidosis, tend to affect the hilar nodes more than the mediastinal, whilst others, e.g. Hodgkin's disease, do the reverse. Lymphadenopathy in sarcoidosis is considered an early manifestation. Lung lesions frequently but not always develop later, but not the reverse. Very occasionally the hilar enlargement in sarcoid is unilateral. The chest film may be the first investigation to demonstrate

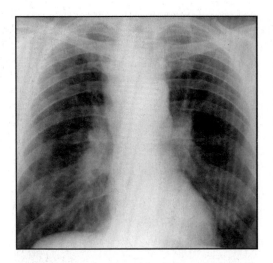

Fig. 2.26 Hilar and mediastinal lymphadenopathy. Note the lobulated hila and 'box-like' widening of the superior mediastinum. Diagnosis: Sarcoidosis.

lymphoma, particularly Hodgkin's, by showing mediastinal, and sometimes hilar node enlargement. Primary tuberculosis, seen mainly in children, is usually associated with unilateral hilar node enlargement, but sometimes mediastinal node enlargement also. There is usually a primary focus visible in the lung. Lung opacities usually accompany node enlargement in metastatic disease and pneumoconiosis. A characteristic of silicosis is the development of peripheral calcification in the nodes often described as 'eggshell' calcification (Fig. 2.28).

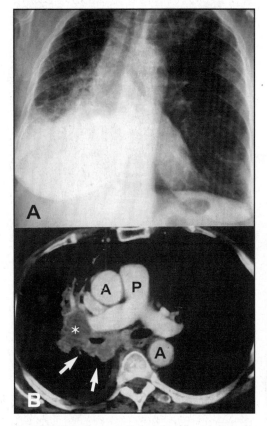

Fig. 2.27 (A) Patchy opacity in the base of the right lung with moderate mediastinal shift and elevation of the right hemidiaphragm indicating collapse in the base of the right lung. (B) Dynamic CT, following intravenous contrast injection, shows a hilar mass (*) and lobulated tissue surrounding the bronchus intermedius, consistent with lymph nodes (arrows). Diagnosis: Bronchogenic carcinoma. Pulmonary artery (P) and aorta (A) are densely outlined with contrast.

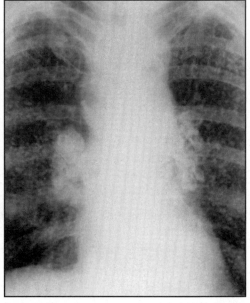

Fig. 2.28 Diffuse bilateral interstitial nodulation and hilar lymphadenopathy. Many lymph nodes have marginal ('eggshell') calcification. Diagnosis: Silicosis.

2.11 Bronchiectasis

The chest radiograph tends to underestimate the extent of this condition in which chronic irreversible dilatation of bronchi is present often with thickened walls (Fig. 2.29). In more severe cases, bronchial outlines can be traced peripherally into the affected segments of lung. Patients present usually because of chronic cough with copious sputum, recurrent pneumonia, or occasionally as a result of haemoptysis. When suspected, high resolution CT is most effective in demonstrating the nature and distribution of bronchiectasis and has replaced bronchography, in which a contrast medium was introduced through the larynx to outline the bronchial tree. CT is of limited value in differentiating the causes of bronchiectasis. The vast majority are idiopathic and considered due to childhood infection disturbing bronchial development. Far less common are broncho-pulmonary aspergillosis, secondary to mucus plugging, often in asthmatics, and ciliary dyskinesia syndrome or late onset cystic fibrosis when seen in adults.

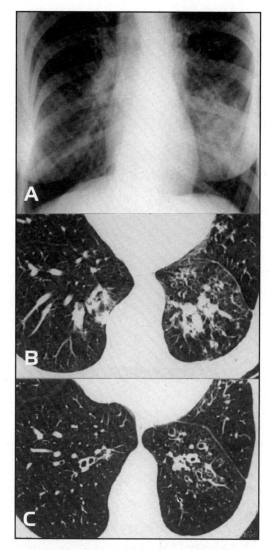

Fig. 2.29 Bronchiectasis. (A) Plain film showing thickened linear markings extending to both bases, left side more than right. (B) CT with the patient supine showing fluid-filled dilated bronchi in cross-section, appearing opaque. (C) CT with the patient prone shows that the dilated thick-walled bronchi have drained and contain air.

2.12 Diffuse Lung Opacities

The uninitiated usually take fright when confronted with a chest film showing extensive opacities throughout both lung fields. This is understandable as there are very many pathological processes which may give rise to such an appearance.

Nevertheless, there are guidelines for interpretation which can be helpful and these are outlined without giving too much detail.

First, the clinical history and examination, as always, are most important. Also, remember tuberculosis in any patient with unusual and extensive pulmonary opacities. It is the one disease in this group with a specific treatment and it is tragic if the diagnosis is missed.

Two major categories of diffuse pulmonary disease are recognized and in most cases, but certainly not in all, a careful inspection of the film will differentiate them.

A. Diffuse alveolar opacities

Accumulation of material within alveolar spaces produces initially small ill-defined mottled areas which later coalesce, forming large homogeneous opaque areas (Fig. 2.30). Air in the bronchi can be seen contrasted by the surrounding parenchymal opacity. The presence of this air bronchogram almost certainly indicates that the widespread abnormality is alveolar in origin (Fig. 2.8).

The clinical setting is all-important in narrowing down the pathological possibilities in diffuse alveolar opacities. The most important differentiating point is whether the patient is acutely and severely ill or whether the illness is of minor nature compared with the extent of the pulmonary opacities. The radiological appearances, per se, are common to all of these causes and are not really helpful in making a differentiation.

Acutely ill patient:

1. Pulmonary oedema.
2. Widespread pneumonic consolidation, e.g. pneumocystis, viral, chickenpox.
3. Goodpastures syndrome (allergic alveolitis).

Not acutely ill:

1. Sarcoidosis.
2. Many unusual causes including alveolar proteinosis and lymphoma.

B. Diffuse interstitial opacities

The interstitium of the lungs extends outwards from the hila and surrounds the vessels and bronchial branches. In the lower portions of the lungs the interstitium can be traced in macroscopic specimens as far out as the pleural surface, where it outlines pulmonary lobules.

Pathological processes which increase the bulk of the interstitial compartment sufficiently will produce changes in the chest film. Diffuse interstitial abnormalities fall very broadly into two categories, although there is considerable overlap and some disease processes show features of both. At one end of the spectrum are nodular opacities consistent with small focal deposits in the interstitium whilst at the other end are the linear or reticular opacities which result from more diffuse infiltrative processes or lymphatic engorgement of the interstitial space.

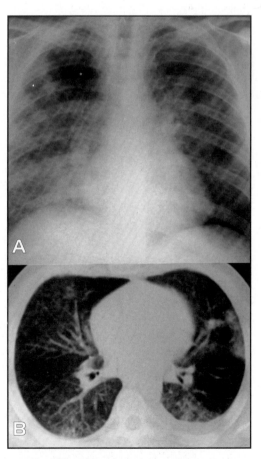

Fig. 2.30 Diffuse bilateral alveolar opacities. (A) The plain film showing ill-defined areas of opacity in both lungs with some air bronchograms (not well shown here). (B) CT shows the patchy airspace consolidation in both lungs. Diagnosis: Alveolar proteinases.

Nodular opacities

Widespread fine nodulation (Figs 2.28, 2.32) may be due to:

1. Miliary TB. Typically, the miliary nodules of blood-spread tuberculosis are only 2–3 millimetres across.
2. Sarcoidosis.
3. Miliary metastases.
4. Pneumoconioses.
5. Histiocytosis.
6. Varicella (chickenpox) pneumonia. Healed childhood infection results in widespread calcified small nodules.

Note: *Very small blood vessels which distend early in heart failure, or are prominent in some normal patients, may be confused with this fine nodular pattern, due to many vessels being seen end on.*

Linear or reticular opacities

A large number of aetiologies have been recorded. The following list includes those more commonly seen.

1. Interstitial oedema from heart failure.
2. Lymphangitis carcinomatosa.
3. Lymphoma.
4. Pneumoconioses.
5. Histiocytosis.
6. Idiopathic pulmonary fibrosis (Hamman-Rich syndrome).

These interstitial opacities result in loss of definition of the hilar shadows centrally and prominent interlobular septa laterally, the so-called Kerley B lines (Fig. 2.31). Sometimes the interstitial linear opacities are associated with lung destruction, giving a 'honeycomb' appearance, e.g. in scleroderma, tuberose sclerosis and cystic fibrosis.

In addition to studying the basic pattern of widespread pulmonary opacities considerable help in diagnosis can be obtained in some cases from changes in surrounding structures. For example, cardiac enlargement as a pointer to pulmonary oedema; calcified plaques in the pleura suggesting asbestosis and focal rib lesions consistent with metastases.

Further tests

Many patients with widespread pulmonary opacities, in the non-acutely-ill group, are

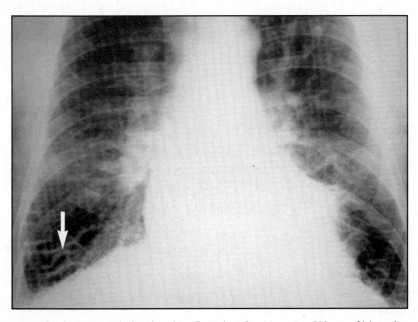

Fig. 2.31 Linear interstitial opacities at the lung base laterally (Kerley B lines) (arrow) and blurring of hilar outlines. Diagnosis: Interstitial oedema following IV fluid overload. The left lung was similar.

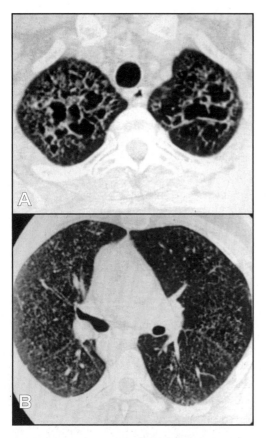

difficult to diagnose. Thin section **high resolution CT (HRCT)** displays the fine anatomical detail of the lung parenchyma with far greater sensitivity than plain radiography (Fig. 2.32). The fine bronchi can be traced out to within 3 cm of the pleura and the detail in pulmonary lobules displayed. Despite the ability to display the pathological anatomy in diffuse lung disease, it remains difficult to diagnose the aetiology in many cases, and pulmonary biopsy may be required. This may be successful when performed bronchoscopically, e.g. in alveolar proteinosis, but usually open surgical biopsy is required and this can now be performed with minimal inconvenience to the patient. Following asbestos exposure pleural plaques are better seen on CT than plain films and are considered benign. For a diagnosis of asbestosis intrapulmonary interstitial changes are required and are best assessed by HRCT.

Fig. 2.32 Langerhan's histiocytosis. High resolution CT. (A) shows apical bullae and (B) the diffuse interstitial nodulation.

2.13 Acute Dyspnoea and Pulmonary Embolism

Radiology has no part to play in the immediate management of the distressed acutely short-of-breath patient, but has an important role soon after.

Causes of acute dyspnoea

1. Bronchospasm.
2. Acute pulmonary oedema.
3. Tension pneumothorax.
4. Pulmonary embolism.

A provisional diagnosis is made clinically of bronchospasm by the presence of stridor, pulmonary oedema by the wet lungs and frothy sputum, and tension pneumothorax by tracheal shift with chest asymmetry. Pulmonary embolism is suspected largely on exclusion of other causes and in some the presence of chest pain and evidence of a site of embolism, ie lower limb DVT.

Investigation

Plain chest x-ray

The chest film is the first study and is used to confirm the clinical diagnosis. In pulmonary embolism the commonest finding, if any, is non-specific areas of vague opacity consistent with patchy atelectasis. Local shrinkage of blood vessels (oligaemia) and a large hilar pulmonary artery are rarely seen. In some patients small peripheral patches of consolidation are consistent with early infarcts.

Ventilation–perfusion radionuclide scan

When pulmonary embolism is suspected two radionuclide scans provide further information and can be performed upright in those dyspnoeic (Fig. 2.33). Patency of pulmonary arteries is demonstrated using an intravenous injection of technetium-labelled albumin macro-aggregates which embolise the pulmonary capillaries for a brief period during which their distribution is recorded by gamma camera. The patency of airways is recorded following the inhalation of radioactive xenon gas. Quantification of the distribution of ventilation (V) and of blood flow (Q) can be obtained and is expressed as the V/Q ratio. Radiologists categorize V/Q scans in terms of the likelihood of pulmonary embolism as high, intermediate, or low probability. For high probability V/Q scans about 90% will be found to have pulmonary embolism. Despite this high specificity there is a low sensitivity and 60% of patients with pulmonary emboli have V/Q scans in the intermediate or low probability range. It is important to correlate V/Q scans with the plain chest x-ray.

Angiography

If further confirmation is required, and particularly in patients with less than high probability V/Q scans in whom clinicians are reluctant, for certain

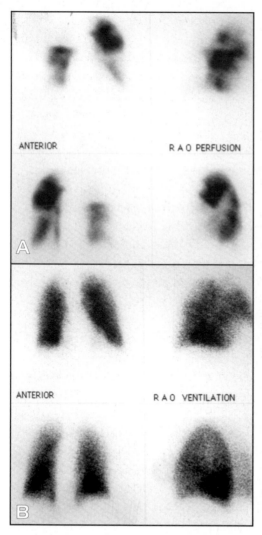

Fig. 2.33 Pulmonary embolism. V/Q radionuclide scan. (A) Perfusion scan. Numerous clear areas consistent with diminished vascularity in both lungs. (B) Ventilation scan shows the poorly perfused areas to be ventilated.

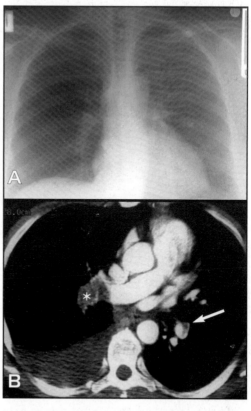

Fig. 2.34 Acute pulmonary embolus. (A) Relative reduction in lung markings in the upper half of the right lung. (B) Dynamic helical CT shows a large embolus in the right pulmonary artery (*). Note embolus also in a left pulmonary artery branch (arrow). A small right pleural effusion is present.

reasons, to use anticoagulation, digital subtraction angiography (DSA) may be used to demonstrate the filling defects within the pulmonary artery tree. Helical CT following contrast i.e. CT angiography (CTA) is a less invasive method of demonstrating the larger pulmonary arteries (Fig. 2.34). Pulmonary emboli which lodge in large pulmonary arteries often fragment early on and pass peripherally. If remaining centrally the embolus becomes incorporated into the wall with resultant dilatation of the vessel which may become apparent later on plain chest films.

With recurrent pulmonary embolism study of the leg veins (see section 3.12) is indicated and in some cases an inferior vena cava filter may be introduced percutaneously through the femoral vein as prophylaxis (Fig. 2.35).

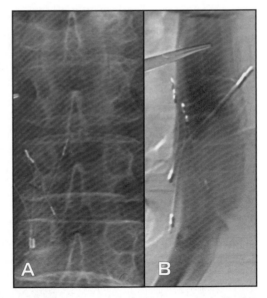

Fig. 2.35 Bird's nest filter in the inferior vena cava. The plain film (A) and contrast study (B) show the filter, which was introduced percutaneously through the femoral vein, in place to trap emboli from the lower limbs and pelvis.

2.14 Neonatal Respiratory Distress Syndrome

A plain chest film may be useful in supplementing the clinical assessment. The rather lengthy list of conditions which can result in respiratory distress can be grouped according to the displacement of the mediastinum.

Mediastinal displacement away from the lesion

Congenital diaphragmatic hernia is more common on the left side and the opacity within the chest may contain gas-filled loops of bowel (Fig. 2.36). These patients frequently have associated pulmonary hypoplasia which is mainly responsible for the distress. Congenital cystic lung may be confused with herniation as it also appears opaque with lucent cystic areas.

Mediastinal displacement towards the lesion

Pulmonary agenesis or hypoplasia and congenital lobar atelectasis, is more common with prematurity, and if unilateral results in mediastinal shift towards the opacity.

With no mediastinal shift

Pneumonia, pulmonary oedema or haemorrhage are difficult entities to diagnose. Hyaline membrane disease, commonly associated with prematurity, produces miliary nodulation throughout the lungs. Meconium aspiration, subsequent to foetal distress in utero with evacuation of meconium into the amniotic fluid, also produces a granular type of appearance to the lung fields, and a pneumothorax may complicate the picture.

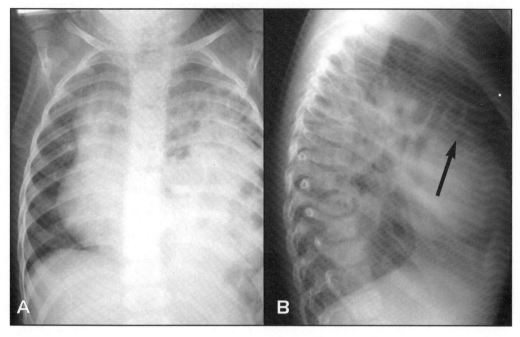

Fig. 2.36 Congenital diaphragmatic hernia. (A) Mediastinal structures markedly displaced with extensive opacity of left hemithorax. (B) Lateral view shows colonic gas pattern (arrow). Hypoplastic lung is often associated.

2.15 Emphysema

Emphysema is a general term meaning 'too much air'. **Compensatory pulmonary emphysema** results from collapse or resection of adjacent lung, whilst localized **obstructive pulmonary emphysema** may result from air trapping in ball-valve obstruction of the feeding bronchus, e.g. foreign body.

Chronic obstructive airways disease (COAD) due to generalized chronic bronchitis and emphysema, when symptomatic, can be diagnosed clinically and assessed by respiratory function tests. Evidence of the disease can be seen commonly in chest films and should be recognized (Fig. 2.37). More advanced changes correlate reasonably well with the clinical picture. Detail of the damaged lung parenchyma is better shown by HRCT.

Chest film appearance in emphysema:

1. Barrel-shaped chest.
2. Flattened diaphragm.

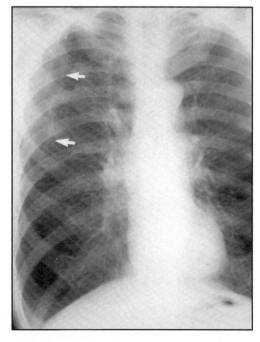

Fig. 2.37 Emphysema. Note the flattened diaphragm, barrel-shaped chest and large bullae laterally in right upper zone (arrows).

3. Altered lung architecture.
   a. presence of bullae
   b. irregular distribution of vascular markings
   c. large hila consistent with pulmonary hypertension.

The lungs are large in this condition resulting in the chest shape and the flattened diaphragm. The low level and flattening of the diaphragm correlate quite well with respiratory function tests. The convention with chest radiology is to make the PA film in full inspiration. If the routine was to film the patient in full expiration patients with emphysema might well be more easily distinguished. On expiration the diaphragm moves very poorly in these patients.

Emphysematous bullae are not seen on chest films unless the bullae become moderately large. They are distributed usually at the apices, along the lateral chest wall, and just above the diaphragm. If they enlarge sufficiently the walls can be made out and the air spaces are seen devoid of vascular markings. It is the distribution of bullae and changes in lung structure which lead to a disturbance in the normal distribution of the pulmonary blood vessels. Some portions of lung appear to have a reduced number of vessels and in other areas a slight crowding. With the development of pulmonary hypertension the hilar shadows tend to increase in size. CT provides a much better display, if required, of the emphysematous bullae and altered lung architecture.

Note: The degree of blackening of the lung fields is not a good indication, per se, of emphysema. Because these patients have a large antero-posterior depth to the chest, the radiographer is encouraged to use a more penetrating beam, when in fact the presence of emphysema requires less radiation. Thus, when requesting chest radiology in these patients, indicate the presence of emphysema in the clinical notes you provide. This will assist the radiographer in not being misled by the large chest dimensions.

Development of heart failure in emphysema

When the heart fails in emphysema changes occur in the chest film which can be confusing unless understood. The development of pulmonary congestion and early oedema has two effects. First, possibly by altering lung compliance and the stretch reflex, the diaphragm adopts a more normal level and shape. The slight cardiac enlargement which occurs may still be within normal limits with the result that some patients who are quite disabled with early cardiac failure, complicating emphysema, can have a relatively normal-appearing chest x-ray. With the development of early interstitial oedema, the enlarged centrilobular air spaces can be seen, giving a 'honeycomb' appearance to the lung field and the peripheral bullae may become visible.

2.16 The Mediastinum

The outlines of the mediastinum are well demonstrated on the plain radiograph because of the air within the lungs. Changes in the cardiovascular outlines (see Chapter 3) are well demonstrated as are masses which extend beyond the confines of the normal mediastinal contour. Within the mediastinum, the position of the trachea and proximal bronchi are visible because of the contained air, and the oesophagus is readily outlined with barium. Dynamic CT following contrast injection provides detailed information of the many vascular structures within the mediastinum. As a result, radiology is accurate in demonstrating the location of mediastinal abnormalities and frequently the nature of the pathology.

Mediastinal lymphadenopathy

The mediastinal nodes are arranged in anterior, posterior, and middle mediastinal chains with the main concentration in the middle mediastinum along the course of the trachea. With generalized enlargement, eg. lymphoma, the superior mediastinum becomes widened (Fig. 2.26) and it is unusual for discrete bulgings to be seen. CT allows assessment of the size of lymph nodes but, unfortunately, provides limited information concerning the internal structure, unless calcification or necrosis is present. In bronchogenic carcinoma, CT has only a 60–70% sensitivity in detecting mediastinal node involvement. However, a lymph node smaller than 10 mm across has a more than 95% chance of being normal in those cases. Mediastinoscopy from the neck allows assessment of nodes as far down as the azygos arch, but mediastinotomy is required for nodes below this level.

Mediastinal masses

It is usual to consider these on the basis of location (Fig. 2.38). The middle mediastinum contains the trachea, oesophagus, the heart and great vessels. The anterior mediastinum lies anterior to this plane and the posterior mediastinum is the plane behind the middle mediastinum.

Anterior mediastinum

The commonest causes for a mass in this region are the 'four T's' (Fig. 2.39).
- Thyroid–retrosternal.
- Thymic tumours and cysts.
- Teratoma.
- 'T' cell lymphoma (Hodgkin's disease).

The presence of thyroid tissue within the chest may be demonstrated with radio–iodine scanning. More commonly the thyroid is a retrosternal extension from the neck, but occasionally completely separate intrathoracic goitres may be found elsewhere in the mediastinum. Thymoma is usually found in those over the age of 40. Most are benign, but some show local malignant spread. About 50% have associated myasthenia

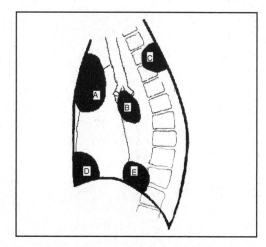

Fig. 2.38 Sites of some mediastinal masses. A: thymus, retrosternal thyroid. B: bronchogenic cysts, lymphadenopathy. C: paravertebral neurofibroma. D: foramen of Morgagni hernia. E: incarcerated hiatus hernia.

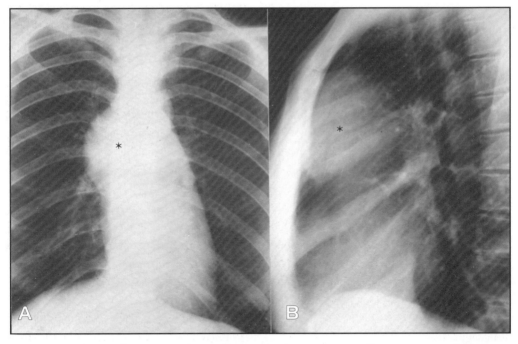

Fig. 2.39 Homogeneous soft tissue mass (*) lying in the anterior mediastinum. Diagnosis: Thymoma.

gravis, although only 15% of patients with myasthenia gravis have a thymoma. Teratomas occur in the younger age groups and they may contain calcification, fat or rarely dental elements.

Middle mediastinum

• Aneurysms of the great vessels.

• Developmental cysts.

• Lymph node masses.

Aneurysms of the ascending thoracic aorta bulge to the right of the mediastinum, and those from the distal arch and descending aorta to the left. Bronchogenic cyst by definition contains

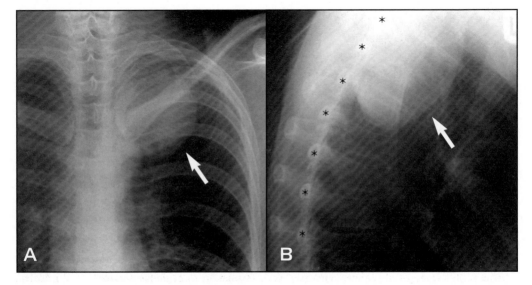

Fig. 2.40 Paravertebral neurofibroma (arrows). Left side ribs are marked (*).

some cartilage, and arises usually below the carina. Enteric cysts may or may not communicate with the gut. These developmental abnormalities, often known as duplication cysts, are shown to be fluid containing on CT.

Posterior mediastinum

- Neurofibroma.
- Meningocoele.
- Phaeochromocytoma.
- Hiatus hernia.

These masses usually involve the paravertebral gutter. Neurofibromas arise from intercostal nerves as they emerge from the intervertebral foramina (Fig. 2.40). Anterior and lateral meningocoeles may also present as mediastinal masses, but the associated bony abnormality in the thoracic spine should indicate the diagnosis. Occasionally a phaeochromocytoma arises in this location close to the sympathetic chain and even a tracking pseudocyst from the pancreas has been detected in this region.

Mediastinal emphysema

Free air in the mediastinum may be seen on the plain radiograph, often in association with

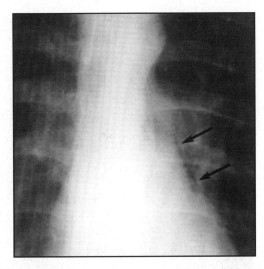

Fig. 2.41 Mediastinal emphysema in an asthmatic. The mediastinal pleura (arrows) is seen as a fine line with air lying medial to it beside the heart.

evidence of surgical emphysema which may be felt in the root of the neck (Fig. 2.41). Usually it results from spontaneous rupture of an air passage into the pulmonary interstitium associated with sudden chest pain. It is said to be more frequent in asthmatics. Of more sinister significance is mediastinal air in the elderly, particularly after vomiting episodes, when it may indicate a rupture of the oesophagus, requiring urgent attention.

2.17 The Diaphragm

On an adult PA chest film in full inspiration the left hemidiaphragm is slightly lower than the right, but not by more than 1.5 cm. In some the right hemidiaphragm may have a double arc to the contour which is a normal variation and does not indicate a mass in the underlying liver. Eventration, considered perhaps due to phrenic nerve dysfunction following birth trauma, is a condition in which a hemidiaphragm, almost always the left, is markedly elevated, displacing mediastinal structures, and shown to be immobile on fluoroscopy (Fig. 2.42). With large pleural effusions the level of the diaphragm may be

obscured on plain films, although the gastric air bubble is a good indicator on the left. US shows the level clearly. Diaphragmatic hernias are of various types. In infancy, a congenital hernia, usually on the left side, is frequently associated with pulmonary hypoplasia and respiratory distress (see section 2.14). In adults an hiatus hernia occurs through the oesophageal opening (see section 6.5). Herniation through the foramen of Morgagni is seen as a rounded opacity in the right cardiophrenic angle and must be distinguished from a pericardial cyst or a fat pad. Herniation through the foramen of Bochdalek, virtually always on the left side posteriorly, results in a soft tissue mass in the posterior costophrenic angle, seen best on a lateral film. Contents include the upper pole of the left kidney, retroperitoneal fat, and sometimes the splenic flexure of the colon or even the spleen. Diaphragmatic rupture, usually the result of blunt trauma, is discussed in section 12.7.

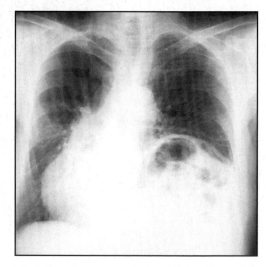

Fig. 2.42   Eventration of the left hemidiaphragm. Asymptomatic patient with no relevant past history. On fluoroscopy the hemidiaphragm showed only passive movement.

Reference

Armstrong, P., Wilson, A. G., Dee, P. and Hansell, D. M. *Imaging of Diseases of the Chest,* 2nd edn, Mosby, 1995.

Cardiovascular System

Cardiac diagnosis is largely a clinical matter and radiology of the heart and lungs is but one of a number of investigations which provide supplementary information. Electrocardiography, cardiac ultrasound (echocardiography) (Fig. 3.1), and radionuclide studies are non-invasive methods which provide information concerning structure and function. The more invasive techniques of cardiac catheterization and angiography may be required in particular cases, but, in future, specialised CT and MRI appear likely to reduce the need for this type of intervention.

3.1 Heart Size and Shape

An enlarged heart is an abnormal heart, but it should be realized that a pericardial effusion may confuse the issue. Pericardial effusions cause a more globular shape with increase to right and left of the midline. The maximum transverse width of the normal adult heart should not be greater than 50% of the width of the thoracic cage in full inspiration. In very early life this ratio is unreliable.

To detect individual chamber enlargement on chest x-rays it is important to know the make-up of the cardiac silhouette as seen in the two standard projections (Fig. 3.2).

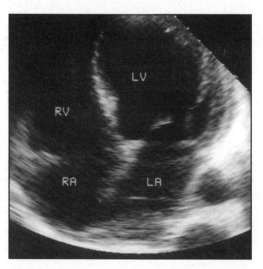

In the PA view from below upwards the right heart border is made up of the right atrium and in young people the superior vena cava extending up to the neck. In adults the ascending aorta bulges slightly to the right to take up a position between the right atrium and the superior vena cava. From above downwards on the left side we see first the distal portion of the transverse arch of the aorta (aortic 'knob' or 'knuckle'), and immediately below it the pulmonary artery trunk. Just below the pulmonary artery is the position of the left atrial appendage but this is inconspicuous unless the left atrium enlarges. The apex is made up by the left ventricle. Note that the right ventricle forms no part of the cardiac border in the PA view.

In the lateral view the lower anterior surface of the heart behind the sternum is made up by the right ventricle and above this the root of the pulmonary artery. Because the lungs meet in the midline, anteriorly aerated lung is seen anterior to the upper part of the heart and great vessels. In older patients the course of the calcified aortic arch

Fig. 3.1 Four chamber view echocardiogram. US displays cardiac movement and this still frame from the study demonstrates both ventricles and atria.

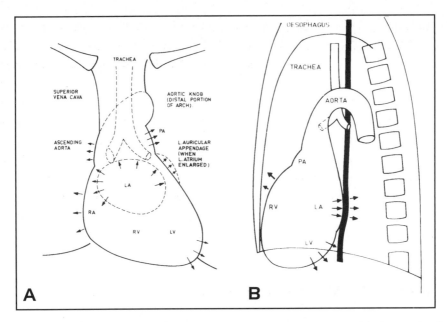

Fig. 3.2 Frontal (A) and lateral (B) diagrams showing the components of the various borders of the heart and mediastinum. Arrows indicate the direction of chamber enlargement.

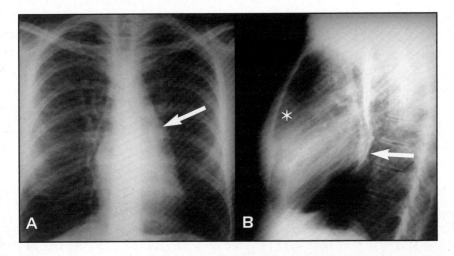

Fig. 3.3 Mitral stenosis. (A) Left atrial appendage prominent on left heart border (arrow). (B) Left atrium indents the barium-filled oesophagus (arrow) and the hypertrophied right ventricle extends upwards behind the sternum (*).

can usually be followed and the air filled trachea traced down to the carina. Also in the lateral view the main stem of the right pulmonary artery is seen end on as a round or oval density just anterior to the carina and its size can be assessed. The left pulmonary artery curves back over the left main bronchus before dividing. Below the carina the posterior margin of the heart is made up by the left atrium which bulges back as the atrium enlarges, e.g. in mitral valve disease (Fig. 3.3). Below the left atrium the left ventricle makes up the lower posterior cardiac margin. Barium in the oesophagus can be used to assess the degree of bulging of the left atrium. With this knowledge of the cardiac contours it is possible to assess to some degree the specific enlargement of various cardiac chambers or great vessels, although it should be realised that this is a rather coarse assessment.

The enlarged right atrium bulges to the right and is easily detected. The enlarging left atrium bulges posteriorly and the left atrial appendage is seen as a bulge on the left heart border in the PA view. The enlarging left atrium also tends to spread the tracheal bifurcation at the carina. Increasing enlargement of the left atrium may result in its right border extending beyond that of the right atrium to give a double cardiac contour on the right side. The left ventricle enlarges downwards and to the left and in the lateral view it extends posteriorly. Right ventricular enlargement is difficult to detect but there may be some expansion upwards detected behind the sternum in the lateral view. Generalized dilatation of the aortic arch results in a prominent aortic knob and the curved outline of the dilated ascending aorta may be clearly evident on the right mediastinal border. As it enlarges the main pulmonary trunk fills in the concavity below the aortic knob resulting in a rather straight upper left heart border. In the lateral view an enlarged right pulmonary artery is seen end on anterior to the carina.

3.2 Pulmonary Blood Vessels

The PA chest film provides useful information concerning the pulmonary, or 'lesser', circulation. Bronchial vessels are not seen in a normal radiograph. The pulmonary arteries branch rapidly in regular fashion, like the branches of a tree. In pulmonary arterial hypertension the peripheral branches become narrower and the central branches more prominent. The pulmonary veins branch less frequently and in a less regular fashion. (Fig. 3.4) In the upper lobes the larger pulmonary artery branches lie medial to the pulmonary veins which become more obvious when congested in heart failure. When studying a normal radiograph, veins in the left upper zone and the right lower zone are more likely to be evident. Frequently quite a large branching arrangement of veins can be seen extending from the right middle and lower lobes. In left-to-right intracardiac shunts a relatively increased volume of blood passes to the lungs causing a general engorgement or plethora of both arteries and veins throughout (Fig. 3.7, 3.8). This generalized distension or **pleonaemia** of

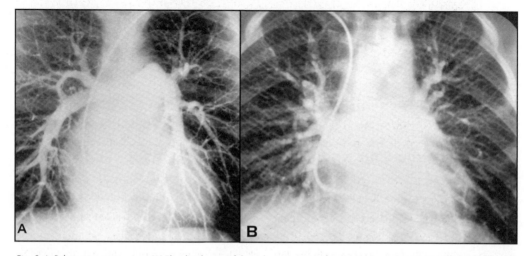

Fig. 3.4 Pulmonary angiograms. (A) The distribution of the pulmonary arteries is clearly demonstrated by contrast medium. (B) The pulmonary veins draining into the left atrium are clearly shown later in the examination. Catheter in the right ventricle.

vessels must be distinguished from the pulmonary venous congestion associated with left heart failure. In many cases of early venous congestion the distension of vessels is more obvious in the upper zones. In right to left shunts, the lungs appear **oligaemic** (Fig. 3.9).

3.3 Congenital Heart Disease (CHD)

Malformations of the heart or great vessels may be symptomless or present clinically through the presence of a murmur, arrhythmia, cyanosis, embolic episodes or the development of heart failure. Significant abnormalities may be present with a normal-appearing chest x-ray, but in most cases the chest film provides useful supportive evidence. Doppler echocardiography frequently demonstrates the disordered cardiac anatomy and function which may require confirmation by cardiac catheterization and angiography. MRI has the potential to replace these invasive techniques in CHD. CHD can be conveniently divided into those with no intracardiac shunt and those with shunting either from the left to the right side or the reverse. Some examples are:

No shunt

- Coarctation of aorta
- Pulmonary valve stenosis

Left to right shunts

- Atrial septal defect (ASD)
- Ventricular septal defect (VSD)
- Patent Ductus

Right to left shunts

- Fallots' tetralogy
- Transposition of the great vessels

CHD without intracardiac shunting

Dextrocardia is rare. A chest film with the heart apex towards the right side marker usually means the side marker on the film has been placed incorrectly! Dextrocardia without transposition of the abdominal organs is more frequently associated with intracardiac abnormalities than is dextrocardia with the abdominal organs also transposed. Normally the aortic arch passes to the left of the trachea before descending on the left side of the spine. Right-sided aortic arch is an important observation on the chest radiograph as it is frequently associated with intracardiac defects (Figs 3.5,3.9). Coarctation of the aorta is associated with notching of the under-surface of ribs bilaterally as a result of the collateral circulation through the intercostal arteries (Fig. 3.6). The aortic valve may be congenitally malformed and stenotic giving rise to symptoms in early adult life. A bicuspid aortic valve, frequently associated with coarctation, may give rise to aortic incompetence. Vascular rings in the mediastinum due to malformation of the great

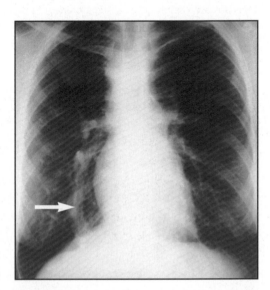

Fig. 3.5 Anomalous venous drainage of the right lung. The large vein draining the entire right lung (arrow) is seen adjacent to the right atrium extending down to enter the inferior vena cava close to its site of entry to the right atrium. The curved vein, becoming wider as it descends, has been designated the 'scimitar' sign. Note right-sided aortic arch.

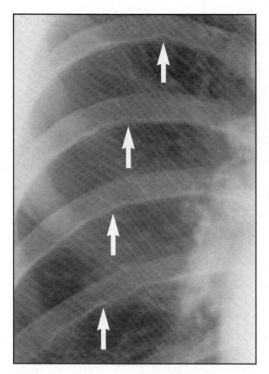

Fig. 3.6 Rib notching (arrows) in coarctation of the thoracic aorta.

vessels may encircle the oesphagus and produce dysphagia. Congenital pulmonary outflow tract obstruction may develop in the ventricular infundibulum below the pulmonary valve, at the valve level, or even distal to the valve as coarctation of the pulmonary artery or its branches. Pulmonary valve stenosis may be an isolated abnormality associated with little disturbance to the pulmonary vascular pattern and is detected by the presence of a murmur in early adult life, or more often it may be associated with an intracardiac shunt.

CHD with intracardiac shunt

Severe disturbances of the cardio-pulmonary circulation due to intracardiac shunting become apparent early in life but less disturbing defects may not be detected until adult life. The presence of a murmur, arrhythmia and, on occasions, paradoxical embolism may be the first evidence of the abnormality. The appearance of the cardiac contour and the mediastinum and pulmonary

vessels provides supportive evidence in making a diagnosis and cardiac catheterization with angiography provides detailed anatomical and functional information.

Left to right shunts

The increased volume in the pulmonary circulation results in generalized engorgement of vessels referred to as pleonaemic lungs (Figs 3.7,3.8). The uniform distribution of the prominent vessels differs from that in venous congestion due to left heart failure when the upper lobe vessels tend to be more distended than the constricted lower lobe vessels. The direction of shunt means the patients are acyanotic. Left to right shunts include:

• Atrial septal defect (ASD).

• Ventricular septal defect (VSD).

• Patent ductus arteriosus (PDA).

• Partial anomalous pulmonary venous drainage.

With congenital left to right shunting the cardiac chambers and great vessels respond according to whether there is a relative increase in

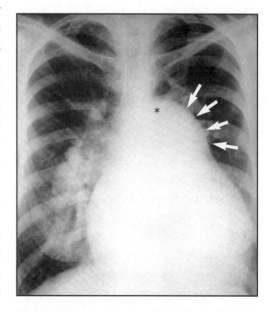

Fig. 3.7 Atrial septal defect with marked left-to-right shunting. Note the small aortic knob (*) and prominent pulmonary artery trunk (arrows) and the vascular dilatation in the lungs centrally. In this case the relatively constricted peripheral lung vessels are consistent with secondary pulmonary hypertension, a common sequel to ASD.

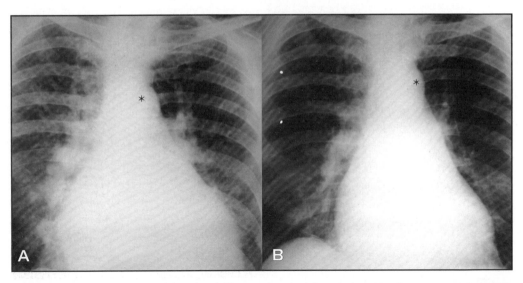

Fig. 3.8 Patent ductus arteriosus. (A) Plethoric lung fields consistent with a left-to-right shunt. Note the prominent aortic knob (*) and moderate cardiomegaly. (B) Post-operatively the lung fields have relatively normal vasculature and the heart size is within normal limits.

blood flow or a relative decrease. In ASD (Fig. 3.7), the increased blood flow affects the right atrium, right ventricle and pulmonary arteries with relative sparing of the left ventricle and aortic arch. Thus, the cardiac silhouette shows a small aortic knob, a prominent common pulmonary artery trunk and no evidence of left ventricular enlargement. However, with PDA (Fig. 3.8) the relative increase in flow affects the pulmonary circulation, the left atrium, left ventricle and aortic arch. Therefore, in PDA a prominent aortic knob is seen with evidence of left ventricular enlargement. The left atrium does not enlarge significantly. Ventricular septal defect (VSD) is more difficult to diagnose from plain films. Pulmonary veins sometimes drain anomalously into the right atrium rather than the left giving rise to what is functionally a left to right shunt. Not infrequently anomalous venous drainage is seen in patients with ASD and requires correction surgically at the time of closing the septal defect. Anomalous venous drainage of an entire lung, almost always the right, is usually into the upper inferior vena cava and the large draining vein has a scimitar-like shape (Fig. 3.5).

Right to left shunts

Shunting of deoxygenated blood to the systemic circulation results in cyanosis. Three of these conditions will be considered:

• Fallot's Tetralogy.

• Transposition of great vessels.

• Eisenmenger syndrome.

The Tetralogy of Fallot (Fig. 3.9) is the classical example of congenital right to left shunt. Severe pulmonary artery stenosis or atresia, an interventricular septal defect, a large aortic root which overrides the septal defect, and an hypertrophied right ventricle make up the tetralogy. The diminished blood flow to the lungs renders them oligaemic on the chest radiograph and the very small pulmonary artery trunk results in an indentation on the left heart border. Bronchial arteries hypertrophy to supply blood to the oligemic lungs and these can be seen sometimes as tortuous irregular vessels particularly in the upper lobes. In recent times the term Fallot's Syndrome has been extended to include all cases with a degree of pulmonary outflow obstruction with an intracardiac septal defect even when cyanosis is not present.

In very early life complete transposition of the great vessels associated with an intracardiac septal defect results in cyanosis but with pleonaemic lungs, and this condition requires surgical correction if the baby is to survive. In patients with left to right shunting due to ASD, VSD or PDA, pulmonary hypertension develops after many years and terminally this can result in reversal of the shunt and the development of cyanosis, a condition known as the Eisenmenger syndrome (Fig. 3.7).

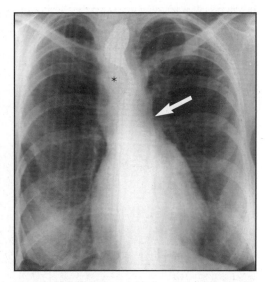

Fig. 3.9 Fallot's tetralogy. Note the right-sided aortic arch indenting the barium-filled oesophagus (*), a common asssociation with congenital heart disease. The pulmonary artery trunk (arrow) and pulmonary vessels in the lung fields and at the hila are relatively inconspicuous (oligaemia).

3.4 Acquired Heart Disease

Acquired diseases may affect valves, myocardium, coronary circulation, pericardium and the great vessels. On plain chest radiography these may be manifest as cardiomegaly, specific chamber (Fig. 3.3) or great vessel enlargement, intracardiac calcification, or by evidence of cardiac failure (Fig. 3.12). Prosthetic heart valves and pacemaker electrodes may be evident on plain films. Function of prosthetic valves, if opaque, can also be assessed by fluoroscopy (Fig. 3.10).

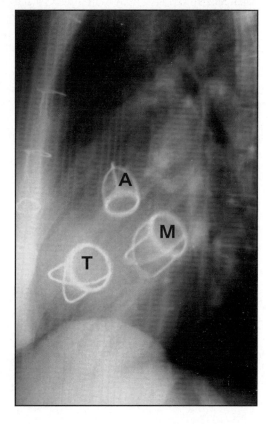

Fig. 3.10 Prosthetic heart valves, aortic (A), mitral (M) and tricuspid (T). Note wire sutures in the sternum.

3.5 Cardiac Calcifications

Image intensifier fluoroscopy is very sensitive in detecting valvular calcification and should be requested in association with chest radiography in patients with suspected valvular lesions.

Calcifications in the coronary arteries can be seen but do not correlate well with the clinical manifestations of coronary disease. Pericardial calcification is seen in constrictive pericarditis (Fig. 3.11).

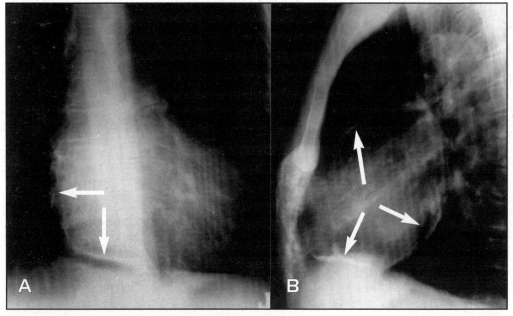

Fig. 3.11 Constrictive pericarditis. The abnormal pericardium (arrows) is heavily calcified particularly over the right side of the heart, with relative sparing over the left ventricle.

3.6 Cardiac Failure, Pulmonary Oedema and Pleural Effusion

As the left ventricle fails it enlarges to a point where the cardiac width exceeds the normal limit of 50% of the chest width in full inspiration. Right heart failure, e.g. as a result of pulmonary hypertension, has less effect on the cardiac silhouette and the heart may not become enlarged. An enlarged transverse diameter to the cardiac silhouette does not necessarily mean ventricular failure. A pericardial effusion can cause it and sometimes in mitral valve disease the right and left atria can become extremely large, widening the cardiac silhouette, whilst the ventricles remain relatively undilated.

A failing left ventricle results in lung changes which can be considered as occurring in three phases, although there is considerable overlap.

1. Pulmonary venous congestion.
2. Pulmonary interstitial oedema
3. Pulmonary alveolar oedema.

1. Pulmonary venous congestion

The first sign of left heart failure is distension of pulmonary veins. For reasons not fully understood the distension is greater in the upper zones than in the lower zones where venous spasm seems to occur. This diversion of blood to

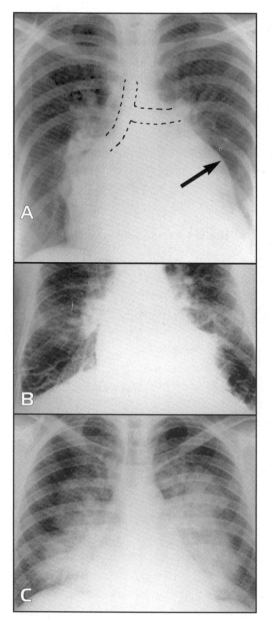

A

B

C

Fig. 3.12 Pulmonary changes of cardiac failure. (A) The earliest phase of venous congestion with prominent veins in the upper zones and relative constriction of veins in the lower zones as a result of diversion of blood in this earliest phase of decompensation. In this case of mitral valve disease the very large left atrium (arrow) is splaying the carina (outlined). (B) Interstitial pulmonary oedema with blurring of the hilar outlines and the presence of Kerley B lines at the lung bases due to lymphatic engorgement of the interlobular septa. (C) Alveolar pulmonary oedema resulting in consolidation, air bronchograms and clinically the production of frothy pink sputum. The central distribution of the oedema is frequently seen but not clearly understood.

the upper zone veins with constriction in the lower zones can be appreciated on chest x-rays although it is a subtle sign (Fig. 3.12A).

2. Pulmonary interstitial oedema

Interstitial connective tissue envelops the branching blood vessels and bronchi. Lymphatics course through the interstitial tissue carrying lymph from peripheral areas centrally. With cardiac failure a bank-up of lymphatic drainage occurs with engorgement of the interstitium. As a result the hilar structures become blurred and peripherally, particularly near the lung bases, the fine interlobular septa become prominent and visible on the chest x-ray as horizontal fine lines, known as Kerley B lines (Fig. 3.12B).

3. Pulmonary alveolar oedema

In the final stage pulmonary oedema fluid accumulates in the alveoli resulting in large areas of homogeneous opacity throughout the lung fields, often more centrally (Fig. 3.12C). The presence of air bronchograms is diagnostic of alveolar opacity.

Although the commonest cause of pulmonary oedema is left heart failure conditions causing it can be grouped as follows:

1. Increased pulmonary arterial capillary pressure: e.g. iatrogenic due to fluid overload.

2. Increased capillary permeability: Toxic gas inhalation; Pulmonary infection; Oedema resulting from central nervous system lesions including subarachnoid haemorrhage and cerebrovascular accidents.

3. Decreased osmotic pressure of blood; Liver disease; Nephrosis.

4. Increased pulmonary venous capillary pressure; Cardiac failure.

It can be seen then that the appearance of diffuse alveolar opacity throughout the lungs on a chest x-ray is non-specific. However, in an acutely ill person with such an appearance the diagnosis will almost certainly be one of the following.

1. Acute pulmonary oedema.
2. Widespread pneumonia.
3. Allergic alveolitis
   (Goodpasture's syndrome).

Cardiac failure is frequently associated with pleural effusions which may develop in the absence of radiographic evidence of pulmonary oedema (see section 2.8). The effusions are often bilateral but when unilateral it is usually at the right lung base. In practice if a pleural effusion is confined to the left base it is unwise to attribute it to cardiac failure until other causes are excluded.

3.7 The Pericardium

The pericardial sac may be the site of a wide variety of disease processes which are manifest clinically by either a pericardial effusion or constrictive pericarditis.

Pericardial effusion

Accumulation of fluid in the pericardial sac widens the cardiac silhouette on chest radiography and this can be confused with dilatation of the heart itself (Fig. 3.13). A large effusion produces a globular shape to the outline and the presence of uncongested pulmonary blood vessels should raise the suspicion, if not suspected clinically. In general, very large hearts are associated with some degree of pulmonary congestion, and if this is not present pericardial effusion should be suspected as the cause of the 'cardiomegaly'. Pericardial effusions can be grouped according to the nature of the fluid.

1. Serous:
   Low serum protein states. Myxoedema. Dressler's Syndrome, i.e. the effusion following a recent myocardial infarct and thought to be auto-immune in nature.
2. Serofibrinous:
   Uraemia; rheumatic fever;
   Viral, usually Coxsachie or Echo;
   Tuberculosis.
3. Suppurative:
   Pneumococcus; Staphylococcus, etc., usually secondary to pneumonia or other infections.
4. Haemorrhagic:
   Dissection of the aortic root; Rupture of the heart following myocardial infarction; Metastases; Trauma.

A pericardial rub may be detected clinically but if confirmation of an effusion is required echocardiography is the simplest test. An echo-free band posterior to the heart is virtually diagnostic of pericardial fluid. CT and MRI, although very sensitive, are rarely required to prove the diagnosis.

Constrictive pericarditis

In time fibrosis of the visceral pericardium may occur leading to impairment of filling of the chambers of the heart, almost always the right heart. Viral and tuberculous pericarditis and haemopericardium are amongst the causes of this

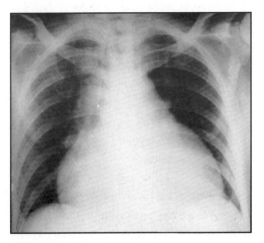

Fig. 3.13 Large pericardial effusion. Note the globular shape to the heart outline and the lack of pulmonary congestion, which differentiates effusion from heart failure.

syndrome, which may be difficult to diagnose. Signs of right heart failure, i.e. raised jugular venous pressure, hepatomegaly, ascites and ankle oedema, in the presence of a relatively normal-sized heart and uncongested lung fields should raise the suspicion of constrictive pericarditis. Calcification may develop in the constricted pericardium and when seen on chest radiographs is diagnostic (Fig. 3.11). Confirmation of the condition usually requires cardiac catheterization and demonstration of an elevated end diastolic pressure in the right atrium. CT scanning will usually identify the thickened pericardium and is a sensitive detector of calcification.

3.8 Coronary Artery Disease

Chest radiography has a limited role in managing patients with angina or myocardial infarction, but coronary arteriography is the definitive examination to display the state of the coronary vessels.

Chest radiography

The heart size remains normal unless myocardial infarction has occurred, when some dilatation of the left ventricle may be seen. The extent of calcification in coronary arteries seen on fluoroscopy does not correlate well with the clinical status of the individual. Severe local infarction in the region of the apex of the left ventricle may lead to myocardial aneurysm formation which can be detected as a localised bulging on the lower left heart border. In the days following an acute myocardial infarction a chest radiograph can assist in assessing the lungs, particularly as pulmonary venous congestion and early interstitial oedema are not detected by the stethoscope.

Coronary arteriography

Special coronary artery catheters are available which are introduced through the femoral artery and, in turn, directed into the ostia of the right and left coronary arteries. In 85% of individuals the left coronary artery divides into the anterior descending and circumflex arteries and the right coronary extends around in the atrioventricular groove to supply the posterior descending artery on the posterior aspect of the interventricular septum (Fig. 3.14A). In about 15% the posterior descending artery is supplied by the circumflex artery so that the entire left ventricular myocardium is dependent on the left coronary artery. It is the left ventricular myocardium which makes up most of the heart muscle and in the majority of patients when an occlusion occurs in the left coronary system anastomoses develop from the right to the left coronary circulation. Injections of contrast medium with the patient in various positions are recorded on cine film or videotape for detailed analysis (Fig. 3.14B,C). Coronary artery occlusions can be bypassed surgically using internal mammary or radial artery or saphenous vein grafts. Many stenoses may be dilated percutaneously using balloon catheters (angioplasty) and their patency maintained by the introduction of metallic stents.

Assessing the myocardium

As part of coronary arteriography a left ventricular injection of contrast medium is made to assess the contractility of that chamber. Previously infarcted muscle may be demonstrated as hypokinetic, akinetic or aneurysmal regions on the ventriculogram. Echocardiography and radionuclide imaging provide non-invasive methods of studying the left ventricular myocardium and even newer techniques, e.g. MRI, are being studied to

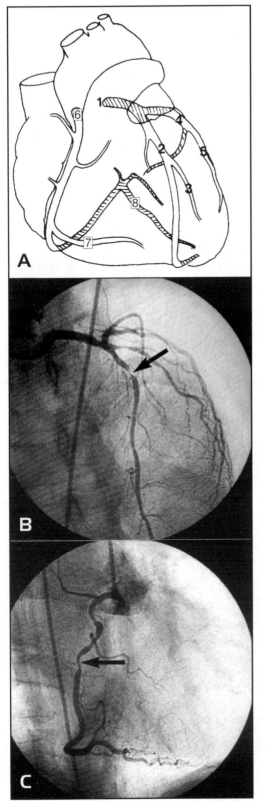

determine their value. Normally, on ultrasound, the myocardial thickness is about 1 cm and the normal left ventricular cavity does not dilate beyond 5.5 cm during diastole. Thallium behaves like potassium and is taken up by the myocardium, so that, if radiothallium is injected, the ischaemic areas will be seen as defects in the myocardial emission images. Thallium myocardial imaging is arranged so as to record perfusion, both during exercise and at rest a short time following. More recently, technetium-labelled sestamibi has been used for the same purpose (Plate 3.15 – see colour plates section).

Fig. 3.14 (A) The coronary artery anatomy. 1 = L main stem, a.; 2 = L anterior descending a.; 3 = Diagonal branch, 4 = Circumflex a.; 5 = Obtuse marginal branch; 6 = R coronary a.; 7 = Acute marginal branch; 8 = Posterior descending a. (B) Selective left coronary arteriogram. Note the tight stenosis (arrow) in the anterior descending branch. (C) Selective right coronary arteriogram. Note the segment of moderate narrowing in the mid-portion of the vessel (arrow).

3.9 Thoracic Aorta

Aneurysms

Most aneurysms of the thoracic aorta fall into one of the following groups:

- Atheromatous aneurysms.
- Dissecting aneurysms.
- Traumatic aneurysms.

Atheromatous aneurysms

With ageing the atheromatous aorta tends to elongate and dilate, sometimes to aneurysmal proportions. The aneurysms are usually fusiform and frequently the lateral margin of the aneurysmal descending thoracic aorta can be seen behind the heart shadow well away from the midline. Likewise dilatation of the ascending aorta is seen as an arc-shaped prominence on the right heart border above the right atrium. Saccular aneurysms are uncommon.

Dissecting aortic aneurysm

Intramural haemorrhage with dissection of the aortic wall over a considerable length is quite common. Hypertension and medionecrosis, as seen in Marfan's syndrome, are predisposing causes of this serious and painful vascular accident which usually has an acute onset. The extent of involvement of the aorta determines the clinical management and on this basis the condition is classified as:

Type A:

Involves the ascending aorta and often the brachiocephalic trunk, carotid and left subclavian arteries and may extend proximally to cause aortic incompetence or haemopericardium which is usually a terminal event. The prognosis is worse than for type B and surgical intervention is often indicated.

Type B:

Does not involve the ascending aorta but only the descending and distal aortic arch. Surgery is usually not indicated.

The dissection frequently extends below the diaphragm to involve the origins of the larger branches, particularly the left renal artery. Various imaging methods have been used to diagnose the condition and its extent. Newer techniques aim to obtain this information with minimal interference to the patient.

Plain radiography

The chest film may show a widened aorta with a prominent aortic knob. If a previous film showed a normal aorta this finding is strongly suggestive of recent dissection.

Transoesophageal echocardiography (TOE)

Passage of an ultrasound catheter into the oesophagus provides diagnosis of dissection in about 97% of cases by demonstrating the intimal

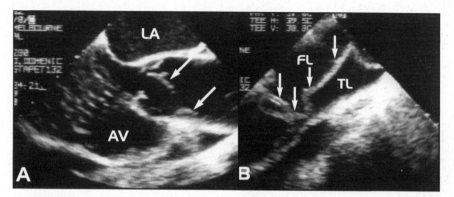

Fig. 3.16 Type A dissection of the ascending aorta. Transoesophageal echocardiography (TOE). (A) Section through aortic root. The intimal flap (arrows) extends down to the aortic valve (AV). (B) Section through the arch showing the true (TL) and false (FL) lumina and the flap (arrows). Left atrium (LA).

flap (Fig. 3.16). Ultrasound also allows assessment of the aortic valve and detection of pericardial fluid. More than 50% of patients with this condition succumb in the first 48 hours and it is important for the diagnosis to be made promptly and treatment instituted. TOE can be performed at the bedside, with experience, causing minimal disturbance to the patient.

Aortography (Fig. 3.17A)

Careful introduction of a catheter from the femoral artery into the ascending aorta for injection of contrast medium usually reveals the diagnosis and the extent of dissection. Often in late films the false sac becomes opacified whilst in other cases the compressed ribbon like true lumen is all that is outlined. The patency of aortic branches can be assessed.

Computed tomography (CT) (Fig. 3.17B)

CT performed during an intravenous injection of contrast medium demonstrates most of the features necessary for clinical management. Scans at three levels usually suffice. Sections through the aortic arch allow classification into type A or type B and sections at the level of the left atrium and the diaphragm demonstrate the extent of downward dissection.

Magnetic resonance angiography (MRA)

MRA, when available, provides all of the information required and avoids the need for contrast medium injection.

Traumatic aneurysms

Decelerating injuries may occur in high speed road accidents. Rupture of the distal portion of the aortic arch may result from such injuries, which are fatal if the mural rupture is complete. In many such injuries a circumferential tear of the intima and media occurs, with the adventitia, the strongest coat of the aorta, remaining intact. An aneurysm results and usually this is in the region of the ligamentum arteriosum just beyond the left subclavian artery origin (Fig. 3.18). Delayed rupture with a fatal outcome may occur or the patient may present incidentally years later because on a chest x-ray the abnormal aortic outline, often calcified, is detected.

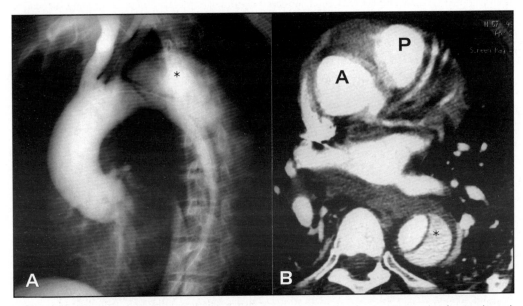

Fig. 3.17 Type B dissection of thoracic aorta. (A) The aortagram shows a large dissection sac (*) extending from just beyond the left subclavian artery downwards to the diaphragm. The compressed true lumen lies anteromedially. (B) Contrast-enhanced CT shows the dissection sac (*) separated from the true lumen by the arc-shaped stripe of dissected aortic wall. A=ascending aorta. P=pulmonary artery.

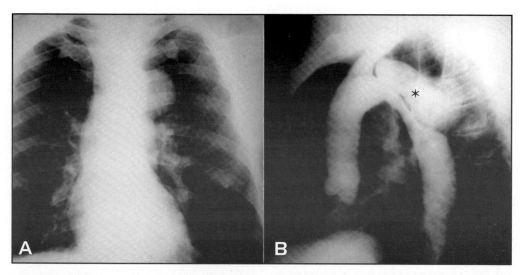

Fig. 3.18 Traumatic rupture of thoracic aorta. (A) The aortic knob is abnormally prominent. (B) Aortogram shows the traumatic aneurysm (*) at the typical site. The patient gave a history of a decelerating injury many years before.

Widening of the upper mediastinum on a chest x-ray of a patient who has experienced a decelerating type of accident with sternal damage should raise the suspicion and, if investigations prove the diagnosis, immediate surgery is indicated because of the risk of delayed rupture.

Patients surviving several days may develop a hoarse voice because of pressure on the left recurrent laryngeal nerve which encircles the aortic arch. The presence of a left-sided haemorrhagic pleural effusion in the days following such an injury should suggest the diagnosis.

Aortography will prove or exclude the lesion and similar information can be obtained nowadays using CT or MRI.

3.10 Abdominal Aorta

Unlike the thorax, where gas in the lungs negates its use, ultrasound is useful, and cost effective, in demonstrating the state of the abdominal aorta. Helical CT following intravenous contrast injection also provides a non-invasive method of assessing the aorta and provides a 3D representation. For detailed study, and in some cases to perform interventional therapy, abdominal aortography following femoral artery catheterization is employed. CT and MRI may be useful in certain cases.

Aneurysm

The vast majority of abdominal aneurysms involve the aorta below the renal arteries although often just below. In general, when an abdominal aortic aneurysm enlarges beyond 5 cm in diameter surgical treatment is considered because of the risk of rupture.

On plain radiography the presence of an aneurysm may be obvious if the calcified aortic intima is detected lying far more laterally than usual. Ultrasound allows definition of the true lumen and mural thrombus (Fig. 3.19) whilst aortography demonstrates only the lumen and may give a false impression if much thrombus is present within a fusiform aneurysm. Conventional axial CT (Fig. 3.20A) shows the lumen and thrombus, whilst helical 3D CT shows calcification and the relationship to the renal arteries (Fig. 3.20B,C).

In selected cases, it is now possible to introduce an endoluminal stent percutaneously by femoral artery catheterization to treat the aneurysm.

Rupture

Spontaneous rupture of the abdominal aorta is amenable to surgical treatment if diagnosed early. It usually results from atheroma or aortic dissection and the leaking blood in the retroperitoneal tissues is a cause of severe pain. On plain radiography the left psoas margin becomes obscured and the left kidney outline, if visible, is displaced upwards and laterally. With this emergency time is of the essence in treatment and US is usually the quickest means of establishing a diagnosis if the clinical picture is uncertain.

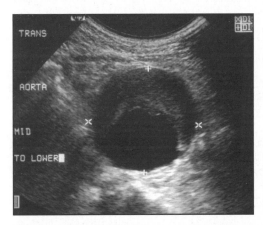

Fig. 3.19 (above) Abdominal aortic aneurysm. Transverse US shows the more echogenic mural thrombus contrasting with the hypoechoic patent lumen.

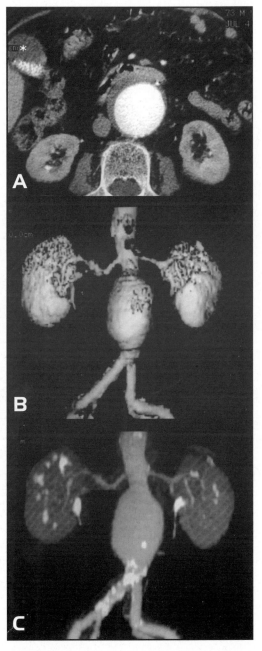

Fig. 3.20 (right) Abdominal aortic aneurysms. (A) Transverse axial CT following intravenous contrast injection shows the aneurysm with a moderate amount of mural thrombus. Note the gallstones in the gallbladder (*). (B) Surface-rendered display following helical CT provides a three-dimensional view of the arterial anatomy. (C) Maximum intensity display following helical CT shows the dense contrast medium in the urinary tract and calcified plaques within the arteries.

3.11 Peripheral Vascular Disease (PVD)

The manifestations of occlusive arterial disease, usually due to atheroma, affect the lower limbs to a much greater extent than the upper limbs. The first complaint is usually of intermittent claudication in the calf and it is only much later in the natural history that patients present with a critical state of ischaemia resulting in rest pain and areas of distal gangrene.

Lower limb arteriography

To fully assess the blood flow to the lower limbs it is necessary to display the arteries from the abdominal aorta to at least the mid-calf. The technique is suitable for ambulatory non-hospital patients. A fine catheter is introduced percutaneously into the femoral artery and guided to the abdominal aorta using fluoroscopy. Using digital subtraction angiography, dilute contrast medium is injected whilst imaging segments of the arterial tree, a procedure which is free from discomfort to the patient.

The arteriograms indicate the presence of atheromatous irregularities and stenoses as well as occluded segments and the presence of collateral circulation. Although lesions may occur at any site atheroma is particularly prone to occur in the adductor canal in the thigh, the distal aorta and common iliac arteries and at the origin of the profunda femoris artery. This procedure, which is generally referred to as **aortography and follow-through** aims to demonstrate the full length of the arterial tree and, when obstructed segments are present, the state of the vessels beyond the obstruction.

When to investigate patients with PVD?

Intermittent claudication is inconvenient for the patient but its onset does not imply that permanent tissue ischaemic changes are imminent. The time-scale leading to rest pain and gangrene is long and previously, when surgical bypass was the only avenue of treatment, the decision to investigate intermittent claudication was delayed. In recent years percutaneous balloon dilatation, or **angioplasty**, has become available as a valuable

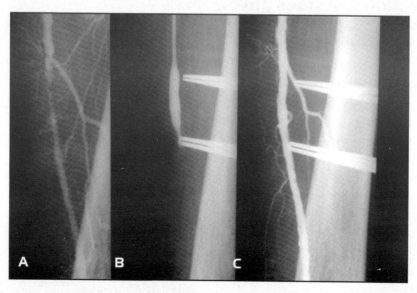

Fig. 3.21 Femoral artery angioplasty. (A) Severe stenosis in the adductor canal. (B) Balloon catheter inflated between skin markers. (C) Satisfactory post-dilatation angiogram.

and effective means of treating localised arterial stenoses (Fig. 3.21). Because of this development, the modern trend is to investigate intermittent claudication early and to perform transluminal angioplasty if significant stenoses are present, particularly as both procedures can be performed on an outpatient basis at the one appointment.

Using similar technique, it is also possible to disobliterate occluded segments of artery. However, initial follow-up indicated that reocclusion frequently occured. To overcome this, the technique of metallic stent insertion has evolved and this ensures longer patency of the recanalised lumen (Fig. 3.22).

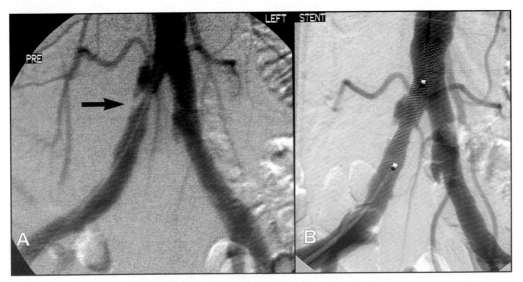

Fig. 3.22 Right Common iliac artery stenosis (arrow) before (A) and after (B) balloon dilatation and mesh wire stenting.

3.12 Deep Venous Thrombosis

Thrombotic occlusion of deep lower-limb veins is commonplace and results in local changes, pain and swelling, or distant pulmonary embolism. Predisposing causes include bed rest, particularly following operations, fractured femoral neck, the presence of abdominal neoplasms such as pancreatic carcinoma, and the later stages of pregnancy. The clinical diagnosis of deep vein thrombosis is notoriously inaccurate and various imaging techniques have been used to clarify the matter. For greatest detail, lower limb venography is the method of choice but should be reserved for those with an inconclusive US examination.

Ultrasound

Colour Flow Doppler (CFD) is the first line of investigation. It has a high sensitivity and specificity in femoral and popliteal vein thrombosis. It can detect occlusive and non-occlusive thrombi. Patency of veins can be tested by compression with the US transducer (Fig. 3.23). An occluded vein is incompressible as well as lacking a colour flow signal. The significance of calf vein thrombosis alone remains controversial, some arguing that there is no risk of pulmonary embolism. Initial examination is often limited to the femoral and popliteal regions, taking about 15 minutes.

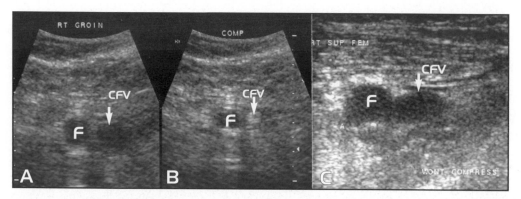

Fig. 3.23 Compression US test. F=Femoral Artery. CFV=Common Femoral Vein. Normal (A) before and (B) after compressing CFV. (C) Thrombosed CFV resists compression.

Lower limb venography

A fine catheter is introduced into a vein on the dorsum of the foot. With a tourniquet around the ankle to direct the contrast medium to the deep veins a moderately large volume of contrast medium is injected and radiographs of the lower limb and pelvis obtained. Films show occluded segments and intraluminal thrombi (Fig. 3.24). Following venography it is wise for the legs to be moved frequently and not kept at rest as the contrast medium may contribute to further thrombosis.

The imaging of suspected pulmonary embolism is discussed in Chapter 2.

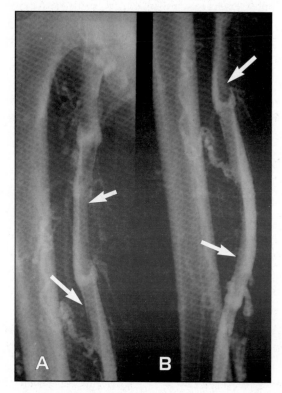

Fig. 3.24 Lower-limb venogram showing an intraluminal clot (arrows) involving the upper (A) and lower (B) femoral vein which remained patent up to the groin where occlusion was demonstrated.

3.13 Lymphatic System, Lymphoma and AIDS

Lymph nodes in the neck, thorax and abdomen, particularly when enlarged, are well demonstrated by CT. **Lymphangiography**, which antedates CT, is a technique of outlining the lymphatic channels and lymph nodes and requires a meticulous dissection to cannulate a lymphatic with a very fine needle. Oily iodine containing contrast medium is then injected, and films made immediately demonstrate lymphatic channels draining the injection site together with the lymph nodes along that chain. By injecting a lymphatic on the dorsum of the foot the inguinal, iliac and para-aortic nodes can be demonstrated together with the lymphatic channels and the thoracic duct. Films made after 24 hours show retention of the medium within the nodes and the nodes remain opaque for several months (Fig. 3.25). Lymphangiography was used extensively in the past to demonstrate neoplastic metastases or lymphoma in lymph nodes and for the investigation of lymphoedema.

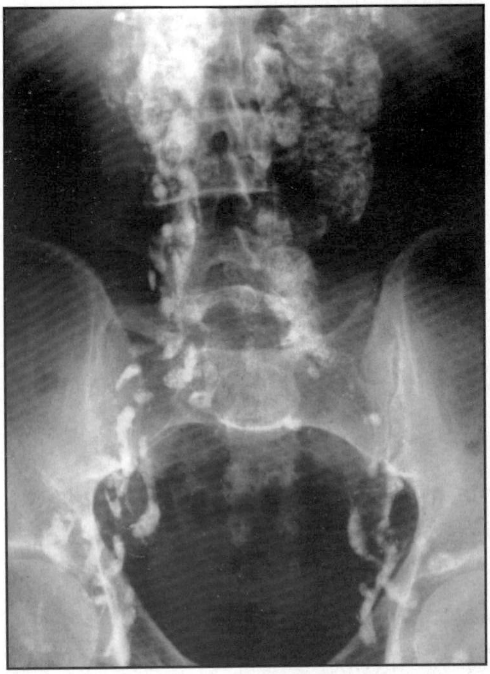

Lymphoma

Hodgkin's lymphoma is usually confined to the lymph nodes and extranodal lymphatic tissue. At presentation Hodgkin's disease is usually supradiaphragmatic and spread occurs from one node group contiguously to the next. Enlarged mediastinal and hilar nodes may be seen on a plain chest film (Fig. 2.26). Staging is important as about 75% of patients are curable with appropriate therapy. Initial staging includes CT of the neck, chest, abdomen and pelvis. Nodes above 1 cm in size are considered abnormal. CT also provides information concerning other relevant organs, particularly the spleen. Lymphoma may cause a homogenous enlargement of the spleen or in some cases there may be patchy involvement with areas of relative radiolucency.

Non-Hodgkin's lymphoma (NHL) also frequently involves the lymph nodes, more so in the abdomen, and the nodes tend to be larger than in Hodgkin's disease (Fig. 3.26). The range of aggressiveness of NHL is broad as is the range of

Fig. 3.25 Abdominal lymphogram. Film made 24 hours after bipedal injection of contrast medium into lymphatics shows normal-sized nodes in the iliac chains and markedly enlarged para-aortic nodes with abnormal architecture. Diagnosis: Non-Hodgkin's lymphoma.

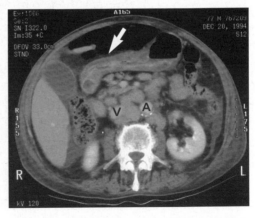

Fig. 3.26 Non-Hodgkins lymphoma. Enlarged mesenteric and para-aortic lymph nodes and thickening of the stomach wall (arrow). Aorta (A). Vena cava (V).

tissues in the various organs which may become involved. As with Hodgkin's disease initial staging involves CT both above and below the diaphragm.

Post-therapeutic assessment of lymphoma patients again depends initially on CT to determine reduction in lymph node size and regression of lesions in extranodal tissues. CT is unable to detect reactivation as opposed to fibrosis, and radionuclide imaging using **gallium 67** (Fig. 3.27) is helpful in making this distinction. With the availability of CT and gallium imaging **staging laparotomy** is rarely used.

AIDS

Acquired Immunodeficiency Syndrome (AIDS), subsequent to human immuno-deficiency virus (HIV) infection, is associated with a wide range of pathology involving virtually all bodily tissues. Radiology only occasionally is first to diagnosis the underlying disease but is required to demonstrate pathological lesions and to diagnosis the aetiology of these if possible, a difficult task

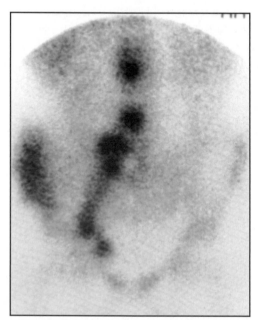

Fig. 3.27 Recurrent abdominal lymphoma. Gallium 67 has been actively taken up by the recurrent enlarged lymphomatous aorto-iliac nodes.

because of nonspecificity. Pathology in HIV infection and AIDS is due to either:

1. HIV infection.
2. Opportunistic infection by a wide range of organisms, bacterial, viral, fungal and parasitic.
3. Neoplasm, particularly Kaposi's sarcoma and lymphoma.
4. Causes unrelated to the HIV infection.

For more accurate interpretation of radiological abnormalities in HIV patients, it is helpful to know not only the symptoms but also the stage of the disease, particularly the CD4 lymphocyte level. With CD4 levels above 200 cells/cubic mm, the level below which a patient is said to have AIDS, infections are more likely to behave like in the general community and be bacterial, including TB. With AIDS patients and lower CD4 levels neoplasms become more likely as do reactivation infections such as toxoplasma and CMV, and other opportunistic infections such as pneumocystis, candidiasis, cryptosporidium and atypical forms of mycobacteria. In AIDS radiology is used for detection of lesions in the chest, brain and spinal cord, abdomen and musculoskeletal system.

Chest

High resolution CT (HRCT) provides detail of the lung parenchyma supplementing plain radiography. In HIV patients lobar or segmental pneumonia and TB with cavitation or pleural effusion predominate, whilst in AIDS patients pneumocystis pneumonia (PCP) is the most common infection. Bilateral perihilar diffuse alveolar opacities are seen on plain films and HRCT usually shows cavitation which may lead to pneumothorax. With low CD4 levels disseminated TB and neoplasms occur. In 50% of AIDS patients with Kaposi's sarcoma (KS) the lungs are involved. Nodular thickening extends along the bronchovascular bundles from the hilum, best shown with HRCT. In more advanced

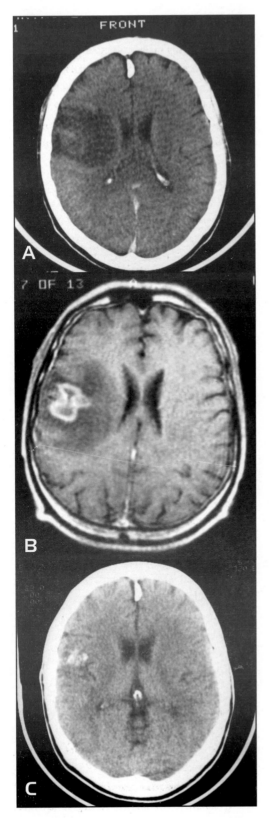

cases, rounded nodules are seen on plain films, having a similar appearance to lymphoma, which is less common than KS in the chest of AIDS patients.

Brain and spinal cord

HIV encephalitis affects predominantly the white matter bilaterally leading to brain atrophy and dementia, often quite rapidly. Toxoplasma (Fig. 3.28) is the commonest cause of focal brain lesions in AIDS, often multicentric and on CT and MRI enhancing following contrast, sometimes showing ring enhancement due to central necrosis. Often the appearance is similar to primary lymphoma, the second-commonest focal mass lesion in AIDS and with a very poor prognosis. Lymphoma is usually solitary. An empirical trial of antibiotic therapy is required to differentiate these conditions, toxoplasma responding well. Other infective agents producing nonspecific changes in the CNS include CMV, TB, cryptococcus and progressive multicentric leucoencephalopathy (PML).

Abdomen

The entire length of the bowel may be affected in AIDS. Infections particularly are seen when the CD4 level is below 100 cells/cubic mm. In the oesophagus HIV and CMV produce localized large ulcers. Candida and herpes have a similar appearance of shallow ulcers involving most of the mucosal surface. These lesions are well shown on barium swallow. Below the diaphragm CT is helpful in showing bowel wall thickening, mucosal changes and the state of the lymph nodes. TB usually involves the ileocaecal region whilst the atypical forms of mycobacteria mainly affect the jejunum accompanied by bulky enlargement of mesenteric nodes. AIDS-related cholangitis considered due to invasion by opportunistic

Fig. 3.28 Toxoplasmosis in HIV-positive patient. (A) contrast enhanced CT and (B) Gadolinium enhanced MRI showing right frontal lesion with surrounding oedema. (C) after one year of treatment showing residual calcification.

organisms results in stricturing of the bile ducts and occasionally the pancreatic duct as well as thickening of the gallbladder wall. Stones are usually not present. KS most commonly involves the duodenum, but also the stomach, where quite large polypoid lesions may be seen. Lymphoma tends to be widespread and aggressive. The renal parenchyma is frequently involved often leading to rapidly progressive renal failure.

Musculoskeletal

Although arthritis may be the first manifestation of AIDS, musculoskeletal lesions are not as common as lesions in other organ systems. Osteomyelitis, abscesses in muscles and various forms of arthritis may occur. Radionuclide bone scan which includes the entire skeleton is helpful in detection of these lesions.

3.14 Hypertension

Hypertension is extremely common and radiology contributes to the management of such patients in various ways. The reasons for investigating hypertension will vary from patient to patient, but include:

- To demonstrate established effects of hypertension.
- To search for a cause of hypertension, if present.
- To establish baselines for monitoring later effects.
- In the management of acute complications of hypertension.

1. To demonstrate established effects of hypertension.

Clinically retinoscopy allows a direct evaluation of the fundus and the state of small arteries. Heart size can be assessed by palpation but chest radiography is more precise.

2. To search for a cause of hypertension, if present.

In most patients with hypertension no cause can be demonstrated and this is referred to as **primary**, or **essential** hypertension. In a minority of hypertensives, a cause can be demonstrated and in some, corrected. If so, in younger patients, a lifetime commitment to hypertensive agents may be avoided. These causes of **secondary hypertension** can be listed as follows.

a. Coarctation of the aorta (Fig. 3.6)
   Coarctation causes rib notching on the chest film, but should be diagnosed by adequate clinical examination.
b. Endocrine causes:
   i.   Cushing's syndrome.
   ii. Phaeochromocytoma.
   iii. Conn's syndrome.

Endocrine conditions should be suspected clinically from the history, examination and basic biochemical tests. If suspected, the adrenals can be clearly demonstrated by CT (see Chapter 5).

c. Renal causes:
   i.   Renovascular. Conditions causing renal ischaemia.
   ii. Parenchymal lesions. Virtually all kidney diseases may be associated with hypertension.
   iii. Constrictive conditions. A rare group of conditions analogous to constrictive pericarditis, e.g. fibrosis following traumatic perirenal haematoma.

The commonest cause of secondary hypertension is kidney disease. Particularly in younger patients it is important to detect renovascular causes which may be reversible using interventional radiological techniques.

Causes of renovascular hypertension

These conditions all result in a degree of renal

parenchymal ischaemia, renin secretion and initiation of the aldosterone cycle.

a. Atheroma.

Occurs at the orifice, in the aortic wall or about 1 cm beyond the orifice in the artery itself (Fig. 3.29A).

b. Fibromuscular dysplasia (Fig. 3.30)

This not uncommon condition affects females to a far greater extent than males. The right renal artery is more commonly affected than the left and typically the kidney is ptosed, i.e. has a long renal artery. Multiple stenoses are often present with intervening small aneurysmal dilatations.

c. A-V fistula.

Sometimes following renal biopsy.

d. Arterial compression from tumours e.g. metastases.

e. Inadvertent ligation of a renal artery branch at surgery.

Investigation

In recent years, the approach to renal assessment in hypertension has changed and the available methods are set out historically.

Intravenous pyelography

The IVP demonstrates renal size and outline and many renal diseases as well as the state of the drainage system. Also, evidence of renal ischaemia consistent with renovascular hypertension can be detected. The presence of renal artery stenosis may be suspected clinically if an abdominal bruit is heard. If the kidney parenchyma and drainage system on IVP appear normal the following subtle signs may indicate unilateral renal ischaemia (Fig. 3.31).

1. Reduced size of the affected kidney.

2. Delayed appearance time of the contrast on the affected side.

3. Increased concentration of contrast medium on the affected side because the ischaemic kidney excretes less sodium and water.

Captopril renography

Using a gamma camera, and after intravenous injection of an appropriate radionuclide, the glomerular filtration rates of the two kidneys can be compared. Beyond a renal artery stenosis, the reduced flow results in a reduced glomerular filtration rate. However, this can be masked by a

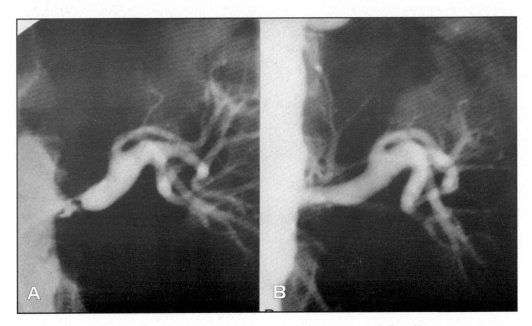

Fig. 3.29 Left renal artery stenosis due to atheroma. (A) Before and (B) after percutaneous balloon dilatation.

compensatory response of the kidney to reduced renal flow. Under such circumstances, the efferent glomerular arterioles go into spasm, an angiotensin effect, increasing the perfusion pressure in the glomeruli and a relative increase in filtration. This effect can be inhibited by the administration of Captopril which blocks the angiotensin cycle and allows the renogram to be more sensitive in detecting the reduced glomerular filtration rate beyond an artery stenosis (Fig. 3.32).

Helical CT scanning

This recently available development is suited to examining the kidneys of hypertensives. Following the intravenous injection of contrast medium, 3D images of the aorta and its branches can be obtained (Fig. 3.20) and at a later stage of the examination the kidney parenchyma and drainage systems can be studied in detail.

Ultrasound

US allows the size, shape, and status of the kidney to be assessed and colour Doppler US allows measurements of flow in the renal artery and its branches. These studies at present are not

sufficiently reliable for the routine demonstration of renal artery stenosis and are very time consuming.

Percutaneous renal arteriography

If renovascular hypertension is suspected from the above tests then generally renal arteriography is indicated to confirm the abnormality (Fig. 3.31B). Renal artery stenoses can be corrected by the interventional radiology technique of balloon dilatation, avoiding open surgery (Fig. 3.29). Dilatation of fibromuscular dysplasia has a good prognosis for remaining patent, but atheromatous narrowings usually require metallic stenting following balloon dilatation.

3. To establish baselines for monitoring later effects.

The plain chest x-ray is also useful as a comparison for assessing cardiomegaly later. However, left ventricular hypertrophy without

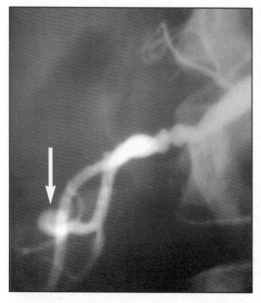

Fig. 3.30 Fibromuscular dysplasia of right renal artery. Typical multiple strictures with dilatations between. Note small aneurysm more distally (arrow).

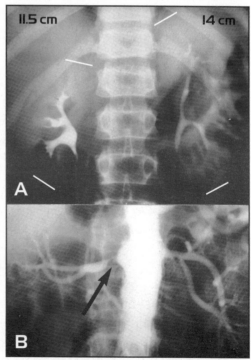

Fig. 3.31 Right renal artery stenosis. (A) IVP shows a reduced right kidney length (see markers) and a denser pyelogram compared with the left. (B) Arteriogram showing tight atheromatous stenosis (arrow) near the right renal artery origin.

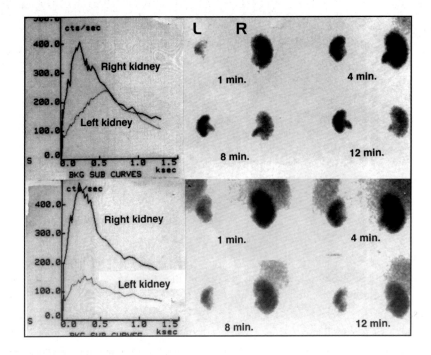

Fig. 3.32 Captopril Renogram. Left renal artery stenosis. Graphs and scans at intervals following radionuclide injection before (above) and after (below) Captopril. The smaller left kidney has a reduced and delayed peak radiation emission compared with the right, which, after Captopril, is further reduced but not delayed, an effect attributed to Captopril reducing compensatory spasm in the efferent glomerular arteriole which accompanies renal artery stenosis.

dilatation does not increase the transverse diameter of the heart.

4. In the management of acute complications of hypertension.

An important role of radiology is in the management of such complications as stroke or myocardial infarction and these matters are dealt with elsewhere.

In summary, in the initial assessment of hypertensives most should have a chest x-ray.

Younger patients should be assessed by IVP or Captopril renography and in certain cases this will lead on to helical CT or renal arteriography. When an endocrine cause is suspected clinically, CT examination of the adrenals is indicated as the next special investigation. In future US may develop to become the initial examination for studying the kidneys of hypertensives.

References

Baum, S.(ed.), *Abrams' Angiography*,
4th edn, Little, Brown and Company, 1997.

Sutton, D. (ed.), *A Textbook of Radiology and Imaging*,
4th edn, vol.1, pt 3, Churchill Livingstone, 1987.

Central Nervous System

Of all the spectacular developments in diagnostic imaging in recent decades the greatest advance has been the ability to display in detail the brain and its blood supply, the spinal cord and cerebrospinal fluid pathways, with minimal inconvenience to the patient.

4.1 Imaging Modalities

Various modalities are used and it is important to appreciate the present status of each of these techniques, some of which are not readily available yet but have significant potential in the future.

Plain radiography

The main application is now in trauma to the face and jaws and cervical spine and also in patients with suspected depressed fracture of the skull vault. It cannot exclude significant brain damage following head injury and CT is required in such cases.

Computed Tomography (CT)

CT demonstrates the skull bones well, but only in axial cross-section except for the face and anterior fossa where coronal sections are possible. The brain tissue is displayed as moderately opaque, but with little differentiation between white and grey matter. The CSF is radiolucent, clearly outlining the ventricles and cisterns. By computer manipulation the CT images may be displayed to show optimally the bones (**bone windows**), or alternatively to demonstrate the soft tissues more clearly (**brain windows**). Because CT is a multisectional technique using x-rays there is the potential risk of damage to the eyes and radiologists plan the angle and extent of CT imaging to avoid the orbits when possible.

In most body tissues the endothelial cells in capillaries have wide junctions which allow the passage of larger molecules into the extra-cellular tissues. This is not the case with brain capillaries, which have tight junctions known as the **blood-brain barrier** which prevents this diffusion. If an iodine-containing contrast medium is injected normally the contrast material does not pass into the brain but remains within the vascular system. However, in many CNS lesions the blood-brain barrier breaks down and contrast passes into the extracellular spaces of the lesion, a process referred to as **contrast enhancement**. In this way the use of contrast medium considerably increases the diagnostic potential of CT. A blood-brain barrier is not present normally in the choroid plexus, the pituitary and pineal glands, which normally enhance with contrast medium. Also, the barrier is lacking in lesions arising from the extra-axial tissues, e.g. meningiomas and Schwannomas, and these lesions enhance markedly. CT images following contrast medium show persisting contrast medium within the cerebral vasculature improving the differentiation between white and grey matter and outlining some of the larger vessels.

Magnetic Resonance Imaging (MRI)

MRI does not demonstrate the bones, because they contain relatively few hydrogen ions or protons, but in other respects MRI has significant advantages over CT in demonstrating the soft tissues. Excellent differentiation of white and grey matter and CSF is obtained, and no ionising radiation is used. To date, no significant harmful effects have been demonstrated. MRI sections can be obtained in any plane and the use of sagittal, coronal and axial images provides detailed definition of the extent of lesions. MRI images are computed reconstructions from radio frequency signals emitted by hydrogen protons in the tissues in response to an incident radio frequency pulse directed into the head from a surrounding coil whilst the head lies in a strong magnetic field. The quality of the displayed MRI image is controlled by the type of incident pulses and this allows for detailed analysis and characterization of lesions. The two commonly employed pulse sequences used are:

- **T_1 weighted spin-echo images**.

This sequence provides optimal display of anatomy (Fig. 4.11A) with structures showing a range of opacity from CSF, which appears black, through the varying shades of grey for brain tissue to subacute haemorrhage, which appears white.

- **T_2 weighted spin-echo images**.

These images, which take longer to obtain than T_1 weighted images, have a greater sensitivity for detecting pathological lesions, which mostly emit a higher signal with this sequence, appearing whiter, aiding their detection. The differentiation between anatomical structures is less clear than with T_1 weighted images and, in particular, CSF appears white on T_2 weighted images (Fig. 4.11B).

Flowing blood appears black on both T_1 and T_2 weighted sequences and this 'signal void' is due to the fact that hydrogen protons are continually moving out of the plane before being able to emit a signal. In similar fashion to the contrast enhancement of CT using iodinated medium, the intravenous injection of paramagnetic gadolinium contrast medium is used in MRI to show evidence of blood-brain barrier breakdown. **Gadolinium** has proven to be safer than iodinated media.

Recent advances in MRI have dramatically shortened exposure times to a point where useful images may be obtained even in disturbed patients unable to keep completely still.

Digital Subtraction Angiography (DSA)

DSA is used for demonstrating cerebral vasculature by injecting iodine-containing contrast medium through a catheter introduced percutaneously into the femoral artery and selectively directed into the appropriate cerebral vessel. The development of computer-based DSA resulted in less contrast medium being required with less patient discomfort and a considerable saving in film and contrast medium costs.

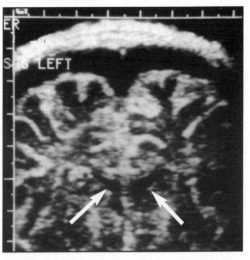

Fig. 4.1 Neonatal US obtained through the anterior fontanelle. The fluid-filled anterior horns of the lateral ventricles are shown (arrows).

Ultrasound (US)

US provides a considerable amount of information concerning the brain of the foetus in-utero. Also, it is the means of demonstrating the brain in the neonatal period whilst the anterior fontanelle remains patent (Fig. 4.1). Following closure the skull bones exclude the use of US except in the neck where US provides important information concerning the cerebral arteries.

Magnetic Resonance Angiography (MRA)

As an extension of MRI technology MRA is now able to demonstrate the cerebral vessels without the use of contrast medium or catheterization. Already quite small aneurysms have been demonstrated and MRA has the potential to replace DSA in many situations (Fig. 4.2).

Positron Emission Tomography (PET)

A PET scanner uses similar technology to the CT scanner with detectors sensitive to the radiation emanating from short-lived radionuclides produced by a cyclotron and injected intravenously. These short-lived isotopes, e.g. fluorine 18, are used to label molecules such as glucose which are taken up at sites of increased cerebral metabolic activity, opening up the field of functional imaging (Plate 1.2; see colour plates section). For example, with the eyes closed very little uptake is seen in the occipital visual cortex but it increases markedly with visual stimulation. More recently the emerging MRI signal has been shown to vary according to focal cerebral activity making functional MRI a potential alternative technique in the future.

Interventional neuroradiology

As in other regions catheter techniques are proving useful in treating particular lesions. Embolisation of vascular malformations, closure of arteriovenous fistulae, lysis of thrombosed vessels, angioplasty of stenoses in vertebral and carotid arteries and closure of some berry aneurysms have been reported.

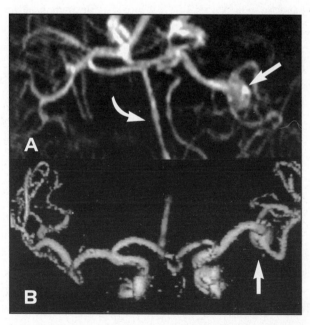

Fig. 4.2 Left middle cerebral artery aneurysm (arrow) shown by magnetic resonance angiography (MRA). (A) Maximum intensity image shows the left middle cerebral artery division and the aneurysm well. The basilar artery (curved arrow) and some branches are included in the section. (B) Surface-rendered image provides a more 3-D appreciation.

Patients with cerebral pathology present in ways which usually allow the clinician to draw up a short list of diagnostic probabilities after obtaining a detailed history and performing a neurological examination. It is in the context of these patterns of presentation that further investigations are requested.

4.2 Subarachnoid Haemorrhage

The sudden onset of severe headache and neck stiffness, sometimes accompanied by neurological signs, is generally easily recognized. Occasionally the onset is more gradual, causing confusion with meningitis and, as a result, some patients are referred to the infectious diseases hospital. Rarely, meningeal irritation is confined to the lumbar region when the bleeding is slow or intermittent resulting in confusion with other causes of backache.

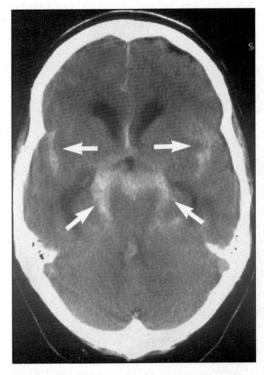

Fig. 4.3 Subarachnoid haemorrhage. CT showing opaque blood in both Sylvian fissures and in the cisterns surrounding the brain stem (arrows).

Causes:

* Berry aneurysm.
  Usually in the region of the circle of Willis. An increased incidence of berry aneurysms is recognised in hypertension, polycystic renal disease and aortic coarctation.
* Arteriovenous malformation.
* Secondary to intracerebral bleeding – spontaneous or into a tumour.
* Trauma.
* Bleeding diseases.

Investigation

1. Computed Tomography (CT)

A CT scan without intravenous contrast is the initial investigation in subarachnoid haemorrhage (Fig. 4.3). Subarachnoid blood is opaque. The site of accumulation usually indicates the site of bleeding. The presence of intracerebral haemorrhage or an arteriovenous malformation (AVM) or even a tumour may be displayed and the degree of ventricular dilatation assessed. Disturbance of CSF circulation is not uncommon after subarachnoid haemorrhage, leading to a degree of hydrocephalus which may require surgical intervention.

If no evidence of bleeding is seen on the CT scan subarachnoid haemorrhage is not excluded and a lumbar puncture may then be indicated for diagnostic purposes. However, the presence of ventricular dilatation on the CT scan should warn the clinician of the risk that lumbar puncture may cause 'coning' of brain tissue.

2. Cerebral angiography particularly when berry aneurysm is suspected

Using DSA, carotid and both vertebral arteries can be selectively studied. The site of subarachnoid blood on CT determines the first artery to be examined. If the causative lesion is found the procedure may be terminated if the patient's condition deteriorates but all four main vessels must be subsequently demonstrated, as aneurysms are multiple in 20–25% of these patients.

Findings

1. Berry aneurysms

These may arise from arterial divisions at any point in the cerebral circulation but the vast majority arise from particular sites around the circle of Willis (Fig. 4.4A).

Berry aneurysms occur at the posterior communicating artery origin (these may compress the third cranial nerve resulting in ptosis), the termination of the internal carotid, the first division of the middle cerebral artery in the Sylvian fissure, or the anterior communicating artery. On the vertebral circulation the majority of aneurysms arise from the termination of the basilar artery or at the origin of the posterior inferior cerebellar artery.

When berry aneurysms first bleed into the subarachnoid space there is usually no neurological deficit, but in some instances severe arterial spasm may develop after three days, leading to cerebral ischaemia and focal signs. In those recovering spontaneously from an initial bleed the aneurysm may become adherent to the brain and a second bleed usually occurs into the brain substance accompanied by neurological signs. Further bleeding may occur into the ventricles.

2. Arteriovenous malformation

These lesions are not uncommon (Fig. 4.4B). They differ from the cerebral capillary haemangioma associated with a 'port wine' stain on the face (Sturge–Weber syndrome) (Fig. 4.24). These abnormalities occur usually in otherwise normal-appearing patients. On angiography an abnormal knot of blood vessels is demonstrated with rapid filling of draining veins. The lesions

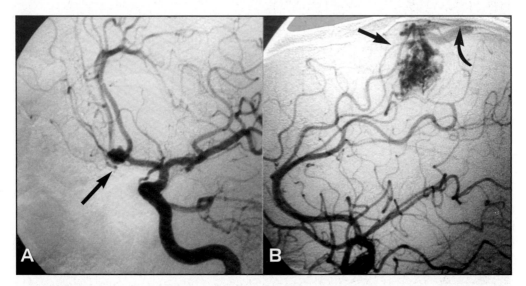

Fig. 4.4 Common causes of subarachnoid haemorrhage. (A) Digital subtraction arteriogram (DSA) showing a berry aneurysm arising at the site of the anterior communicating artery (arrow). (B) DSA showing a parasagittal arteriovenous malformation (AVM) (straight arrow). The AVM is supplied mainly from a calloso-marginal branch of the anterior cerebral artery. Note the early filling of the draining vein (curved arrow).

vary in size from a few millimetres to malformations involving a large portion of brain. The usual pattern for a patient with an AVM is for bleeding to occur only occasionally over many years. The haemorrhage may be confined to the brain or involve the subarachnoid space and, although the patient may be severely disturbed initially, recovery is not uncommon with a return almost to the previous state.

4.3 Strokes

The term **stroke** implies the sudden onset of focal neurological signs with or without diminished consciousness. The acute onset implies a vascular accident consistent with one of the following:

- Cerebral haemorrhage: Spontaneous or into a tumour or AVM.
- Embolism.
- Cerebral thrombosis.
- Transient ischaemic attack or 'mini-stroke'.

Investigation

For most patients, following an acute stroke CT should be performed soon after the event, particularly if anticoagulant therapy is proposed. CT differentiates infarction, for which anticoagulation may be indicated, and haemorrhage, when it is generally not. CT may indicate underlying pathology and provides prognostic information.

Cerebral haemorrhage

Extravasated blood is very opaque on CT and, if present, is seen immediately following an acute stroke (Fig. 4.5A). The clot may be well-defined having no significant radiolucent zone around it. Spontaneous haemorrhages are frequently associated with hypertension and are seen in the

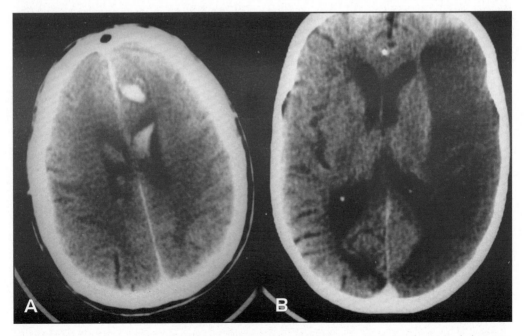

Fig. 4.5 CT scans in two stroke patients. (A) Haemorrhage in the left frontal lobe connects with the lateral ventricle which contains blood. (B) Large low-density area on the left typical of infarction due to left middle cerebral artery occlusion.

basal ganglia area, cerebellum or in the brain stem. If a clot is seen at an unusual site it raises the possibility of an underlying lesion such as an AVM or a neoplasm.

Cerebral infarction

Ischaemic infarcts result from thrombosis or embolism and the site depends on the vessels involved. Immediately following an acute infarct CT may be normal, but by about four hours oedema in the infarct appears as a radiolucent area which is usually well seen by 24 hours. On follow-up small infarcts may clear almost completely on CT but larger areas remain as well-defined radiolucent areas as a result of degeneration of neural tissue (Fig. 4.5B). Occasionally haemorrhagic infarcts are seen in which some opaque blood is seen in the central portion of an infarct, but the surrounding zones of radiolucency point to infarction as the primary lesion.

The future

MRI has the potential to display the intrinsic nature of infarcted brain tissue differentiating the central necrotic and irreversibly damaged area from a surrounding zone of tissue with a precarious blood supply, referred to as the **ischaemic penumbra**. The size of the penumbra, which MRI can demonstrate soon after a stroke, influences the prognosis and is thought likely to act as a guide as to whether therapy, e.g. anticoagulation, may be helpful.

Transient Ischaemic Attacks (TIAs)

A TIA is really a mild stroke which clears rapidly and may be episodic over days or weeks. The cause is usually atheroma of the carotid artery bifurcation, which disturbs flow by causing stenosis leading to occlusion or produces tiny platelet emboli. The neurological deficit may be of various types. Transient blindness, often described as a curtain drawing down over the eye, is a common manifestation but transient hemipareses or sensory disturbances may also occur.

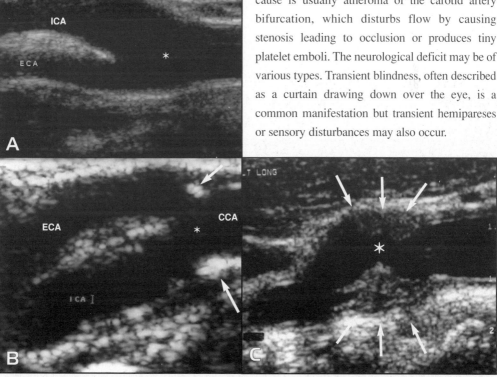

Fig. 4.6 Carotid artery bifurcation US. (A) Showing normal patency of vessels at the point of division (*) into external (ECA) and internal (ICA) arteries. (B) Highly echogenic foci (arrows) represent calcific atheroma. (C) Moderate narrowing of the lumen (*) at the bifurcation due to protruding atheromatous plaque (arrows).

Investigating the patient with TIAs

It is accepted that such patients may suffer an irreversible stroke and investigation is necessary without delay. Surgical correction of carotid artery stenosis, when indicated, is generally regarded as valuable and early treatment of those patients may obviate the need for long term nursing resulting from an established stroke. A bruit is usually heard in the neck and should be carefully looked for clinically. The NASCET controlled study in the USA has shown a definite benefit from carotid artery surgery in patients having a 70% or more narrowing of the carotid artery, and more recently those with 50–70% stenosis have shown a benefit from endarterectomy.

Cerebral CT

Usually TIA patients show no major abnormality but small cortical infarcts are consistent with an extracranial atheromatous source of emboli.

Ultrasound

Currently US is the method most frequently used initially to study the carotid arteries in the neck.

1. Imaging

US can measure the calibre of vessels at the bifurcation. Plaques appear hyperechoic and if calcified may produce acoustic shadowing (Figs 4.6, 4.7).

2. Flow

Doppler US allows quantification of flow, which increases significantly with stenosis. A velocity of 120 cms/sec beyond a stenosis correlates well with narrowing greater than 50% (Plate 4.8; see colour plates section).

3. Turbulence

On colour flow Doppler display laminar flow appears red or blue, if flow is towards or away from the transducer, but at a site of stenosis turbulence is indicated by yellowish colouration. On a Doppler graph the frequency pattern is disturbed in a turbulent zone and appears as spectral broadening (Plate 4.9; see colour plates section).

DSA

US is unable to demonstrate the intracranial portion of the carotid artery and if surgery is contemplated following CT and US, DSA is usually used to confirm

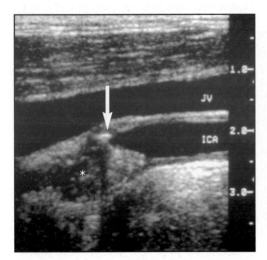

Fig. 4.7 Total occlusion of the internal carotid artery at its origin. Note: a calcific plaque anteriorly (arrow) and echogenic thrombosis (*). The jugular vein (JV) lies anteriorly.

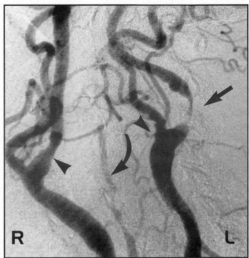

Fig. 4.10 DSA following aortic arch injection of contrast. The left external carotid artery is tightly stenosed (straight arrow) and both internal carotid artery origins are irregular (arrowheads). The right vertebral artery (curved arrow) contains two stenosed segments. The left vertebral artery has not filled consistent with occlusion.

the findings by injecting selectively the major arteries supplying the circle of Willis or injecting into the aortic arch (Fig. 4.10) outlining the major arteries in the neck simultaneously.

The future

MRI is ideally suited for the investigation of TIAs. At the one examination the cerebral tissue can be studied and using MRA the full extent of the arteries in the neck and the head can be outlined. When available MRI is already the method of choice for investigating TIA patients.

4.4 Brain Tumours and Mass Lesions

Space-occupying lesions in the brain are characterized clinically by the gradual but unrelenting development of symptoms and signs of a focal neurological abnormality. Signs of raised intracranial pressure may also be detected, e.g. papilloedema. If a lesion develops in a relatively silent area, such as the frontal lobe, symptoms may be non-specific, e.g. headache, and the clinical signs, if present, subtle.

Causes

A wide range of focal space-occupying lesions may be found in the brain but the majority are included in the following list.

Neoplasms

Primary (based on cell or tissue of origin)

- Glial cells (glioma)   astrocytoma, oligodendroglioma, ependymoma.
- Neuronal cells   medulloblastoma.
- Meninges   meningioma*(benign)*, haemangiopericytoma *(varying grades of malignancy)*.
- Nerve Sheaths   Schwannoma *(benign)*.
- Lymphoreticular cells   primary lymphoma.

Metastatic Common primary sites are:

- Bronchus   60–75%
- Breast   20–25%
- Melanoma   2–10%
- Others   < 2% kidney, G.I. tract.

Cysts   e.g. epidermoid, dermoid, hydatid, arachnoid, colloid.

Abscesses

Surface Collections e.g. subdural haematoma.

Whilst in adults most neoplasms are supratentorial, in the paediatric age group 70% lie below the tentorium with 75% in the cerebellum and 25% in the brain stem. In this group medulloblastoma and ependymoma tend to seed along the CSF pathways, whilst the juvenile pilocytic astrocytoma is relatively benign. Gliomas are the commonest primary brain tumours in adults and prognosis varies from less than twelve months for the very malignant glioblastoma multiforme to many years for some well-differentiated astrocytomas. Lymphomatous tumours vary in response to therapy but if associated with HIV infection (see section 3.13) the prognosis is poor.

Investigation

When a cerebral space lesion is suspected clinically radiological investigation is indicated. The aim is to demonstrate the site and size of the lesion, whether it is single or multiple, suggesting metastases, and to display the intrinsic characteristics of the lesion in an endeavour to determine the pathology. Also, imaging aims to demonstrate the effects of the lesion on surrounding tissues by demonstrating perifocal oedema, hydrocephalus, and herniation of brain which may be subfalcine, uncal through the tentorial hiatus, or tonsillar through the foramen magnum. CT when first introduced was a major advance in detecting these lesions but the capability of radiology has been further advanced significantly by the advent of MRI.

Magnetic Resonance Imaging

MRI is the method of choice for investigating these patients. It is extremely sensitive in detecting focal lesions. Metastases only several millimetres across may be demonstrated. MRI clearly demonstrates the effects on surrounding tissues and provides a considerable amount of information concerning the internal pathological anatomy of focal masses. Even so the specificity in characterizing these abnormalities remains relatively low and biopsy is frequently required for a definitive diagnosis. The multiplanar facility of MRI allows accurate localization of lesions. The availability of a range of techniques, by varying the radiofrequency pulse sequences, allows for detailed analysis of these abnormalities (Fig.

4.11). The basic sequences employed are the T_1 weighted spin-echo sequence which clearly demonstrates the anatomy and the T_2 weighted spin-echo sequence which highlights pathological tissue. Intravenous gadolinium is used to demonstrate enhancement of pathological tissues which lack the normal cerebral capillary blood brain barrier. Cerebral metastases, which contain capillaries akin to the primary tissue and extra-axial lesions, for the same reason, readily enhance, whilst gliomas which contain a mix of normal and abnormal capillaries usually enhance to some extent. Low-grade astrocytomas generally show no contrast enhancement. Cerebral abscesses typically show wall or 'ring'enhancement but this is a non-specific finding shared with necrotic tumours (Fig. 4.12) and lymphoma.

MRI differentiates masses which are intra-axial, i.e. within the CNS, from extra-axial, arising from meninges or surrounding structures (Fig. 4.15). It can determine the cystic nature of lesions and detect necrosis within tumours, which generally indicates a poorer prognosis. Gliomas

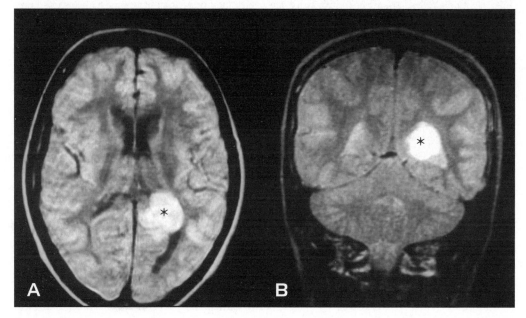

Fig. 4.11 MRI of ependymoma. (A) The axial T_1 weighted scan shows a well-defined tumour (*) of high signal lying close to the trigone of the left lateral ventricle. (B) The T_2 weighted coronal section again shows the well-defined tumour (*). Note the CSF has a higher signal than on T_1.

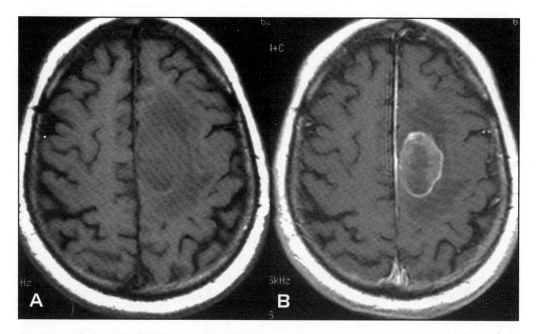

Fig. 4.12 Cerebral Tumour. Glioblastoma multiforme. (A) T_1 weighted MRI shows a central zone of higher signal with surrounding low signal. (B) T_1 weighted MRI after IV gadolinium shows dense ring enhancement of the central zone consistent with necrosis.

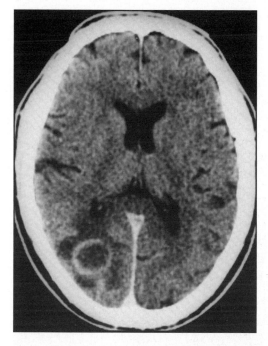

Fig. 4.13 Cerebral tumour. Glioblastoma multiforme. CT following contrast showing central ring enhancement with surrounding low density oedema.

and certain metastases, e.g. melanoma, have a tendency to bleed and MRI can detect haemorrhage within these tumours and in most cases can differentiate it from non-neoplastic haematoma. Fat-containing focal lesions, e.g. teratoma, dermoid, lipoma, are easily identified on MRI as fat gives a high signal on T_1 and T_2. Vascularity of lesions may be apparent on MRI because the moving blood is seen as a void, i.e. black on the image, in all sequences. Calcification, because of its low hydrogen proton content may not be seen at all, or may be seen as a void, and this is one of the few disadvantages of MRI.

Computed Tomography (CT)

CT is used to supplement MRI by demonstrating the skull bones if necessary. Also, if MRI is not available CT may be used initially. The sensitivity for detecting focal lesions is very much less than with MRI, particularly in the posterior fossa, but is significantly improved by using intravenous iodinated contrast enhancement, which is mandatory when using CT in these patients (Fig. 4.13).

4.5 Hearing Loss

The causes of deafness can be divided into **conductive hearing loss** where there is impairment of air conduction due to disease in the external auditory canal, the tympanic membrane, or the middle ear, and **sensorineural hearing loss** in which the defect lies in the labyrinth, the internal auditory canal or the brain stem. In some conditions, e.g. otosclerosis, the hearing loss is of mixed aetiology. Clinical examination and audiometric tests usually allow categorization of the type of loss. Radiology is important in the further investigation of some patients and nowadays CT and MRI have almost completely replaced plain radiography and plain film tomography.

Conductive loss

Auroscopy allows visualization of the lumen of the external canal and the tympanic membrane but CT is indicated if congenital atresia or stenosis is present and to demonstrate the extent of an acquired exostosis or, on occasions, the extent of invasion of a squamous cell carcinoma. In the middle ear CT is able to demonstrate the malleus and incus, the lateral semicircular canal, canal for the facial nerve, the mastoid antrum and air cells, the tegmen, i.e. the bony plate between the middle ear and the cranial cavity, and also the posterior recesses of the middle ear. Inflammatory or post-traumatic effusions in the middle ear may be demonstrated, and also ossicular abnormalities, either congenital or following head trauma. Cholesteatomas, although non-malignant, are locally invasive and the extent can be well displayed pre-operatively by CT (Fig. 4.14).

Sensorineural loss

In young children when sensorineural hearing loss may be due to labyrinthine dysplasia CT is indicated to demonstrate the bony labyrinth, and also in adults suspected of otosclerosis, a condition which causes ossification of the oval and round windows of the middle ear extending to the cochlea and resulting in a mixed hearing loss. In adults with progressive sensorineural hearing loss, MRI is indicated as the most sensitive means of detecting an acoustic neuroma, a lesion which usually can be surgically removed successfully. Brain stem neoplasms or multiple sclerosis may

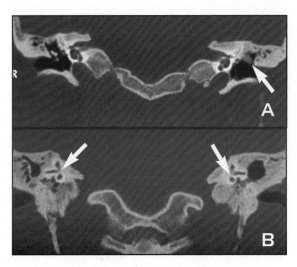

Fig. 4.14 CT. Cholesteatoma in left middle ear extending into the mastoid. (A) Compared with the normal right side the bony ossicles are absent on the left and a small soft tissue mass (arrow) can be seen. (B) This section posterior to (A) shows the semicircular canals (arrows). The mastoid antrum on the left has been eroded and may involve the horizontal canal.

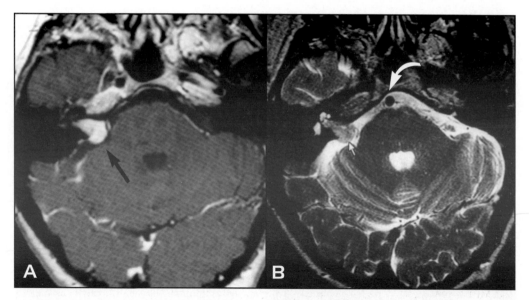

Fig. 4.15 Right acoustic neuroma shown by MRI. (A) T_1 weighted image showing the tumour (arrow), with high signal, extending anterolaterally to the internal auditory canal. (B) T_2 weighted image shows the tumour (straight arrow) surrounded by the high signal CSF. The basilar artery (curved arrow) can be seen surrounded by CSF anterior to the pons.

also be shown by MRI and meningiomas in the cerebellopontine angle also.

Acoustic neuroma

The tumour (Fig. 4.15) is misnamed, being a Schwannoma which arises from the upper or lower branch of the vestibular division of the eighth nerve and presses on the acoustic division. Most acoustic neuromas are sporadic but in some it is a manifestation of neurofibromatosis I, i.e. von Recklinghausen's syndrome, which may be associated with changes in other organs, including optic nerve glioma. The presence of bilateral acoustic neuromas is the hallmark of neurofibromatosis II, also autosomal dominant and associated with the development of meningiomas, ependymomas and other Schwannomas. Sporadic cases usually present in middle age or beyond whilst the genetically determined abnormalities present earlier.

4.6 Disturbance of Vision

Normal sight depends on the integrity of not only the structures within the globe and the muscles attached externally to it, but also on lengthy neural pathways to the visual occipital cortex with connections upwards to higher centres and downwards to the brain stem nuclei of the third, fourth and sixth cranial nerves which supply the extraocular muscles. Most visual problems result from intraocular abnormalities which can usually be accurately diagnosed clinically. In patients with pathology situated in the orbit or in the extensive neural pathways posterior to the globe the anatomical site and sometimes the nature of the lesion can be predicted clinically but radiology is required in most cases for detailed diagnosis.

The globe

When the light-conducting media are opacified by cataract, haemorrhage or membranes preventing ophthalmoscopy, contact US, with the transducer placed on the eyelid, is the most practical method of demonstrating the posterior segment. Retinal detachment, haemorrhages and tumours, as well as other pathology may be well seen.

The orbit

The large amount of intraorbital fat favours CT as the method of choice for displaying the extra-ocular muscles, the optic nerves, the lacrimal glands, the larger blood vessels and the bony boundaries of the orbit. Optic nerve enlargement is seen in optic nerve glioma, meningioma arising

from the nerve sheath (Fig. 4.16), and the demyelinating condition called optic neuritis. Gliomas affect younger patients more than meningioma. In only half of those with optic neuritis does further evidence of multiple sclerosis develop later. Optic neuritis without nerve enlargement can be detected by special MRI techniques.

Various neoplasms arise in the retrobulbar tissues and CT findings are usually non-specific. The commonest is a cavernous haemangioma, which enhances with IV contrast but others include lymphoma, and metastasis. Swelling of extra-ocular muscles, and increase in orbital fat associated with exophthalmos may occur in hyperthyroidism and is well shown by CT (Fig. 4.17). Orbital pseudotumour,

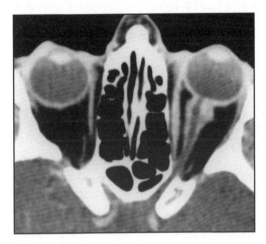

Fig. 4.16 Optic nerve sheath meningioma. The axial contrast enhanced CT scan shows the tumour encircling the left optic nerve.

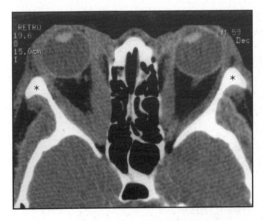

Fig. 4.17 Thyroid eye disease. Bilateral proptosis is present. Normally the posterior margin of the globe should lie at least 1 cm behind the line joining the anterior extent of each zygomatic bone (*). The intraocular muscle bellies are clearly swollen but the tendons anteriorly are relatively spared.

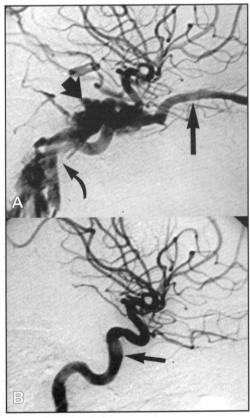

Fig. 4.18 Carotico-cavernous fistula. (A) The cavernous sinus (short arrow), an ophthalmic vein (long arrow) and petrosal veins (curved arrow) have filled with contrast following internal carotid artery injection. (B) Internal carotid injection following percutaneous transfemoral catheterization and balloon occlusion of the fistula site (arrow).

a strange condition usually considered inflammatory, may affect virtually all of the soft tissues, causing proptosis, but has a non-specific appearance on CT. Biopsy is generally required.

Juxtasellar region

Chiasmal lesions cause bitemporal hemianopia. The region is best demonstrated by MRI but CT is frequently required for bony detail. Pituitary tumours (see Chapter 5), meningiomas, and large berry aneurysms, which enhance vividly with contrast, may all impinge on the optic chiasm.

Carotico-cavernous fistula between the internal carotid artery and the cavernous sinus results in unilateral proptosis, sometimes pulsating, and a detectable bruit (Fig. 4.18). A direct type arises from rupture of a small intracavernous aneurysm or is post-traumatic. An indirect type secondary to a

dural arteriovenous fistula typically develops spontaneously in middle-aged women. CT shows a distended sinus and superior ophthalmic vein. The diagnosis is confirmed by DSA and interventional radiological techniques are usually successful in closing the fistula.

Cerebrum and brain stem

Homonymous hemianopia results from optic tract interference. MRI is the best modality for demonstrating lesions in the brain which interfere with the optic pathways. The commonest extraocular pathology causing impaired vision is vascular insufficiency, particularly in the basilar artery territory, which supplies the brain stem and occipital lobes. Arteriography may be indicated in these patients and in acute stroke with severe visual loss thrombolysis via the catheter may help in some cases.

4.7 Diffuse Brain Pathology

The high sensitivity of MRI in showing subtle abnormalities in the brain, particularly the white matter, is proving invaluable in the investigation of patients with syndromes which suggest diffuse or multifocal pathology. CNS infection has increased

rapidly in recent years due primarily to the high incidence of infection in HIV related disease. The specificity in diagnosing the various viral, bacterial, fungal and parasitic infections is low, but the sensitivity is high. Most show evidence of

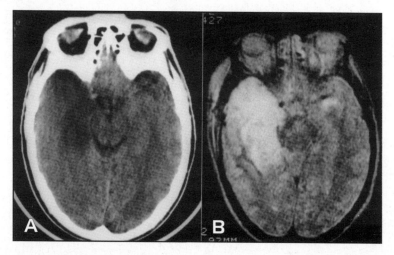

Fig. 4.19 Herpes simplex encephalitis. (A) Axial CT showing low density consistent with oedema in the right temporal lobe with a small patch anteriorly in the left temporal lobe. (B) T$_2$ weighted MRI shows high signal in the affected areas.

cerebritis and sometimes meningitis with the pathological tissue giving a high signal, appearing white, on T_2 weighted images (Fig. 4.19).

The sensitivity in detecting demyelination allows MRI to monitor activity of multiple sclerosis more accurately, it seems, than clinically. MS plaques have a high signal on T_2 weighted images, but appearances are non-specific and shared by other demyelinating conditions. Plaques may be seen anywhere in the CNS tissue including the cranial nerves. They are particularly frequent in periventricular white matter, the corpus callosum and the brain stem (Fig. 4.20).

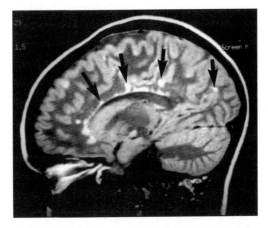

Fig. 4.20 Multiple sclerosis. Sagittal T_2 weighted MRI at the level of the corpus callosum shows numerous discrete foci of high signal consistent with plaques of demyelisation (arrows).

4.8 Cerebral Symptoms without Signs

The yield of abnormalities from radiology of the brain is generally low for patients presenting with such symptoms as headache, vertigo, or 'blackouts' who show no abnormality on careful clinical neurological examination. If persistent it is reasonable to perform CT, which is readily available, to detect the occasional pathology and, if negative, to satisfy the patient. Headache may be the only manifestation of midline obstructive lesions which produce ventricular dilatation, i.e. hydrocephalus. In time papilloedema should be seen but occasionally this is equivocal. The dilated ventricles are readily seen on CT and the level of obstruction also. Colloid cyst at the foramen of Monro (Fig. 4.21), congenital or acquired stenosis of the aqueduct of Sylvius, and congenital or acquired fourth ventricular outflow obstruction can all be shown by CT. Because very small lesions in the region of the aqueduct may be missed by CT, all new cases of hydrocephalus

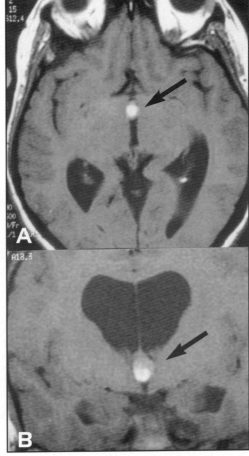

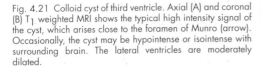

Fig. 4.21 Colloid cyst of third ventricle. Axial (A) and coronal (B) T_1 weighted MRI shows the typical high intensity signal of the cyst, which arises close to the foramen of Munro (arrow). Occasionally, the cyst may be hypointense or isointense with surrounding brain. The lateral ventricles are moderately dilated.

should be screened at least once by MRI. In childhood until the anterior fontanelle closes the size of the ventricles can be shown by US.

Late onset epilepsy due to cerebral tumour is usually associated with clinical evidence of a focal neurological abnormality. Radiology may not be necessary in younger epileptics although MRI is usually advised in post-traumatic cases and those with complex partial seizures. The ability of MRI to demonstrate the lesion of **mesial temporal sclerosis** has led to correction of temporal lobe epilepsy following resection of the lesion (Fig. 4.22). The principal role of neuro-imaging of patients with dementia is to rule out treatable lesions, e.g. a meningioma in a silent area such as the frontal lobe, or hydrocephalus which may be revealed by CT. MRI can aid the distinction between Alzheimer's disease and multi-infarct dementia, the two commonest dementia causes, by demonstrating disproportionate atrophy of the mesial temporal structures, e.g. the hippocampi, in Alzheimer's.

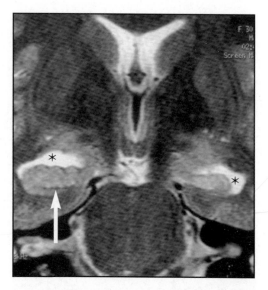

Fig. 4.22 Mesial Temporal Sclerosis. Coronal T$_2$ weighted MRI through the anterior tips of the temporal horns (*) shows the normal hippocampus on the right (arrow). Note the undulating soft tissue outline giving an appearance suggesting toes on end, consistent with its name, Pes Hippocampus. On the left the Pes Hippocampus is shrunken and of slightly higher signal than the right.

4.9 Head Injuries

Head trauma is extremely common ranging from the trivial to the life threatening, and careful clinical assessment is necessary in each case. Head trauma may damage the skull and intracranial contents, the facial bones, or the upper cervical spine. Radiology is usually indicated to confirm or exclude injuries and CT and plain radiography are the methods of choice.

Computed Tomography (CT)

If intracranial damage is suspected CT is mandatory and, medicolegally it is unacceptable to perform only plain radiography as it does not exclude intracranial damage which may be present in the absence of skull fractures

(Fig. 4.23). The decision to perform CT will depend on individual circumstances but certain conditions are clear indications for CT including loss of consciousness, fitting, neurological signs, bleeding or CSF discharge from ear or nose, and extensive soft tissue damage. In unconscious patients it is advisable to continue the CT examination downwards to include the upper cervical spine. Intravenous contrast enhancement is generally not necessary.

Findings

In head injury patients the CT data is displayed using a soft tissue window to show the brain tissue and CSF and a bone window to show the calvarium. Traumatic haemorrhage in the brain is

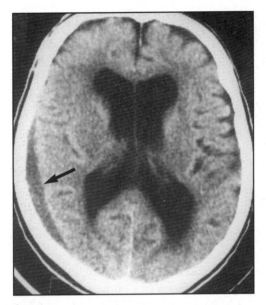

Fig. 4.23 Subdural collection. The low density convexity collection (arrow) compressing the right parietal region is shown on CT.

opaque and easily detected and subarachnoid bleeding also. Acute unclotted surface collections, either sub or extradural, may be isodense with brain tissue initially but their presence may be indicated by shift of midline structures if the bleeding is unilateral. Air within the skull vault is readily detected. Depressed skull fragments are usually well seen and linear fractures through the skull base also. Linear fractures in the vault occasionally may not be detected.

Plain radiography

It is important to specify the exact region when requesting these studies to ensure that the appropriate views are obtained.

Skull:

This examination will include the skull vault, i.e. the integument of the brain. As stated CT is required if intracranial damage is suspected.

Facial bones:

The views are specifically for the maxillary region and zygomatic arches. In severe facial injuries CT may be preferred initially to provide more detailed information.

Mandible:

The views will demonstrate the entire bone but are inadequate for the maxilla and orbits. Orthopantomography requires special equipment and produces on a single strip of film an elongated and somewhat distorted view of the jaws.

Cervical Spine:

In unconscious patients, a single lateral view of the cervical spine is indicated if skull CT is not available to include the area.

Findings

1. *Skull vault*

Linear fractures usually extend from the vault to the skull base (Fig. 4.24) and over time blurring of the outline with slight sclerosis allows ageing of the fracture. Fractures of the base are usually very

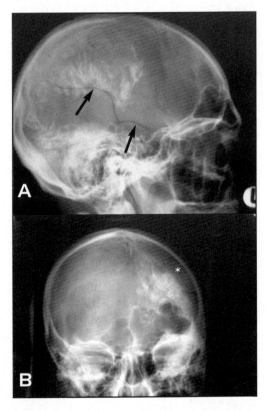

Fig. 4.24 Linear skull fracture (arrows) in a patient with Sturge–Weber syndrome. The lateral (A) and AP (B) films show the typical cortical calcification, the hypoplasia of the left side of the skull with increased size of the left frontal sinus. The patient sustained the fracture following a seizure and the clear space lateral to the calcified cerebral cortex (*) raised the possibility of a subdural collection.

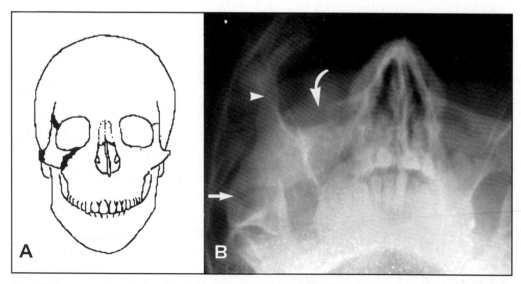

Fig. 4.25 Fractures involving the lateral third of the face. (A) Diagram. (B) The plain x-ray shows a fracture line through the right maxillary antrum (curved arrow) with depression of the lateral portion of the orbital floor. A second fracture is seen in the fronto-zygomatic suture (arrowhead), and a third fracture (arrow) through the zygomatic arch.

difficult to detect and CT is preferred. A depressed fracture usually has a rim of increased density along part of the fracture line due to slight overlap of the depressed fragment and a tangential view is used to display this better.

2. Facial bones

The commonest facial injury, after nasal bone fractures, involves the lateral third with depression of the zygoma or malar bone resulting from three fracture lines, one through the lateral aspect of the maxillary antrum, the second through the zygomatic arch and the third through the fronto-zygomatic suture (Fig. 4.25). Elevation of the depressed zygoma may be necessary and is performed using a lever introduced through a small incision in the adjacent hairline.

Fractures involving the middle third of the face may extend right across through both maxillae resulting in instability and are usually treated by wiring the jaws. Le Fort described three lines of weakness in the region (Fig. 4.26). Type 1 extends transversally above the alveolar margins. Type 2 passes through both maxillary antra and the orbital floors and base of the nose. Type 3

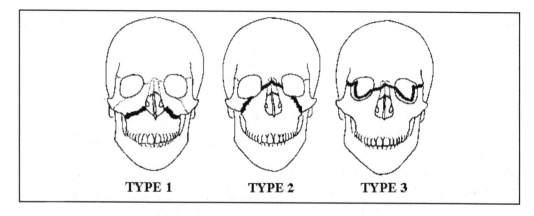

Fig. 4.26 Le Fort types of fractures involving the middle third of the face.

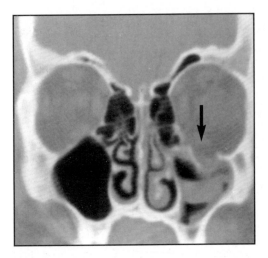

Fig. 4.27 Blow-out fracture of the floor of the left orbit. Coronal CT shows the depressed bony fragment with extrusion of soft tissue into the left maxillary sinus (arrow).

extends from one fronto-zygomatic suture to the other running through both orbits and the base of the nose.

A direct blow to the orbit may result in a 'blow-out' fracture of the orbital floor or medial wall (Fig. 4.27). Orbital tissues, including muscle fibres, may be trapped in the fracture line. Clinically a blow-out fracture should be suspected if the patient has failure of convergence of the eyes on upward gaze, and CT is recommended in such cases.

3. Mandible

Mandibular fractures most commonly occur through the region of the canine teeth and through the condylar neck. Intra-oral dental films or pantomography may be necessary to show the relationship of fractures to the dental roots.

4. Nasal bones

Fractures are very common and the majority can be managed without radiology. Because of the prominence of suture and vascular markings linear fractures are not readily detected. Nasal deformity can usually be detected and corrected clinically.

4.10 Spinal Cord Abnormalities

Dysfunction of the spinal cord and the emerging nerve roots may result from disease in the spinal column, the surrounding meninges, or within the spinal cord itself, or from interference with the blood supply to the neural tissue. Abnormalities of the spinal CNS can be divided broadly into **myelopathies**, in which there may be interference with descending and ascending tracts resulting in upper motor neurone lesions, and **radiculopathies**, in which emerging nerve roots are disturbed resulting in lower motor neurone lesions and sensory changes confined to the appropriate dermatomes.

Myelopathies
Adults

Most conditions leading to spinal cord disturbance are included in the following:

Spinal column

• Fracture–dislocations.

• Intervertebral Disc Disease (IDD).

• Metastases.

• Osteomyelitis.

• Cervical canal stenosis.

Meninges

• Meningioma.

• Lymphoma.

• Abscess metastases.

• Haematoma.

Blood supply
- Arteriovenous malformation (AVM).
- Infarction.

Spinal Cord
- Tumours: astrocytoma, ependymoma.
- Transverse myelitis.
- Multiple sclerosis.

Nerves
- Neurofibroma, Schwannoma.

Childhood

Additional to conditions listed above certain congenital abnormalities may result in cord dysfunction.
- Spinal dysraphism.
- Tumours: dermoid, teratoma.

Investigation

The acute onset of a myelopathy is an emergency because if the myelopathy is due to cord compression immediate surgery is indicated because the damage becomes irreversible in a few hours. The gradual onset of a myelopathy may be unsuspected clinically particularly if the spinal cord lesion is in the lumbo-sacral segments. Bladder or bowel dysfunction which may be the presenting symptom in these cases may be attributed to local pathology, e.g. prostatism. The lower sacral dermatomes are in the peri-anal region and are not usually tested clinically so that the associated sensory disturbance is missed.

1. Magnetic Resonance Imaging (MRI)

If available MRI should be the initial study in all myelopathy patients. MRI is very sensitive in detecting focal abnormalities in the region. It is able to differentiate cystic and solid lesions, haemorrhage and areas of cord softening or myelomalacia. MRI can determine the site of tumours accurately but is unable to differentiate the various types of neoplasm (Fig. 4.28). The typical appearance of a syrinx is easily recognised (Fig. 4.29). Plaques of multiple sclerosis are seen

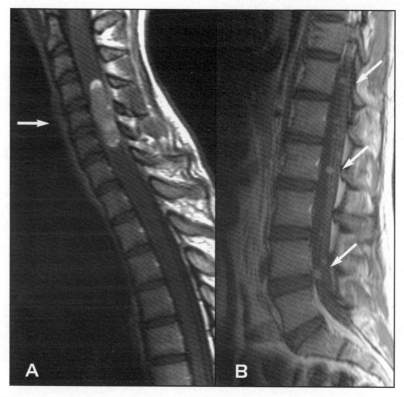

Fig. 4.28 (A) Cervical cord ependymoma (arrow) T_1 weighted MRI. (B) Tumour seeding to the lumbar nerve roots (arrows).

and usually evidence of spinal AVM also, but spinal angiography may be needed for confirmation.

2. Plain radiography

Vertebral body disease may lead to bony collapse and compression of the spinal cord. Metastases involve the vertebral bodies but do not extend across the intervertebral disc. Fracture dislocations and osteoporosis may also lead to cord compression (see Chapter 14). Osteomyelitis involves the vertebral bodies immediately adjacent to the intervertebral disc and typically bony destruction on both sides of a narrowed disc suggests strongly an infective process.

In the cervical region the antero-posterior depth of the spinal canal, determined developmentally, influences the likelihood of developing spinal cord compression in later life due to the added factor of bulging of intervertebral discs. Such compression is unlikely in persons with a depth of more than 12 mm (Fig. 4.30). Neurofibroma may have a dumb-bell shape, partly within and partly outside the spinal canal. In such cases unilateral enlargement of an intervertebral foramen may point to the diagnosis (Fig. 4.31).

3. Radionuclide scan

In patients known to have had cancer and presenting with slow onset myelopathy the whole body bone scan may show the extent of bony metastases which appear as 'hot' spots.

4. Myelography

If MRI is not available myelography is usually indicated. Following lumbar puncture a water soluble, isotonic with CSF, contrast medium is injected. The contrast medium is totally absorbed following examination. If an obstructive lesion is

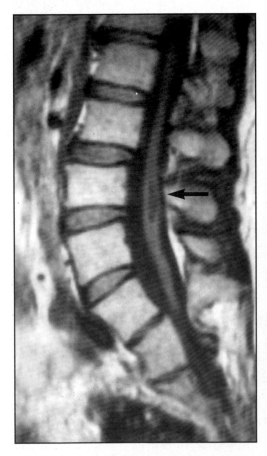

Fig. 4.29 T₁ weighted MRI. Sagittal section shows a 'tethered' cord extending down to S2 vertebra and a syrinx (arrow) expanding the cord at L4–5. A developmental abnormality. The normal spinal cord ends at L2.

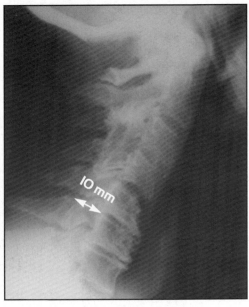

Fig. 4.30 Cervical spondylosis. Lateral view shows narrow discs at C5–6–7 with osteophytes on the adjacent disc margins. Note the narrowed spinal canal (normal > 12 mm).

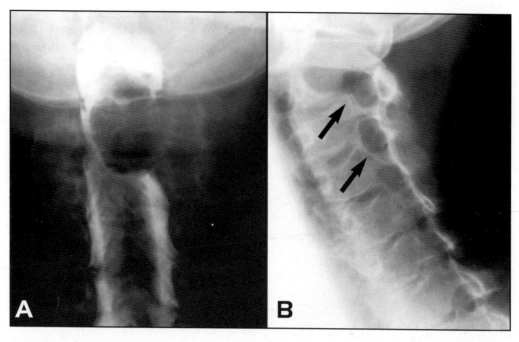

Fig. 4.31 Large upper cervical tumour displacing the cervical cord slightly towards the right in the myelogram (A) and extending outside the spinal canal (B) through the adjacent expanded intervertebral foramina (arrows). Diagnosis: Neurofibroma.

causing the myelopathy the upper extent of the column of contrast medium in the subarachnoid space will have a particular shape at the level of obstruction allowing diagnosis as to whether the obstructing lesion is extradural, intradural but extramedullary, or intramedullary (Fig. 4.32).

Radiculopathies

Disease of emerging nerve roots is usually due to intervertebral disc abnormalities (IDD), most commonly in the lumbar and cervical regions. The following section is devoted to IDD. Other conditions which cause a radiculopathy include arachnoiditis, and nerve sheath tumours.

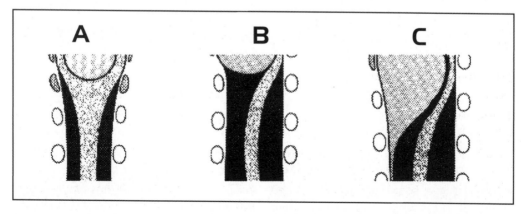

Fig. 4.32 Types of tumour blockage on myelography. Appearance of the contrast column (black) at the level of obstruction in (A) intramedullary (B) intradural extramedullary and (C) extradural masses. Note the relationships of the contrast to the line of the rounded pedicles.

4.11 Intervertebral Disc Disease (IDD)

About 50 years ago the importance of intervertebral disc disease (IDD) as a cause of symptoms was first realized. Before that the various aches and pains in the back and limbs were attributed to soft tissue changes and descriptive terms such as lumbago, sciatica, neuralgia and myositis were commonplace diagnoses. The socio-economic impact of IDD has been enormous and it is important to understand the anatomy and ageing process in discs as well as the pathology.

In young people a relatively high pressure exists in the nucleus pulposis which bears the weight in the erect position. During ageing the water content of the nucleus reduces and the weight bearing is taken by the annulus fibrosis. Whilst in the elderly the discs may remain of normal appearance, in most the ageing process causes degeneration and the annulus tends to bulge. At the point of attachment to the vertebral body bony spurs, or osteophytes, develop and may become very large.

Disc degeneration

Degeneration of discs, in which a radial tear develops in the annulus, usually posteriorly, may occur at any age, often in the third and fourth decades. The relationship to trauma is unclear although a traumatic episode is frequently associated with the onset of symptoms. The nomenclature of disc disease is confused but the following classification is of practical value.

1. Protruding disc

With degeneration the radial tear in the inner annulus fibres is filled by the spreading nuclear material. The annulus bulges, i.e. protrudes, and this bulging may be generalized over a broad segment of the disc or localized at a point where the remaining annulus is very thin.

2. Extruded disc

Rupture of the annulus allows nuclear substance to extrude into the spinal canal, usually into the epidural space. This process is sometimes referred to as herniation but it is an inappropriate term which suggests extruded material may be reduced, like a hernia, and this is not so. Differentiation between an extruded disc and a local protrusion may be difficult but is usually insignificant.

3. Sequestrated disc

The extrusion may pierce the posterior longitudinal ligament, become separated and move away from the disc level, usually downwards. In time it may calcify.

In time degenerate discs lose height and usually develop osteophytes on the vertebral margins.

Clinically IDD may present as a myelopathy due to spinal cord pressure, a radiculopathy due to nerve pressure, or with pain arising from the degenerate discs themselves. Most commonly cervical and lumbar IDD cause symptoms of radiculopathy and occasionally cervical IDD presents as a myelopathy. Cord pressure from thoracic disc herniation is far less common.

Low back pain and sciatica syndrome

IDD may produce pain of two types and it is important to differentiate between them. **Discogenic pain** arises from degenerative changes within the disc and is localized to the lower back and buttocks and is not considered due to pressure on emerging nerve roots. **Neurogenic pain** results from nerve root pressure and is usually manifest as sciatica with pain extending into the dermatomes of the lower limb. Assessing whether nerve root pressure exists may be difficult clinically. However, if a reflex, knee jerk or ankle jerk, is diminished this is strong supporting evidence of such pressure.

Investigation

A conservative attitude is advocated as the majority of patients with low back ache and sciatica recover given time. It is important to set a time scale for investigation of these conditions and, except in cases of severe acute sciatica in which early surgery may be indicated, the program should extend over some weeks of conservative management and the patient informed. Failure to set such a program is a cause frequently for patients to seek alternative medicine.

Plain radiography

If investigation is indicated plain x-rays of the lumbosacral spine and pelvis should be obtained first.

Findings

1. Osseous disease

Vertebral metastases, myeloma or osteomyelitis may present clinically as a radiculopathy with backache. Osteoarthritis of the hip may also.

2. Developmental anomalies

Developmental abnormalities producing asymmetry in the lumbosacral spine may render the discs more prone to degeneration because of abnormal weight distribution, e.g. unilateral fusion of the fifth lumbar transverse process to the sacrum producing scoliosis. Spondylolisthesis, i.e. a defect in the pars interarticularis, most often of L5, may be demonstrated and this may be associated with IDD (Fig. 4.33). Spina bifida of lumbar neural arches is usually insignificant but occasionally may be associated with intraspinal abnormalities, e.g. tethered spinal cord (Fig. 4.29).

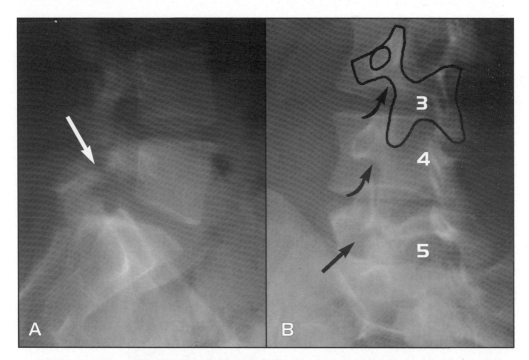

Fig. 4.33 Spondylolisthesis of fifth lumbar vertebra. (A) Bilateral defects in the pars interarticularis (arrow) have allowed L5 to slip forward on S1. In the oblique view (B) the normal appearance of the neural arch components at L3 (Black outline) have an appearance suggesting a scottish terrier. The neck (curved arrows) is the intact pars interarticularis. The appearance at L4 is also normal. The pars defect at L5 (arrow) is seen as a lucent band or 'collar' across the neck.

3. Evidence of intervertebral disc disease

Narrowing of the intervertebral disc space is a late result of disc degeneration, taking months to develop. Normally the lumbar disc spaces increase very slightly in depth from above down to the L4–5 level but the normal L5–S1 space may be quite narrow developmentally (Fig. 4.34A). Calcification or a small amount of gas may be seen on rare occasions within degenerative discs. A Schmorl's node results from a disc protrusion or extrusion through the developing vertebral body end plate. These nodes are seen as small rounded lucencies projecting into the vertebral bodies from the discs and usually they have a fine sclerotic margin (Fig. 4.35).

Magnetic Resonance Imaging

MRI is the method of choice in these patients if further investigation is required. About 90% of lumbar disc extrusions occur at L4–5 or L5–S1 levels. Because a considerable amount of epidural fat exists in this area standard T_1 and T_2 weighted spin-echo (SE) MRI sequences clearly show the extrusions (Fig. 4.36), which have a low signal appearing dark, against the high white signal of fat on T_1 weighted images. The detailed anatomy of the discs is clearly seen. Normally the central portion of the disc can be differentiated from the outer annulus which has a lower signal. A normal appearance of a disc on a T_2 weighted SE image in which the central disc gives a bright white image virtually excludes protrusion or extrusion (Fig. 4.34B). With progressive degeneration the central disc loses signal as it becomes more fibrosed (Fig. 4.36B). MRI also shows the emerging nerve roots in great detail and in some cases osteophytic lipping on the facet joints can be seen encroaching on the intervertebral foramina.

Computed Tomography

If MRI is unavailable then CT may provide useful information (Fig. 4.37). Because CT provides limited information concerning the discs the

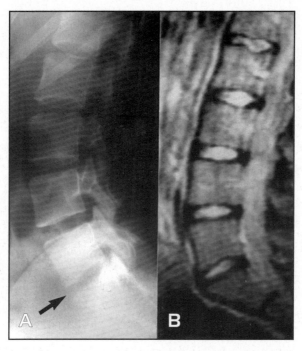

Fig. 4.34 Normal lumbar spine. (A) Plain film shows normal discs. Note narrower L5–S1 disc (arrow). (B) T_2 weighted MRI. Normal high signal nucleus pulposus with surrounding low signal annulus at each level.

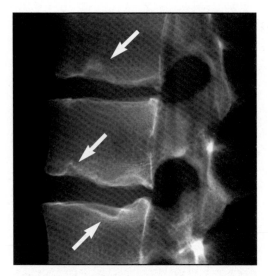

Fig. 4.35 Schmorl's nodes (arrows).

indication should be persisting neurogenic pain rather than discogenic low back pain. The usual CT examination includes angled single sections directly through each of the lowest three discs and a detailed axial series extending from L3 to S1 bodies. The detail shown by CT is considerably less than with MRI. However, protrusions and extrusions can usually be detected.

Myelography

Injection of contrast medium into the lumbar subarachnoid space is unnecessary if MRI is available but may be necessary to clarify the findings on CT. The contrast medium outlines the nerve root sheaths clearly and pressure from extruded discs or other swellings can be demonstrated (Fig. 4.38). However, a laterally-placed disc extrusion may be beyond the filling of the root sheath and missed. CT performed following myelography may give more information.

Discography

In this technique fine needles are introduced into the centres of each of the lower three lumbar discs and contrast medium injected. The main use has been in cases of discogenic pain, without evidence of disc bulging or extrusion, to demonstrate disc degeneration and to assess the patients pain reaction on injection. The availability of MRI has largely replaced discography for the demonstration of structural abnormalities of the disc, but the pain-provocative aspect of discography is still occasionally used to diagnose discogenic disease.

Cervical spondylosis and brachial pain

Disc degeneration is extremely common in the mid-cervical region and most older people show evidence of it. About 90% of cervical disc extrusions occur at C5–6 and 6–7 levels. Apart from causing discogenic pain, IDD may produce myelopathy due to spinal cord pressure or a radiculopathy due to nerve root pressure.

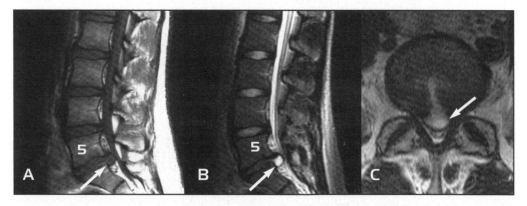

Fig. 4.36 Extruded nucleus at L5–S1. (A) T$_1$ weighted MRI shows low signal extrusion (arrow) contrasting with high signal fat. (B) Low signal L5–S1 disc indicating degeneration. The extrusion (arrow) is associated with a low signal osteophyte. (C) Axial view shows the extrusion (arrow) compressing the theca.

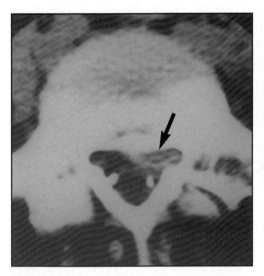

Fig. 4.37 Large intervertebral disc protrusion. CT shows the extruded disc material as relatively dense (arrow) and occluding the left lateral L4 root sleeve. The patient presented with acute sciatic syndrome.

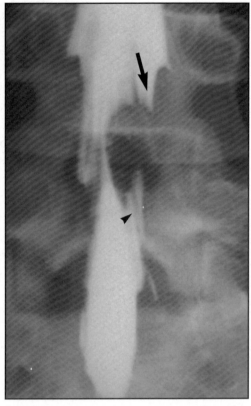

Fig. 4.38 Large disc extrusion at L4–5. The L5 nerve root (arrow) is compressed and the S1 root (arrowhead) is deviated medially.

Radiculopathy

Brachial pain is a common manifestation of cervical IDD. Most extrusions occur laterally. The upper surface of a cervical vertebra is curved because of the uncinate processes laterally and the disc also curves up at each side. At this point disc extrusion impinges on the emerging nerve root.

Myelopathy

Central extrusion of a cervical disc is uncommon and cord pressure usually results from a general protrusion. Whether protruded discs impinge on the cervical spinal cord very much depends on the antero-posterior depth of the canal, which can be assessed radiologically and normally should be 12 mm or more. Pressure on the anterior portion of the spinal cord results in an upper motor neurone lesion to the lower limbs or both upper and lower limbs, generally manifest as spastic weakness. Interference with the anterior spinal artery may also contribute to the syndrome.

Investigation

Plain radiography

The typical changes of cervical disc degeneration, referred to as cervical spondylosis, are disc space narrowing and the presence of osteophytes on the vertebral margins (Fig. 4.30). Oblique views are usually obtained to demonstrate the extent of osteophyte encroachment on the intervertebral foramina. The antero-posterior depth of the bony canal should also be measured. Plain films may show evidence of bony disease, e.g. metastases, the presence of a cervical rib, and in rare instances the apical lung opacity of a Pancoast tumour, all of which may present with brachial pain.

Films made soon after cervical spine injury may appear normal, but a film made some months later may show evidence of disc narrowing, an indication of degeneration following the injury.

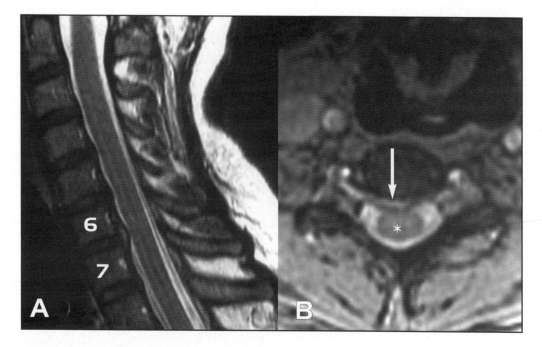

Fig. 4.39 Cervical disc protrusion. (A) Gradient echo MRI shows high signal (whitish) protrusion at C6–7, differentiating it from osteophytes, which would be low signal. (B) Axial view shows the protrusion (arrow) is central. No pressure on spinal theca(*).

Magnetic resonance imaging

MRI is the method of choice for studying these patients. Because very little epidural fat is present in the region special pulse sequences are used to demonstrate anatomical detail. Using gradient echo (GE) sequences it is possible to differentiate bulging discs from bony osteohytes (Fig. 4.39). When MRI images of the nerve root sheaths and intervertebral foramina are suboptimal or equivocal, myelography followed by CT is used to investigate radiculopathies. In cervical myelopathy MRI demonstrates the degree of pressure on the cord from the protruding disc anteriorly and the ligamenta flava posteriorly, which tend to hypertrophy in the elderly.

Myelography

Contrast medium introduced by cisternal puncture outlines the cervical nerve root sheaths and also the degree of cord compression (Fig. 4.40). The use of CT following the introduction of contrast medium provides better definition. CT alone is of very limited value in the cervical region compared with its use in the lumbar region.

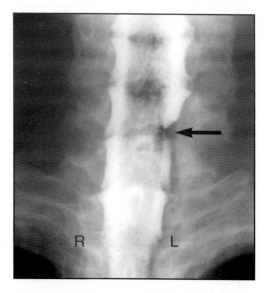

Fig. 4.40 Acute left brachial pain. Myelography shows filling defect of the left 7th root sleeve due to lateral disc herniation (arrow).

Reference

Osborn, A. G., *Diagnostic Neuroradiology,* Mosby, 1994.

Modern techniques allow detailed imaging of most endocrine organs. The pituitary, thyroid, adrenal glands and the gonads can be demonstrated. The parathyroids and islet cell tissue of the pancreas are not normally seen but abnormalities, usually neoplastic enlargement, in those sites may be displayed.

5.1 Pituitary

Magnetic Resonance Imaging (MRI) provides exquisite detail of the pituitary and adjacent structures. The anterior and posterior lobes can be identified and the infundibulum or pituitary stalk also (Fig. 5.1). In the suprasellar region the optic chiasm and the adjacent hypothalamus can be clearly seen and laterally the cavernous sinuses with the contained carotid arteries and neural structures can be identified. MRI has shown physiological variation in size of the pituitary, which reaches its maximum size during the later stages of pregnancy.

Normally the pituitary lies centrally within the sella turcica beneath the diaphragma sellae. A normal variant is seen when the diaphragma is deficient allowing CSF to enter the sella. The pituitary gland becomes flattened against the floor

of the sella, a condition referred to as an **'empty sella'** (Fig. 5.2).

Clinical indications

Patients are referred for detailed imaging of the pituitary region:

1. When a functioning pituitary adenoma is suspected

The anterior lobe secretes growth hormone (GH), prolactin, adrenocorticotropic hormone (ACTH), thyroid stimulating hormone (TSH), follicle stimulating hormone (FSH), and luteinizing hormone (LH). The posterior lobe stores, but does not produce, antidiuretic hormone (ADH). Pituitary adenomas make up 10–15% of all intracranial neoplasms and are well defined by a pseudocapsule and are almost always benign. Carcinoma is a rarity. 25% of adenomas are non-functional. 50% of functional tumours secrete prolactin presenting as amenorrhoea and galactorrhoea in premenopausal women. Adenomas producing GH and ACTH are less common and those producing TSH, FSH and LH rare. 10% of adenomas are plurihormonal, most commonly secreting prolactin and GH. Evidence of acromegaly may be seen on plain radiography (Fig. 5.3).

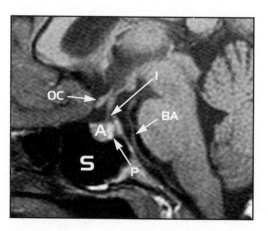

Fig. 5.1 Normal T_1 weighted MRI of pituitary. I = Infundibulum. A = Anterior pituitary lobe. P = High signal posterior lobe. OC = Optic chiasm. BA = Basilar artery. S = Sphenoidal sinus.

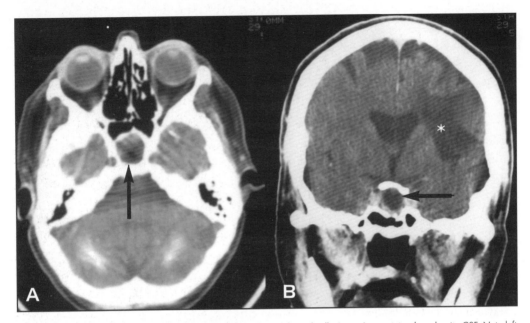

Fig. 5.2 Empty sella turcica. Axial (A) and Coronal (B) CT show enlarged sella (arrow) containing low density CSF. Note left cerebral infarct (*) and bilateral cerebellar dentate nucleus calcification of no particular significance.

Pituitary hyperfunction may occur without an adenoma. Anything which suppresses the production or transport of inhibitors from the hypothalamus to the pituitary through the infundibulum may cause this. Tumours arising in the suprasellar region which compress the stalk may be responsible for this so-called 'stalk section effect'.

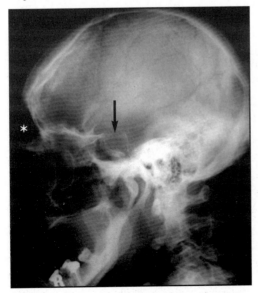

Fig. 5.3 Acromegaly. Note the expanded pituitary fossa (arrow), the large frontal sinuses (*) and the obtuse angle to the mandible.

2. When clinical evidence suggests a mass lesion in the pituitary region

Pressure on the optic chiasm is suggested by the presence of bitemporal hemianopia. Masses may become large enough to obstruct the foramen of Monro causing hydrocephalus and raised intracranial pressure with papilloedema. Pressure on the pituitary stalk area and posterior pituitary lobe may result in decreased ADH and diabetes insipidus, or in a few cases increased secretion of anterior lobe hormones. Suprasellar masses include craniopharyngiomas, large pituitary adenomas, usually nonfunctioning and presenting later than functioning tumours, gliomas of the optic tracts or hypothalamus, meningioma, germ cell tumours, chordoma arising from the clivus or a large carotid aneurysm.

3. When an acute pituitary complication is suspected

Pituitary apoplexy is the term used to describe haemorrhage or infarction of a pituitary adenoma resulting in sudden increase in size and clinically severe headache, acute visual loss and profound hypotension.

Findings

Adenomas

Appearances are divided into those small adenomas less than 1 cm with insignificant alteration in pituitary size or shape and referred to as **microadenomas** (Fig. 5.4), and larger tumours greater than 1 cm and reaching up to several centimetres in size referred to as **macroadenomas** (Fig. 5.5). Macroadenomas are clearly demonstrated on MRI and CT and an enlarged sella may be seen also on plain x-rays. Microadenomas, of which the ACTH adenoma is the smallest, measuring on average 3 mm, are more difficult to show. On MRI and CT, with the use of contrast medium intravenously and serial imaging, so called dynamic studies, microadenomas are usually demonstrated.

Inferior petrosal sinus blood sampling

Passage of a percutaneous catheter from the femoral vein via the jugular to the inferior petrosal sinuses allows blood sampling of anterior lobe hormones. With microadenomas the secretion favours one or other side depending on the situation of the tumour. The method is useful in cases where imaging is equivocal (see Cushing's syndrome).

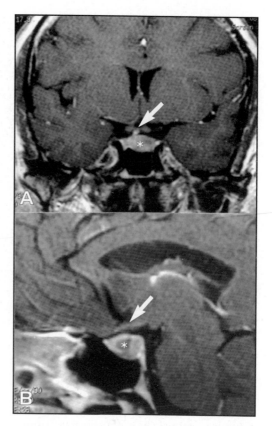

Fig. 5.4 Microadenoma of the pituitary. T_1 weighted MRI following intravenous gadolinium contrast shows a well defined rounded low signal mass (*) within the pituitary bulging the diaphragma slightly upwards. The optic chiasm (arrow) is not affected.

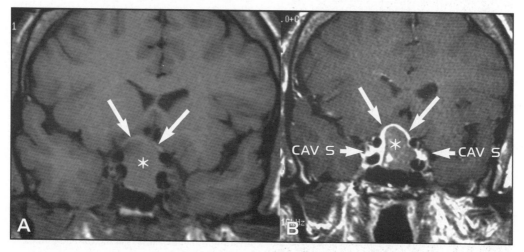

Fig. 5.5 Macroadenoma of the pituitary (A) Coronal T_1 weighted MRI shows the adenoma (*) pressing on the optic chiasm (arrows). (B) Following IV gadolinium the cavernous sinuses (Cav. S) developed a high signal. The carotid syphons appear as black (signal voids). The adenoma is heterogenous and the vascular capsule (arrows) is well shown.

Craniopharyngioma

These benign tumours arise from Rathke's pouch remnants within the sella or in the immediate vicinity above. Usually cystic and containing calcium they can usually be distinguished from other pathologies in the region. They have a bimodal age distribution being predominant in the first two decades with a second peak beyond middle age.

5.2 Adrenals

A major advantage from the development of CT, and later MRI, has been the ability to clearly demonstrate the adrenal glands. The soft tissue of these organs, although small, is clearly shown with both techniques in contrast to the surrounding fat.

Clinical indications

1. When adrenal hyperfunction is present

The three layers of the adrenal cortex produce corticosteroid hormones and three clinical conditions are recognized resulting from overproduction, **Cushing's syndrome, adrenogenital syndrome**, and **Conn's syndrome**. From the medulla the overproduction of noradrenaline and adrenaline by a phaeochromocytoma, usually presents clinically with episodic hypertension, pallor and sweating.

2. To detect the presence of metastases

The adrenals are a common site of metastasis particularly from bronchogenic lung cancer. CT performed to assess the primary lung cancer is always extended down to include the adrenals.

3. As part of other radiological examinations of the abdomen

When the upper abdomen is examined for any purpose by CT the adrenals are well seen and an unsuspected adrenal mass is not infrequently detected, the so-called **'incidentaloma'**. Most of these are benign, non-secretory adenomas.

4. In childhood to detect a neuroblastoma

This is the most common solid malignant tumour in children under four years of age, occurring earlier than Wilm's tumour of the kidney. It may be present in the newborn and can be confused with acute adrenal haemorrhage. The tumour arises anywhere within the sympathetic neural chain but most commonly in the adrenals (70%). Frequently the mother detects an abdominal swelling but in others the first symptoms relate to metastases or the effects of catecholamines, which are secreted in large amounts from the tumour.

5. When adrenal hypofunction is present

Addison's disease is uncommon and usually considered due to atrophy with an auto-immune basis. CT shows atrophic glands in these patients without calcification, but appearances do not distinguish between primary adrenal failure and that secondary to hypopituitarism. Some cases result from tuberculosis or opportunistic infections and these adrenals may appear swollen and calcified. An acute Addisonian crisis, usually resulting from shock, sepsis or a bleeding diathesis, may be fatal and CT will usually demonstrate large rather dense adrenals due to adrenal haemorrhage.

Cushing's syndrome

The condition should be suspected from the faeces, body habitus, diabetes, hypertension and osteoporosis and is confirmed by high cortisol levels in the urine.

Causes

1. Increased pituitary ACTH secretion – 65%
   Due to pituitary microadenoma, macroadenoma or pituitary – hypothalamic dysfunction.

Cushing's syndrome due to pituitary overproduction of ACTH is known as Cushing's disease, named after Harvey Cushing, the famous Boston pioneer neurosurgeon.

2. Adrenal tumour – adenoma – 20%
                    – carcinoma – 10%

3. Ectopic source of ACTH – 5%
   Lung carcinoma, carcinoids, phaeo-chromocytomas and pancreatic islet cell tumours and others may secrete ACTH.

4. Administration of steroid drugs

Investigation

1. Adrenal CT

If the adrenals are responding to increased ACTH secretion they may appear hyperplastic bilaterally. If an adrenal tumour is present the contralateral

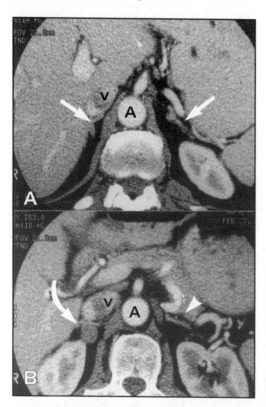

Fig. 5.6 (A) CT through normal adrenal glands (arrows). The right adrenal lies immediately posterior to the vena cava (V) and the limbs of the left adrenal are seen above the upper pole of the left kidney. (B) A small 1 cm soft tissue mass is seen in the right adrenal (curved arrow) consistent with an adenoma. The left adrenal (arrowhead) appears small.

gland may appear atrophic due to feedback ACTH suppression (Fig. 5.6). Carcinoma is suspected with tumours larger than 4 cm, with heterogeneous tissue and often calcifications (Fig. 5.7).

2. Chest x-ray

The chest is the commonest site of ectopic ACTH production and a chest film should be obtained particularly if the adrenal glands are hyperplastic.

3. Pituitary Magnetic Resonance Imaging

MRI is the best means of demonstrating micro and macroadenomas and other relevant pathology in the region.

4. High dose dexamethasone
   suppression testing

If the imaging tests do not reveal the cause, suppression tests may distinguish pituitary from ectopic sources of ACTH. Pituitary overproduction is partly suppressed but ectopic sources not.

5. Inferior petrosal sinus sampling

If tests point to the pituitary as the source but no tumour is demonstrated, bilateral sinus sampling may localize the source of ACTH within the pituitary and surgery may be performed despite the absence of imaging evidence of a microadenoma. The average size of the microadenoma is only 3 mm in Cushing's disease.

6. CT of chest and other possible ectopic sites

It may be necessary if tests suggest an ectopic site. CT is more sensitive than plain films of the chest in detecting small tumours.

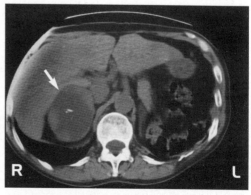

Fig. 5.7 Right adrenal carcinoma. The tumour (arrow) is 7 cm across, heterogeneous with calcification.

Adrenogenital syndrome

Overproduction of adrenal androgens causes virilism in females and precocious puberty in males. On CT the adrenals may be hyperplastic or there may be an adenoma or carcinoma. **Congenital adrenal hyperplasia** is the most common adrenal disorder of infancy and childhood and may be present at birth when the adrenals appear grossly enlarged and nodular.

Conn's syndrome

First described in 1956, primary aldosteronism results from excessive secretion of mineralocorticoid from the outer glomerular layer of the adrenal cortex. The hormone causes retention of sodium and water and patients usually present with hypertension. A persistently low serum potassium, prior to antihypertensive therapy, is the clue to diagnosis. The cause is an adrenal adenoma in 80%, bilateral hyperplasia in 20% and carcinoma is rare. On CT the adenomas are very small, being less than 2 cm in size, and may be multiple. In one third of cases the adenoma is undetected on CT. If adrenal CT demonstrates a probable adenoma bilateral exploratory surgery is performed. If CT is

negative bilateral adrenal venous sampling may indicate the side of the adenoma. The venous sampling catheter is introduced percutaneously from the femoral vein selectively into the adrenal draining veins.

Phaeochromocytoma

About 80% of these catecholamine-producing tumours occur as solitary adrenal masses. Bilateral tumours are present in 10% and in a further 10% the tumour is extra-adrenal. Noradrenaline and adrenaline secretion lead to hypertension which is often episodic and the diagnosis is suggested by an increased level of metabolites in the urine. In less than 10% the tumour is malignant (Fig. 5.8). Occasionally the tumour is part of a multiple endocrine syndrome. On CT the tumour appears solid and may calcify. The larger the tumour the more likely is malignant change. If a tumour is not seen in the adrenals on

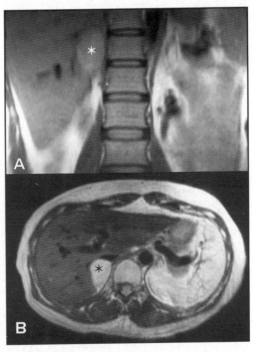

Fig. 5.9 Phaeochromocytoma of right adrenal. (A) T_1 weighted MRI shows the moderately high signal tumour (*) due to lipid content. (B) T_2 weighted axial image shows the tumour having a similar high signal to subcutaneous fatty tissue.

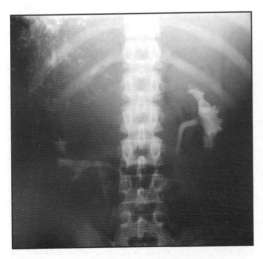

Fig. 5.8 Large calcified malignant phaeochromocytoma. The tumour, 20 cm across, is displacing the upper pole of the right kidney in the usual way for adrenal masses.

CT or in the tissues immediately adjacent then an ectopic site is suspected. Ectopic tumours may occur along the length of the sympathetic neural chain, even in the bladder wall, and coronal MRI should be performed from the mediastinum to the bladder base. These tumours have a distinctive MRI appearance because of the lipid content giving a high signal particularly on T_2 weighted spin-echo images which makes them appear white (Fig. 5.9). Iodinated contrast medium may provoke an hypertensive crisis in these patients and angiography should be avoided.

Adrenal masses

Most causes of an adrenal mass are included in the following:

- Cortical:
    Adenomas *(functional and non-functional).*
    Carcinomas.
- Medullary:
    Phaeochromocytoma.
    Neuroblastoma, Ganglioneuroma.
- Metastases.
- Myelolipoma.
- Cysts and pseudocysts.

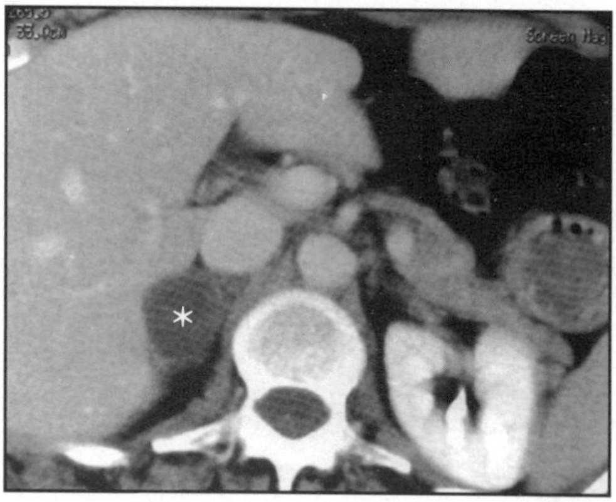

Fig. 5.10 Right adrenal tumour (*). In this patient with primary bronchogenic carcinoma the low density of the adrenal mass consistent with a fatty content favours an incidental non-functioning adenoma rather than metastasis.

Myelolipoma is a benign lesion which can be identified radiologically because of the presence of fat. Cysts are frequently the result of previous haemorrhage. A common problem with small masses detected incidentally is to differentiate between a non-functioning adenoma and a metastasis. Based on the relatively high fat content within adenomas MRI, and sometimes CT, is able to make the distinction between these two lesions in most cases (Fig. 5.10).

5.3 Thyroid

Patients present clinically because of a thyroid lump or with manifestations of hyper or hypothyroidism. In cases of abnormal thyroid function radiology has a supplementary role, but is helpful in assessing thyroid masses.

Abnormal function

Hyperthyroidism

The functional state of the thyroid gland is routinely assessed using laboratory assays of thyroxine, tri-iodothyronine (T4 and T3 respectively) and thyroid-stimulating hormone (TSH). If required, thyroid-stimulating hormone-

releasing hormone (TRH, secreted by the hypothalamus) may also be assessed. This allows patient classification as hypothyroid, hyperthyroid or euthyroid (normal levels of circulating thyroid hormone).

In the hyperthyroid patient nuclear imaging has a role in differentiating Graves' disease, i.e. diffuse goitre, multinodular goitre or solitary hyperfunctioning nodule. Radioiodine and pertechnetate are radioactive tracers which are trapped by the thyroid in a similar manner to circulating iodine. Radioiodine is synthesized to thyroglobulin, the precursor of thyroid hormone, and allows assessment of thyroid metabolism. Pertechnetate is technically simpler to use and delivers a lesser radiation dose, but demonstrates uptake only. These tests document thyroid metabolism and allow identification of thyroid tissue, but they do not assess the patient's thyroid functional status.

Thyroid eye disease

Lid retraction usually accompanies hyperthyroidism. Potentially more threatening to vision is the swelling of ocular muscles and great increase in orbital fat which causes proptosis, loss of globe motility and, in some, optic atrophy. CT or MRI document these changes well (see section 4.6).

Hypothyroidism

In childhood the features of cretinism can be recognized clinically, but in less obvious cases of hypothyroidism the radiologist may be the first to suggest the diagnosis because of delayed appearance of secondary epiphyseal centres in the skeleton.

In the mature adult hypo or hyperthyroidism have no specific systemic radiological manifestations.

Thyroid masses

A diffusely enlarged thyroid is most likely due to:

- Simple idiopathic goitre.
- Multinodular goitre.
- Graves' disease.
- Autoimmune thyroiditis.
- Iodine deficiency goitre (rarely).

Palpable lumps in the thyroid are common and may be due to:

- Multinodular goitre.
- Cysts:
  usually due to haemorrhage into or
  degeneration of a colloid nodule.
- Neoplasms:
  adenoma or carcinoma.

- Lymphoma.
- Metastasis.

Plain radiography, ultrasound, radionuclide scanning and biopsy all contribute to reaching a diagnosis in a particular case.

Plain radiography may demonstrate a soft tissue mass and displacement or compression of the trachea (Fig. 5.11). Curvilinear calcifications are frequently seen in degenerating thyroid nodules. When the anatomical extent of a goitre is an issue CT is indicated and can demonstrate any retrosternal extension.

*Note: iodinated contrast medium **must not** be administered if radionuclide scanning is contemplated, as the small amount of free iodine liberated from the contrast will interfere with radionuclide uptake in the thyroid for a number of weeks.*

The patient presenting with a solitary lump in the thyroid needs characterization of the lump's malignant potential. This at present cannot be reliably achieved by any one test in isolation, and a logical approach is as follows.

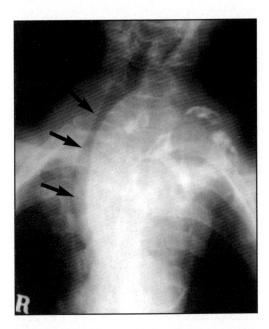

Fig. 5.11 Multinodular goitre. The large thyroid mass extends below the sternal notch into the anterior mediastinum and displaces the trachea (arrows) markedly towards the right. Calcifications are consistent with degeneration of nodules.

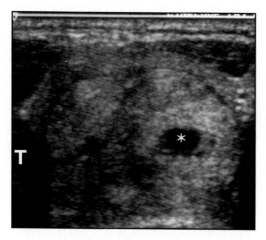

Fig. 5.12 Multinodular goitre. US of the left side of the thyroid shows marked enlargement with large nodules. Cystic degeneration (*) is seen centrally within the largest nodule. The trachea (T) is displaced to the right.

US is a useful first line of investigation, and will reliably differentiate cystic from solid masses (Fig. 5.12). Only a very small percentage of cystic thyroid lumps are neoplastic, the majority being degenerate colloid nodules in a multinodular goitre. If required, these may be aspirated under ultrasound control, and resolution is expected in benign cysts.

If US shows the lump to be solid, radionuclide studies may be used to characterize the lesion as 'hot' or 'cold' (Fig. 5.13). Hot nodules which take up the isotope are virtually ruled out as being malignant neoplasms, and may represent adenomas or hyperfunctioning non-neoplastic tissue. A cold nodule (mass with poor radionuclide uptake relative to normal tissue) may be malignant, and most proceed to biopsy. CT is used to show spread to lymph nodes and surrounding tissue (Fig. 5.14).

Metastatic and ectopic thyroid

Lingual thyroid, substernal extension of a goitre and intrathoracic goitre can all usually be demonstrated by radionuclide scanning. The ability to demonstrate metastatic thyroid carcinoma varies with the degree of tumour differentiation. Well-differentiated papillary or follicular tumour metastases can be shown with radioiodine following thyroidectomy. This may require cessation of thyroxine suppression treatment for a few weeks. Less differentiated tumours and medullary carcinoma do not take up radiotracers. Over 90% of thyroid carcinomas are papillary type.

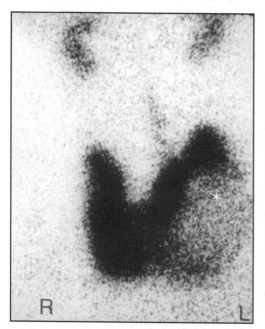

Fig. 5.13 Thyroid carcinoma. The pertechnetate radionuclide scan shows poor uptake in the palpable left-sided thyroid nodule(*), shown to be solid on US. This 'cold' nodule was biopsied to provide the histological diagnosis of carcinoma.

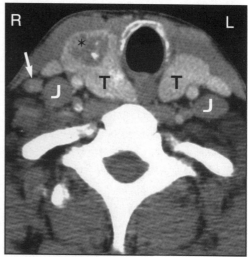

Fig. 5.14 Thyroid carcinoma. The heterogeneous mass (*) shows patchy contrast enhancement in this dynamic CT. Note the metastatic lymph node (arrow). Compare with left side. T=Thyroid. J=jugular vein.

5.4 Parathyroids

Hyperparathyroidism

Patients with overproduction of parathormone present with symptoms resulting from hypercalcaemia, such as lassitude, weakness, thirst, polyuria, anorexia and nausea, or as a result of the renal or bone complications of the condition.

Radiology plays a part in demonstrating parathyroid pathology and in demonstrating the complications of the condition in the urinary and skeletal systems.

Causes:

1. Primary

Due to adenoma in about 80%, carcinoma in 2% and hyperplasia of the glands in the remainder.

2. Secondary

The parathyroids respond to conditions causing hypocalcaemia by hyperplasia and increased parathormone production. Renal failure with resultant phosphate retention and low blood calcium is the commonest stimulant but malabsorption syndrome may have the same stimulating effect.

3. Tertiary

This term is used for those cases of secondary hyperparathyroidism in which an adenoma develops in response to long-standing hypocalcaemia and parathyroid hyperplasia.

Renal complications of hyperparathyroidism are far more common than extensive bone changes and it is interesting that it is unusual for an individual patient to have both kidney and skeletal changes.

Renal lesions

Opaque calcium oxalate calculi commonly complicate hypercalciuria. Calcification may also occur within the renal pyramids and can be detected on plain radiography. **Nephrocalcinosis**, the term given to this pattern, may also occur in forms of papillary necrosis, sponge kidney, and sarcoidosis (Fig. 5.15).

Bone lesions

Widespread bone changes are unusual and occur in only 15%. These changes are of three types:

* Changes of osteomalacia. Loss of bone density. Thinning of trabeculae and cortex.

* Evidence of osteoclastic activity. This can be well-shown in the fingers where the subperiosteal osteoclastic activity produces a fine irregular erosion of cortex, particularly along the margins of the phalanges (Fig. 5.16). The demonstration of this change is highly specific for the condition. The bone absorption due to osteoclastic activity may also result in erosion of the outer ends of the clavicles. Intense mineral loss in the skull vault results in a granular appearance, the so-called **pepper pot** skull (Fig. 5.17).

* Bone cysts. These localized lucent areas in bone gave rise to the old name for the condition, described by Von Recklinghausen, 'osteitis fibrosa cystica'. The cystic lesions are considered to be osteoclastomas and haemorrhage may occur within them to produce so-called **brown tumours**. Radiologically these cysts may expand the bone (Fig. 5.18).

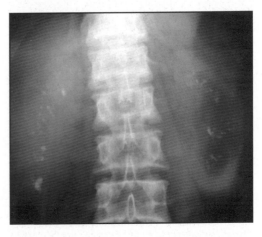

Fig. 5.15 Nephrocalcinosis in primary hyperparathyroidism. The calcifications are in the medullary pyramids.

Secondary hyperparathyroidism may result from malabsorption syndrome or from renal failure. In addition to the features described renal failure patients may show:

- Bone sclerosis. The reason for this is uncertain. The **rugger jersey** appearance of the spine is due to relative density adjacent to the intervertebral discs (Fig. 5.19).
- Metastatic calcification. Calcification in the walls of blood vessels may be extensive, a feature not usually seen in primary hyperparathyroidism.

The differentiation of osteoporosis, osteomalacia and hyperparathyroidism may not be possible in a particular case radiologically. Osteoclastic activity in the fingers may be present and help to distinguish hyperparathyroidism when other radiological manifestations of that condition are not present.

Diagnosing the parathyroid lesion

1. Serum calcium levels

Although parathormone can be estimated in the blood the diagnosis is usually dependent on showing elevated serum calcium levels. It should be noted, particularly in the investigation of

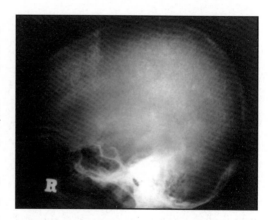

Fig. 5.17 Hyperparathyroidism. Osteoporotic ('pepper pot') skull.

patients with recurrent urinary calculi, that the hypercalcaemia due to hyperparathyroidism may be episodic and a number of estimates should be obtained over an extended period in such patients.

2. Surgical neck exploration

A skilled surgeon is favoured over expensive and sometimes equivocal radiology as the first line of management in these cases. To counter the widely held view that radiological demonstration of an adenoma is a necessary prelude to operation it has been said 'the only localization study required in patients suspected of hyperparathyroidism is to locate an experienced parathyroid surgeon'! Radiology is used generally for the small percentage of patients in whom exploration is negative, suggesting an ectopic site. The widespread use of x-ray bone densitometry machines for osteoporosis assessment is now contributing about one-third of the patients for neck exploration. In primary hyperparathyroidism over 80% of cases are due to a single adenoma in one of the four normally situated glands posterior to the thyroid lobes.

3. Tc–99m sestamibi scintigraphy

Technetium-labelled sestamibi, a complex molecule, is taken up by thyroid and parathyroid tissue but is retained in parathyroid adenomas for longer. Using **single photon emission CT** (SPECT) sestamibi scanning is reported to be

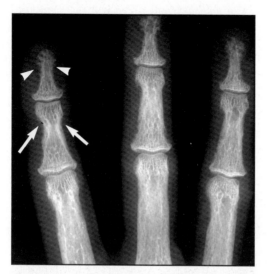

Fig. 5.16 Hyperparathyroidism. Marked osteopaenia. Osteoclastic activity has eroded the margins of the shafts of the middle phalanges (arrows) and also the terminal tufts (arrowheads) of the distal phalanges.

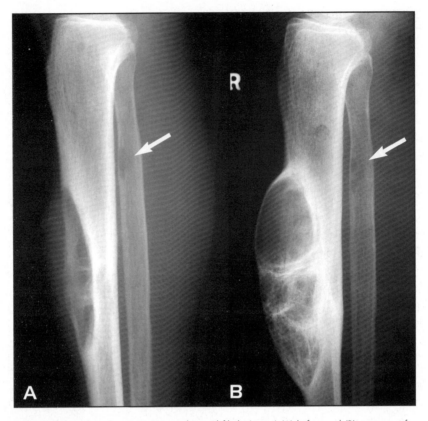

Fig. 5.18 Hyperparathyroidism. Brown tumours in tibia and fibula (arrow) (A) before and (B) one year after removal of a parathyroid adenoma.

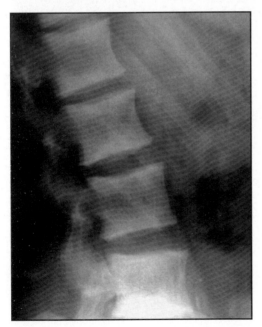

Fig. 5.19 Renal osteodystrophy. The vertebral bodies show increased density adjacent to the disc spaces ('rugger jersey' spine).

more sensitive in adenoma detection than other previous agents (Fig. 5.20).

In a small number of cases the adenoma is ectopic, usually in the mediastinum. SPECT scanning with sestamibi is the first technique used to find the ectopic tumour, but CT or MRI or parathormone assay of venous blood samples collected from mediastinal and neck veins may be required.

Other endocrine organs are discussed elsewhere: **pancreas** (Chapter 10), **testis** (Chapter 11) and **ovaries** (Chapter 13).

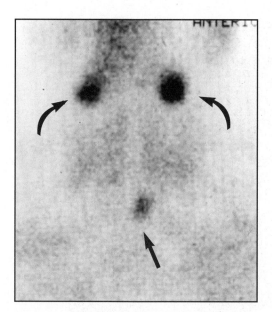

Fig. 5.20 Parathyroid adenoma. This delayed technetium 99m sestamibi radionuclide scan shows clearly a left-sided adenoma (arrow) after the sestamibi had cleared from the thyroid. Radionuclide is retained also in the submandibular glands (curved arrows).

Reference

Sutton, D., *Textbook of Radiology and Imaging*, 6th edn, Churchill Livingston, 1998.

Within a year of the discovery of x-rays in 1895, Walter Cannon, then a first-year medical student, researched the development of a contrast medium to demonstrate the upper gastro-intestinal tract. He considered both bismuth and barium salts as possibly suitable and produced radiographs of bismuth outlining the oesophagus in a goose. By 1910 barium sulphate was adopted as the agent for contrast studies of the gastro-intestinal tract. Advances in technology have resulted in barium which effectively coats the mucosa, gas to produce double-contrast imaging, drugs to temporarily paralyse the portion of gut being studied, and sophisticated imaging equipment to provide fine detail. The past 15 years has seen the rapid development of upper gastro-intestinal endoscopy and it vies with barium studies as the primary means of investigation. Endoscopy has the advantage of obtaining a biopsy but is invasive, with specific complications, and is about three times as expensive as the barium meal. Neither method is infallible in diagnosis and there is a need for careful evaluation of both methods, particularly in times of cost consciousness.

6.1 Salivary Glands

About one litre of saliva is secreted per day by the three pairs of major salivary glands and hundreds of minor salivary glands dotted throughout the mucosa of the sinuses, oral cavity, nasal cavity, pharynx and trachea. Although plain radiography may demonstrate calculi, and **sialography**, in which contrast is injected into the parotid or submandibular ducts, may provide useful information, computed tomography (CT) is now preferred for most clinical problems. MRI may provide useful additional information in determining the extent of neoplasms, particularly perineural extension. Pain, suggesting duct obstruction, or a swelling are the commonest clinical presentations.

Calculi

About 90% of salivary gland stones occur in the submandibular gland (Fig. 6.1) and around 80% are radio opaque on plain films and virtually all are on CT. Mucus plugs and duct strictures are other causes of obstruction and sialography is indicated to demonstrate the obstruction and the degree of duct dilatation. An obstructed sublingual gland swells forming a so-called **ranula** which is seen as a low density well-circumscribed mass on CT in the floor of the

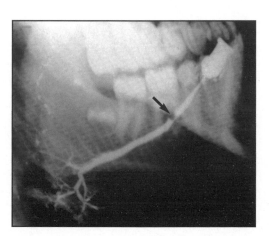

Fig. 6.1 Submandibular duct calculus. The sialogram shows a small filling defect (arrow) due to a nonopaque calculus.

mouth, and in some cases, a 'plunging' ranula extends into the neck.

Sjogren's syndrome

This condition, considered of autoimmune origin, includes in its manifestations salivary gland swellings, particularly the parotids, and a dry mouth. Metaplastic changes in the ducts result in sialectasis and sometimes stricturing as shown on sialography.

Neoplasms

CT and MRI are sensitive in detecting salivary tumours and showing their extent but have limited specificity. In general the larger the gland swelling the greater the chance the neoplasm is benign. About 80% of parotid tumours are benign and the vast majority of those occur in the superficial portion of the gland (Fig. 6.2). 60% of submandibular tumours and 25% of minor salivary gland tumours are benign.

Pleomorphic adenoma (benign mixed salivary tumour) is the commonest salivary gland tumour and is benign. On CT it is well circumscribed, usually heterogeneous, and may contain calcification. The parotid is the only salivary gland to contain lymphoid tissue and is the site of adenolymphoma (Warthin's tumour), which is also benign and typically occurs in middle-aged men. Lymphoepithelial cysts and nodules in the

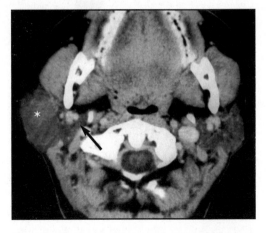

Fig. 6.2 Pleomorphic adenoma of right parotid gland. Contrast-enhanced CT shows the well-defined heterogeneous tumour (*) in the superficial portion of the gland. The deep portion of the gland (arrow) is not involved.

parotid are seen in seropositive HIV patients and these swellings may be the initial symptom in AIDS.

Malignant tumours have varying histology and frequently arise in salivary tissue remote from the major glands. They are less well-defined on CT and the adenoid cystic carcinoma (cylindroma), most commonly arising from the minor glands, tends to spread by perineural invasion, which is best shown on MRI with gadolinium enhancement.

6.2 The Barium Meal

When a barium meal is requested the radiologist examines oesophagus, stomach and duodenum. The clinical notes provided should indicate clearly the nature of the problem. To obtain double-contrast images, the mucosa is first coated with swallowed barium and then gaseous distension is obtained by swallowing effervescent solutions. The upper gastro-intestinal tract is paralysed for a short period,

using Buscopan, to avoid motion and to obtain detailed images.

Barium sulphate is a safe contrast material and is not absorbed. However, if it leaks to the peritoneal cavity, dense adhesions form. If such a possibility exists, the examination should be performed with a water soluble contrast medium, e.g. Gastrografin.

The role of the barium meal

1. Dysphagia

A barium study should be performed initially and in appropriate cases should be followed by oesophagoscopy.

2. Dyspepsia and epigastric discomfort

This is a common presentation and suggests the presence of peptic ulceration or, far less likely, gastric carcinoma. In recent times, the cause of peptic ulceration is better understood and effective drugs have been developed for treatment. An argument used in favour of endoscopy as the primary investigation for these patients has been that the barium meal is not sufficiently sensitive in detecting gastric cancer. Recent studies negate this and indicate a sensitivity of 96% for double-contrast barium meal in detecting gastric carcinoma. Furthermore, only 3.7% of the cases were referred for endoscopy to determine the specific nature of the abnormality; of those referred, 19% turned out to be cancer and the others benign. The barium meal does miss superficial acute ulceration, but the significance of making that diagnosis is doubtful given the availability of drug therapy which could be tried empirically. In this particular group of patients with dyspepsia and epigastric discomfort, a reasonable program of management would be to perform a barium meal with the knowledge that it would show the presence of chronic ulceration and gastric carcinoma. If negative, upper abdominal ultrasound would be indicated to exclude gallstones, which may have a similar presentation. If no relief results from empirical drug treatment directed at acute peptic ulceration, then endoscopy may be indicated.

3. Haematemesis and melaena

In acute cases, endoscopy is the primary investigation and should be performed as soon as feasible. In those patients in whom no abnormality is seen or doubt exists, a barium meal should be performed when the patient is fit to attend the department.

4. Epigastric mass

To provide accurate localization of the mass and, in some cases its nature, CT is indicated. Preparation for the examination includes outlining the upper gastro-intestinal tract with contrast medium to make identification of bowel as opposed to soft tissue optimal.

5. Persistent vomiting

In adults suspected clinically of pyloric stenosis it is wise to hospitalize the patient and empty the stomach using a gastric tube in severe cases. The commonest causes are chronic duodenal ulcer and carcinoma of the distal stomach. In some ulcer patients the stenosis relaxes with treatment. Endoscopy is the preferred initial study as it allows for biopsy of the stenotic lesion.

6.3 Dysphagia

In neonates, particularly those with polyhydramnios, dysphagia accompanied by coughing and excessive salivation is indicative of a **congenital tracheo-oesophageal fistula**. The majority have a blind-ending oesophagus which can usually be demonstrated on a lateral film by passing a soft feeding tube to the blockage and injecting air. Contrast medium is rarely necessary.

Dysphagia acquired in later life has numerous causes which are set out as for obstruction in other tubular structures in the body.

Mechanical:

In the lumen
- Foreign body. Food.

In the wall
- Carcinoma. Stricture. Web.

Outside the wall

- Mediastinal mass.
- Vascular ring.

In the lumen beyond

- Carcinoma of stomach.

Functional:

- Cricopharyngeus achalasia.
- Scleroderma.
- Cardiospasm or gastro-oesophageal achalasia.
- Presbyoesophagus ('corkscrew oesophagus').

True dysphagia is present when the patient feels food sticking at a particular level and is to be differentiated from difficulties in initiating swallowing and the feeling of a 'lump in the throat' (globus hystericus). Patients may accurately indicate the level of the obstructing lesion and true dysphagia should not be dismissed without a cause being found. There is virtually always a demonstrable cause found by thorough radiological and endoscopic investigation.

Mechanical Obstruction

Foreign body (Fig. 6.3)

Acute obstruction due to food, usually meat, is most often secondary to an underlying partial obstruction. Patients with high oesophageal acute obstruction present with cough, due to tracheal aspiration and copious sputum, because the daily saliva (about one litre) cannot be swallowed.

Carcinoma (Fig. 6.4A)

Over 80% are squamous cell carcinomas and the majority occur in the lower oesophagus below the carina. About 80% of these patients are male. Squamous carcinoma of the upper oesophagus is much less frequent and has a higher incidence in females. The findings are:

1. Localized constant segmental stricture.
2. Abrupt change from normal oesophagus to abnormal.
3. Evidence of tumour proliferation ('shouldering').
4. A surrounding soft tissue mass is sometimes seen.

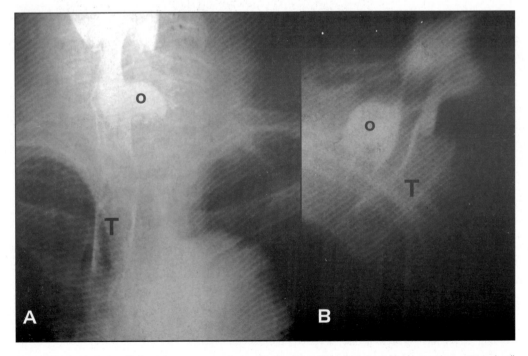

Fig. 6.3 Foreign body (steak) obstructing upper oesophagus. AP view (A) and lateral (B) show dilated oesophagus (O) and spill of contrast to the trachea (T).

These findings are classical but it is important to note that the appearance of oesophageal carcinoma may simulate a benign lesion, e.g. stricture. Adenocarcinoma of the stomach not infrequently infiltrates the lower end of the oesophagus producing dysphagia.

Oesophageal carcinoma occasionally escapes detection early on despite careful investigation. In many cases, the radiologist can be highly confident in diagnosing carcinoma when the specific features are present. When an apparently benign stricture is demonstrated, however, the confidence level in excluding carcinoma is very much lower and the diagnosis should not be accepted without confirmation by oesophagoscopy. Even then, and using biopsy, the presence of a carcinoma may be missed.

Staging the extent of carcinoma is crucial in determining the feasibility of surgery. CT is recommended to detect distant metastases in liver and lungs, and can assist in demonstrating direct involvement of the airways, aorta, and pericardium. CT also demonstrates abnormally large lymph nodes, particularly mediastinal, coeliac and gastro-hepatic, but is unable to detect metastases in normal-sized nodes. Also, CT fails to demonstrate the extent of invasion of the oesophageal wall by smaller tumours, but this can be shown using **endoscopic ultrasound**, so long as the probe can pass through the lesion.

Stricture (Fig. 6.4B)

Benign stricture due to reflux oesophagitis usually occurs below the level of the carina and has the following features:

1. Segmental stricture – less well demarcated than carcinoma.
2. The normal lumen tapers into the stricture.
3. No evidence of proliferation of tissue.
4. Gastro-oesophageal reflux, with an associated hiatus hernia. (see section 6.5).
5. An ulcer crater may be present in the oesophagus.

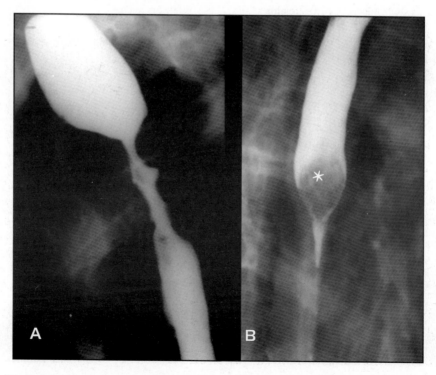

Fig. 6.4 (A) Carcinoma of the upper oesophagus. Note the abrupt change from normal calibre to stenosis and indentations consistent with neoplastic tissue. (B) Oesophageal benign stricture with impacted meat (*). Note the smooth tapering of the lumen.

Functional obstruction

Cricopharyngeus achalasia (Fig. 6.5A)

The cricopharyngeus muscle passes transversely across the posterior aspect of the upper end of the oesophagus and is a recognizable band within the inferior constrictor muscle. It may hypertrophy and not relax adequately during swallowing so that dysphagia is experienced. Gastro-oesophageal reflux is frequently present and may be the stimulus to the muscle hypertrophy. The obstruction due to cricopharyngeus spasm is considered nowadays to be responsible for the development of a pharyngeal pouch (Zenker's diverticulum). Immediately above the cricopharyngeus in the posterior wall of the pharynx there is a deficiency of muscle and a small pouch of mucosa may protrude, eventually reaching a size which may be palpable.

Presbyoesophagus (Fig. 6.5B)

This term is used particularly in the USA for the abnormal contractions of the oesophagus very frequently seen in the elderly (presby = old), causing minor dysphagia. Normally, oesophageal peristalsis is a co-ordinated stripping action from above downwards. In the elderly, tertiary contractions are a prominent feature. These result in localized constrictions giving the lumen a 'corkscrew' appearance with a disorganized peristaltic action.

Cardiospasm or achalasia of the cardia (Fig. 6.5C)

In this condition the lower end of the oesophagus fails to relax, particularly during swallowing which normally causes relaxation. The features are:

1. Tapering of the terminal oesophageal lumen.
2. Marked dilatation of the oesophagus above. The oesophagus may be seen on PA chest films extending out to the right of the cardiomediastinal shadow and containing a fluid level in the erect position.
3. Little, if any, peristalsis in the dilated oesophagus.
4. Absence of the gastric air bubble, consistent with the 'sump' effect of the fluid-filled dilated oesophagus.

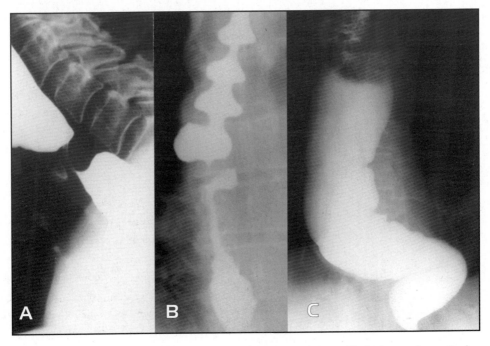

Fig. 6.5 Functional oesophageal obstructions. (A) Cricopharyngeus achalasia. (B) Presbyo-esophagus ('corkscrew' oesophagus). (C) Achalasia (cardiospasm).

5. Changes consistent with carcinoma of the oesophagus, which frequently complicates the condition.

Scleroderma

Diminished motility and dilatation resulting in a degree of dysphagia may be an early manifestation in this condition.

6.4 Dyspepsia and Epigastric Pain

The initial decision to be made by the clinician in such cases is whether to investigate or not. Varied symptomatology within this category is commonplace and frequently there is nothing to find on clinical examination except perhaps for some tenderness. If organic disease is present it most likely stems from the stomach, duodenum, gall bladder, or pancreas and in most cases the distinction cannot be made with confidence clinically. Sheer logistics make it unreasonable to investigate every patient who presents and it is more acceptable to proceed initially with a period of empirical treatment to determine whether the syndrome is persistent requiring further diagnostic investigation. When the decision to investigate is made, it is important that the protocol should be comprehensive. Barium meal

is a logical first step but upper abdominal ultrasound should be performed also. Patients are on record with four negative barium meals before a diagnosis of gallstones was made! The pancreas is shown on US and further detail is provided by CT and ERCP (endoscopic retrograde cholangio-pancreatography) (see Chapter 10). In patients with persistent symptoms and negative contrast studies, endoscopy is indicated and also, in some cases, CT. The radiological appearances on barium meal of the most common lesions presenting with these symptoms will be described.

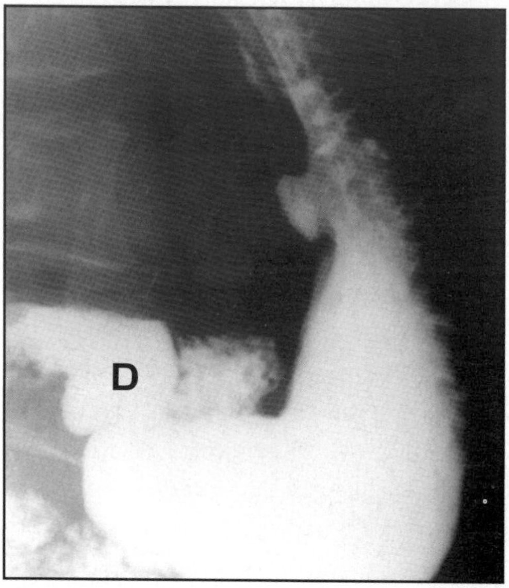

Chronic gastric ulcer

1. An ulcer niche projecting most often from the line of the lesser curvature (Fig. 6.6).
2. A well-developed neck to the ulcer.
3. Radiating rugae from the ulcer margin seen through the air-filled stomach (Fig. 6.7).

When these features are present, the diagnosis can be made with confidence. With ulcers on the greater curvature and in the fundus the degree of certainty is much less and endoscopy with biopsy is recommended.

Chronic duodenal ulcer (Fig. 6.8)

The vast majority lie in the first part which is suspended on a mesentery. The radiological evidence of ulceration is:

1. Constant deformity of the first part (i.e. the duodenal 'cap') even following Buscopan. Scarring in the cap usually results in the production of a trefoil appearance due to drawing in of opposite margins of the cap.

Fig. 6.6 Chronic benign gastric ulcer. The ulcer crater projects from the lesser curvature and has a well-defined neck. D=duodenal cap.

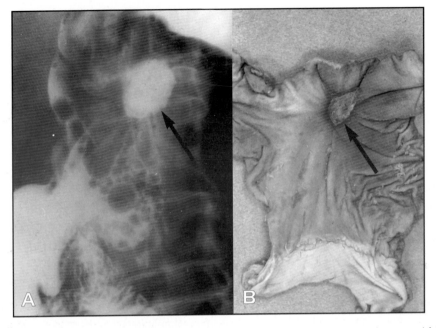

Fig. 6.7 Gastric ulcer on lesser curvature. Double-contrast barium meal. (A) Crater (arrow) and radiating rugal folds seen through the gas-filled stomach. (B) Resected specimen.

2. An ulcer niche. Ulcers arise mostly on the anterior or posterior surface and it may be difficult to demonstrate them in profile. Posterior wall ulcers retain barium when the

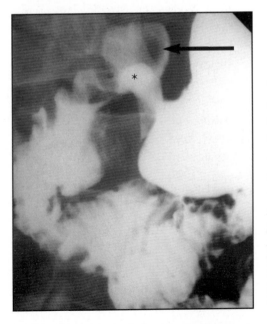

Fig. 6.8 Chronic duodenal ulcer. The duodenal cap is contracted. The ulcer crater (*) is seen as a density just beyond the pylorus. Pseudodiverticulum (arrow).

patient is lying supine and are well seen with double-contrast filling of the cap.

3. Pseudodiverticulum formation. Scarring in the mid-portion of the cap results in ballooning of the unaffected base of the cap on one or other margin, producing a relatively large pouch in some cases.

Acute peptic ulcers

Acute peptic ulcers or erosions in gastritis involve the mucosa and are usually 2–3 mm across. In the gas-distended double-contrast gastric studies, they are seen most often in the pyloric antrum and may be multiple. No doubt the detection rate of these erosions, which occur frequently, is considerably less with barium meal compared with endoscopy. However, the significance of actually demonstrating these erosions can be questioned, particularly now that effective drug therapy is available. A negative double-contrast barium meal examination of stomach and duodenum should suffice to exclude chronic peptic ulceration and carcinoma of the stomach.

Follow-up barium meals in peptic ulcer patients

The barium meal provides an easy means of checking on the healing of a typical chronic gastric ulcer. If prompt reduction in size does not take place endoscopy and biopsy should be carried out. With established chronic duodenal ulcer, however, follow-up barium meals to assess the effects of therapy are generally unhelpful. It is difficult to assess ulcer niche size and the scarring of the duodenum tends to be permanent.

Carcinoma of the stomach

Unfortunately, the vast majority of patients first present to the clinician when the tumour is well advanced. Recent studies have shown that double-contrast barium meal detects 96% of gastric carcinomas and the features on the barium meal are sufficiently specific for the radiologist to diagnose carcinoma with confidence. Endoscopy is required to confirm the diagnosis in only very few cases, but does provide biopsy material. Dyspepsia and epigastric pain are common in carcinoma patients and there is usually severe loss of appetite.

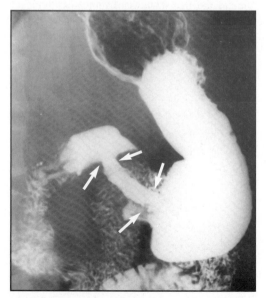

Fig. 6.9 Gastric carcinoma. The pyloric antrum between the arrows is narrowed and on fluoroscopy lacked peristalsis consistent with an annular constricting carcinoma.

The radiological appearance of these adenocarcinomas depends on the macroscopic type.

1. Annular constricting

As with similar lesions elsewhere in the gut there is a consistent irregular narrowing of the lumen of the stomach with evidence of proliferation of tissue at the limits of the lesion ('shouldering'). This type is frequently seen in the pyloric antrum (Fig. 6.9).

2. Linitis plastica

The wall of the stomach is infiltrated and the scirrhus nature of the lesion results in an overall shrinkage of the stomach.

3. Fungating

A large intraluminal polypoid mass of tumour fungation may be seen without evidence of obstruction.

4. Ulcerating

It is likely that ulcer cancers are neoplastic from the outset and malignant change in a benign peptic ulcer is considered most unusual. Clues to an ulcer crater being neoplastic are:

a. The crater does not project from the adjacent line of the stomach lumen.

b. A well-defined narrow neck is not present.

c. The lesion is away from the lesser curvature.

d. Radiating rugal folds do not continue to the edge of the ulcer in double-contrast views.

Detailed preoperative staging of gastric carcinoma is rarely required as the prognosis is poor and some form of palliative surgery usually required. CT demonstrates distant metastases, usually to liver, lungs or adrenals, and also intraperitoneal seeding including the Krukenberg tumour seeded to the ovaries (Fig. 6.10).

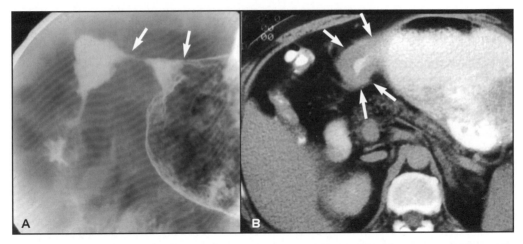

Fig. 6.10 Gastric carcinoma. (A) Double-contrast barium meal showing constant narrowing of the pyloric antrum (between the arrows). (B) CT shows the encircling mass of neoplastic tissue (arrows) around the gastric lumen.

6.5 Hiatus Hernia and Gastro-Oesophageal Reflux

The physiology of the gastro-oesophageal junction and the diaphragmatic hiatus is complex and not well understood. Normally the junction lies below the hiatus and there is a considerable resistance to gastro-oesophageal reflux. In some the resistance is low, resulting in gastro-oesophageal reflux, oesophagitis and symptoms

often referred to as 'heartburn'. In most of these patients the gastro-oesophageal junction and a small pouch of stomach moves above the diaphragm, a so-called **sliding hiatus hernia** (Fig. 6.11). In some a pouch of stomach adjacent to the gastro-oesophageal junction protrudes through the hiatus, known as a **para-oesophageal**

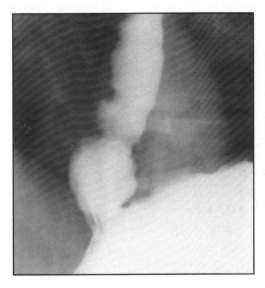

Fig. 6.11 Sliding hiatus hernia. Barium refluxed freely from the filled stomach to the oesophagus with manual abdominal pressure.

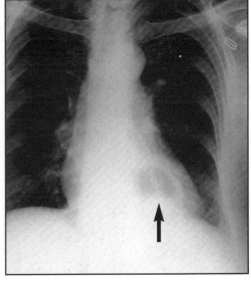

Fig. 6.12 Incarcerated hiatus hernia (arrow) seen as air-fluid level behind the heart. Asymptomatic patient.

hiatus hernia but most of those cases have a degree of sliding hernia also.

Testing for gastro-oesophageal reflux is easily performed by the radiologist during barium meal. With the oesophagus emptied and the stomach full of barium manual abdominal pressure is applied and the oesophagus checked for reflux. Occasionally, a large hiatus hernia containing an air-fluid level and incarcerated is detected behind the heart on a chest film (Fig. 6.12). Most of these patients are elderly females and most have no symptoms referrable to the hernia.

6.6 Haematemesis and Melaena

Bleeding from the gut may be severe, acute and life-threatening, or may be slower, episodic and leading to anaemia. The blood may be vomited, known as **haematemesis**, or passed per rectum as bright red blood or tarry stools due to altered blood, called **melaena**.

Acute severe gastro-intestinal haemorrhage is considered in section 12.6. This section deals with less severe bleeding, particularly from the upper gastro-intestinal tract.

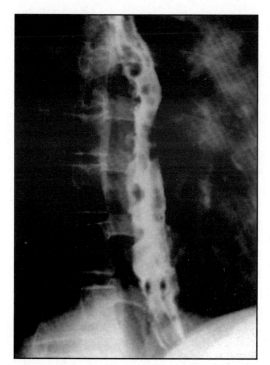

Fig. 6.13 Oesophageal varices in portal hypertension. The varices are seen as filling defects in the barium column.

Haematemesis

The main causes are:

1. Peptic ulceration.
2. Oesophageal varices.
3. Mallory-Weiss oesophageal tear.
4. Carcinoma of the stomach.

Upper gastro-intestinal bleeding is best studied by endoscopy initially if bleeding is not severe. In patients with lesser degrees of bleeding a preliminary barium meal in the department may provide valuable information.

Oesophageal varices (Fig. 6.13)

Demonstration of varices indicates the presence of portal hypertension, which is discussed in section 10.5. The mucosa of the normal empty oesophagus, lightly coated with barium, is seen as a series of roughly parallel opaque lines due to barium within the folds. When submucosal varices are present the folds are displaced in a manner consistent with the presence of small rounded submucosal swellings. Varices may also be demonstrated in the gastric fundus, where they may become quite large, and when few in number may cause confusion with other lesions.

Melaena

The main causes are:

1. Chronic duodenal ulcer.
2. Meckel's diverticulum (see Chapter 7).
3. Carcinoma of the right side of the colon occasionally.

It is important to be aware that administration of iron tablets orally can cause a similar appearance in the faeces. Endoscopy and barium meal are the investigations initially in melaena patients. Unless a definite cause for the bleeding is found in the stomach or duodenum, it is important to check the colon by barium enema and if negative the small intestine should be studied.

6.7 Epigastric Masses

In many cases, the likely cause will be apparent from the clinical information. However, in others the nature of the mass will be uncertain. It might arise from stomach, liver, pancreas, para-aortic nodes, or the lesser sac, or even transverse colon. Because the majority of upper-abdominal masses are neoplastic, and more often malignant, the most cost-effective imaging investigation is CT. In many instances the nature of the mass will be clearly indicated and a considerable amount of valuable additional information obtained concerning the pathology and its site of origin.

Reference

Gore, R. M., Levine, M. S. & Laufer, I.
Textbook of Gastrointestinal Radiology.
W. B. Saunders Co., 1994.

Small Intestine

The small bowel is an unusual tubular structure. It not only transports but has important digestive and absorptive functions. Large volumes of fluid are secreted into its lumen daily and even larger absorbed. The length of the small bowel, its movements, and the fluid content make it a difficult structure to demonstrate radiologically in detail. Fortunately, apart from acute obstructive lesions, abnormalities of the small intestine are relatively uncommon compared with the large bowel so that imaging studies are only required occasionally. Acute small bowel obstruction and acute gastro-intestinal haemorrhage are considered in Chapter 12.

7.1 Imaging Modalities

The main imaging modalities for studying the small intestine electively are:

1. Barium studies.
2. Computed Tomography (CT).
3. Angiography.
4. Radionuclide studies (see Chapter 12).

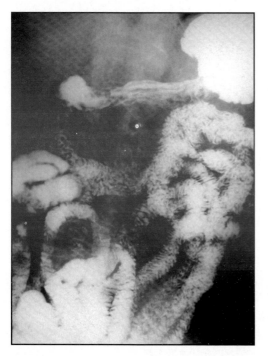

Barium studies

A detailed barium study of the small intestine cannot be adequately performed at the same time as an upper gastro-intestinal series and should be scheduled on a separate occasion. Most radiologists when requested to perform 'Barium meal and follow-through' concentrate on the upper gastro-intestinal tract unless the clinical notes clearly indicate possible small bowel pathology. Three methods of examining the small intestine are available. First, the radiologist may follow the passage of barium, given orally, on fluoroscopy making spot films of the various segments of small bowel down to the caecum (Fig. 7.1). To obtain adequate coating of the mucosa in the face of the very large amount of fluid, the radiologist employs special barium and takes precautions to avoid too much overlapping of small bowel loops which may obscure detail. The second method, referred to as **small bowel enema** or clysma, introduces the barium directly into the upper small bowel through a

Fig. 7.1 Normal small bowel pattern. The mucosal folds (valvulae semilunares) produce a delicate 'herringbone' barium pattern.

nasoduodenal tube. The small bowel is distended as the barium is followed and imaged throughout. Generally, this method is reserved to provide more detail should the oral method be equivocal. The third method is to reflux the barium into the small intestine using the barium enema. This is useful for demonstrating the distal small bowel in some cases.

Barium demonstrates the calibre of the small intestine which generally should not exceed 3 cm in the jejunum narrowing to a maximum of about 2 cm in the ileum. Peristaltic activity can be seen on fluoroscopy and video recorded. Films show the distribution of small bowel loops which may suggest the presence of an hernia. Separation of barium-filled loops suggests thickening of the bowel wall. More specific appearances such as intussusception may be demonstrated. Mucosal abnormalities may be demonstrated but the appearances have low specificity.

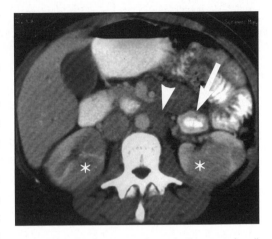

Fig. 7.2 Abdominal lymphoma. The involved segment of small bowel (arrow) shows a 'double halo' surrounding the intraluminal barium. Note lymphomatous tissue within both kidneys (*) and enlarged para-aortic lymph nodes (arrowhead).

Computed Tomography (CT)

CT provides valuable information concerning the wall of the small intestine and the state of the mesentery. Ascites is well shown and relevant organs such as the liver and the abdominal lymph nodes are demonstrated. In certain clinical situations CT should be the initial diagnostic examination supplemented in certain cases with bowel opacification or intravenous contrast enhancement. On CT the normal bowel wall should not exceed 4 mm in width and it has a homogenous appearance. Most benign intestinal lesions cause circumferential and symmetrical wall thickening but usually less than 1 cm. The bowel wall generally is slightly less dense than other soft tissues, particularly the abdominal wall muscles, and after intravenous contrast injection the thickened wall may show circular zones of different density consistent with enhancement of the epithelium or the serosa (the **double halo** sign) (Fig. 7.2). Adhesion of bowel loops,

abscesses, and occasionally fistulae may be demonstrated. Asymmetric small bowel wall thickening is more suggestive of neoplasm, particularly if more than 2 cm thick.

Angiography

The jejunum receives arterial supply from the coeliac axis by way of the gastroduodenal and pancreaticoduodenal arteries. The remainder of the small bowel receives arterial supply from the superior mesenteric artery which also supplies the right side of the colon. The venous drainage by way of the superior mesenteric vein blends with blood from the splenic vein to enter the liver by the portal vein. Both coeliac and superior mesenteric arteries are readily catheterized via the femoral artery. Delayed films following arterial injection display the venous drainage.

Radionuclide studies

Technetium-labelled red blood cells injected intravenously are used initially in the investigation of bleeding from the small intestine. Even with very slow bleeding the radioactive blood cells, having entered the bowel, tend to pool and be seen as a 'hot' spot. However, the site of the isotope may be considerably lower down in the gut than the site of bleeding. Sodium pertechnetate is taken up by ectopic gastric mucosa which is present in over 50% of Meckel's diverticula (Fig. 7.3).

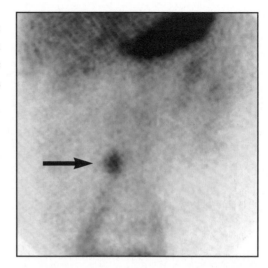

Fig. 7.3 Meckel's diverticulum. The radionuclide scan shows intense uptake in the gastric-type mucosa of the diverticulum (arrow) following intravenous injection of pertechnetate.

7.2 Clinical Indications

Problems for which elective imaging of the small intestine may be indicated include:

1. Chronic intermittent small bowel obstruction

Although barium studies are well-established as the initial investigation, evidence shows that CT in certain patients is more informative. In patients with a history of cancer and clinical symptoms suggesting intestinal obstruction CT has the primary role (Fig. 7.2). In patients with a history of abdominal surgery, but without cancer, or those in which a stricture following non-steroidal anti-inflammatory drug therapy is suspected, CT has a secondary role to barium studies. However, if the clinical findings suggest an abscess or a palpable abdominal mass then CT is the logical first investigation in these patients also.

2. Obscure chronic gastro-intestinal haemorrhage

In these cases the small intestine is studied after excluding a significant lesion in the large intestine or upper gastro-intestinal tract. Radionuclide studies may indicate the small bowel as the site of bleeding and barium studies are used initially to demonstrate the lesion. In the very young, when Meckel's diverticulum is the likely site of bleeding, radionuclide studies are indicated initially (Fig 7.3).

3. Malabsorption syndrome

Clinically the features of malabsorption may include diarrhoea, steatorrhea, flatulence, abdominal distension and weight loss. Malabsorption may occur at various levels and may be classified.

a. Maldigestion, e.g. chronic pancreatitis.
b. Mucosal abnormality, e.g. coeliac disease.
c. Malassimilation at the enterocyte level, e.g. lymphangiectasia.
d. Due to stasis and bacterial overgrowth, e.g. diverticulosis (Fig. 7.4), blind loops, fistulae, scleroderma and idiopathic pseudo-obstruction.

Radiology has a very limited role in the diagnosis of malabsorption states, for which biochemical tests and small bowel biopsy are

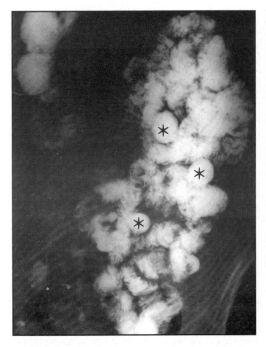

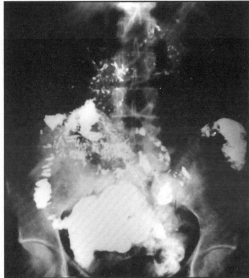

Fig. 7.5 Malabsorption syndrome. The barium is clumped resulting in poor coating of the mucosa due to excess mucus.

Fig. 7.4 Multiple small bowel diverticula (*).

important diagnostic tools. Barium studies allow assessment of the small bowel mucosa but appearances are nonspecific in most instances (Fig. 7.5). Dilated loops of bowel and stasis as a site for possible bacterial overgrowth may be shown with barium and CT may be indicated to demonstrate the width of the bowel wall.

7.3 Intussusception

Telescoping of one section of the bowel into another adjacent segment accounts for about 90% of bowel obstruction in infants, ranking second only to appendicitis as the most common cause of an acute abdomen in childhood. Most of these cases begin in the distal ileum and are idiopathic, occurring between 3 to 18 months of age. Barium enema is used not only to confirm the condition but to reduce the intussusception using the hydrostatic pressure of the barium column. If the diagnosis is evident clinically with a typical palpable mass, reduction may be achieved by injecting air rather than barium. In adults intussusception is relatively uncommon. In the colon it is usually due to a primary carcinoma whilst small bowel intussusception in adults usually results from a benign tumour. On barium studies an intussusception typically has a characteristic appearance, referred to as 'coil spring' (Fig. 7.6). On CT the lesion has a target-like appearance due to layers of mesenteric fat and higher attenuating bowel wall (Fig. 7.7). A similar appearance may occasionally be seen with ultrasound with alternating hyper- and hypoechoic layers within the mass.

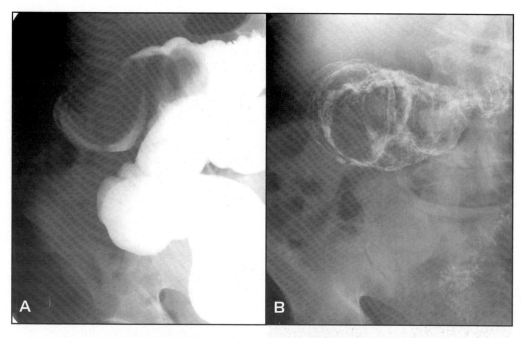

Fig. 7.6 Intussusception of colon carcinoma. Barium enema. (A) Filling defect at the hepatic flexure. (B) After evacuation barium is retained between the intussusceptum and the intussuscipiens ('coiled spring' appearance).

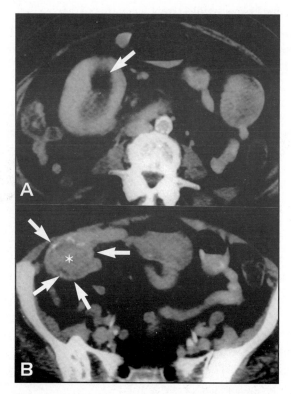

Fig. 7.7 Intussusception secondary to ileal polyp. CT shows (A) radiolucent mesenteric fat (arrow) as part of the intussusceptum. (B) More distally at the head of the intussusception. The intussusceptum is seen as a filling defect (*) within the intussuscipiens (arrows) with traces of barium between the two.

7.4 Crohn's Disease

Although any part of the gastro-intestinal tract from the mouth to the anus may be affected by this chronic idiopathic inflammatory disease, the small bowel is by far the major site of involvement. The terminal ileum is the commonest site where it is sometimes referred to as **regional ileitis**. The disease may be protracted with long periods of remission.

The early changes effect the mucosa and may be shown by detailed barium studies. The mucosal folds become thickened and the mucosa has a coarse villous pattern. Small shallow mucosal erosions surrounded by a small halo of oedema, known as 'apthoid ulcers' may be identified. Although non-specific these changes occurring in the ileum are very strongly suggestive of the disease. With progression of the disease to involve the deeper layers of the bowel wall strictures develop and an ulceronodular pattern is seen in the mucosa on barium studies (Fig. 7.8). Deep ulcers, resembling rose thorns, project from the lumen into the thickened wall. Wall thickening, usually symmetrical and sometimes showing a double halo appearance after contrast medium is seen on CT, which also demonstrates changes in the mesentery, adherent loops and abscess formation (Fig. 7.9). Sometimes fistulae are shown to other bowel loops, the skin or occasionally the urinary bladder. Characteristically, several segments of the gastro-intestinal tract may be involved with Crohn's disease with normal intervening segments, the so-called 'skip' lesions. Colonic Crohn's disease is referred to in Chapter 8.

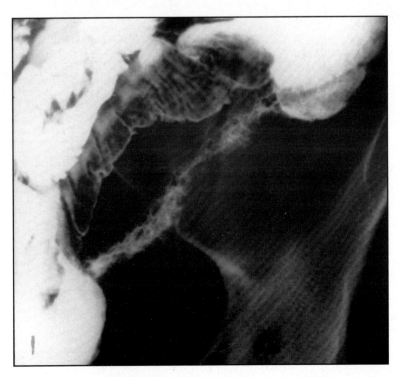

Fig. 7.8 Regional enteritis (Crohn's disease) of the ileum. Barium outlines a long segment of abnormal ileum which is narrowed, rigid and has an abnormal nodular mucosal pattern.

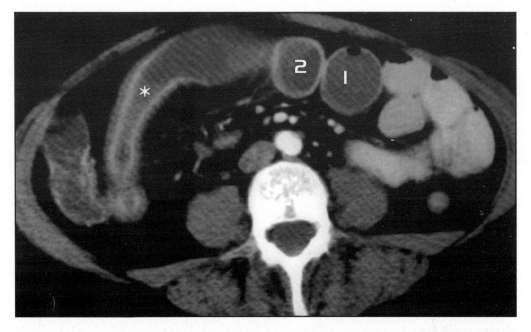

Fig. 7.9 Regional enteritis (Crohn's disease). CT following intravenous and oral contrast shows a segment of involved ileum in longitudinal section (*) with stenosis and wall thickening. Two non-barium filled loops are shown in cross-section; one (1) has a normal wall and the other (2) shows the beginnings of wall thickening.

7.5 Neoplasms

Surprisingly in view of its length, neoplasms of the small bowel are relatively uncommon. Benign and malignant tumours occur with about equal frequency. Benign tumours, most commonly leiomyoma, lipoma or adenoma may present because of bleeding or intermittent obstruction, frequently as a result of intussusception. On barium studies these tumours may be seen as intraluminal filling defects arising from the wall.

Carcinoid tumours are potentially malignant and usually occur in the distal ileum. The commonest site for these tumours is the appendix but the second commonest site is the small bowel where carcinoids account for 25% of small bowel tumours. On barium studies the tumour is rarely detected until measuring 2 cm in size by which time 90% have metastasised. On penetrating the muscle wall the tumour serotonin provokes an intense desmoplastic effect resulting in a tumour mass best shown by CT. Adenocarcinoma is more common in the upper small bowel and usually obstructs early on. Lymphoma is slower to obstruct and extends along the bowel wall, often at multiple sites (Fig. 7.2). Haematogenous metastases from melanoma or bronchogenic carcinoma result in multiple polypoid lesions, sometimes with central ulceration. Serosal metastases usually obstruct and may be associated with ascites.

Reference

See Chapter 6.

Patients with large bowel pathology may present with symptoms of gradual onset or more acutely. Altered bowel habits, blood in the faeces, or lower abdominal discomfort, may be the first indications of disease in the large intestine. Acute intestinal obstruction and gastro-intestinal haemorrhage are discussed in Chapter 12. Further investigation of the large intestine after an adequate clinical examination, including digital rectal examination, may be performed by barium enema or endoscopy. These methods are considered complementary. Barium enema provides a total overview of the large intestine, whilst endoscopy allows for inspection of the mucosa and biopsy, and if necessary, removal of polyps. The flexible sigmoidoscope allows for inspection of the distal colon, where most carcinomas are found and the colonoscope allows for the entire length of the colon to be studied in most cases. Barium enema and colonoscopy both require careful bowel preparation to minimise faecal retention.

8.1 Barium Enema

Double-contrast barium enema is the primary diagnostic investigation for the large intestine following thorough clinical examination, including digital and visual examination of the distal sigmoid and rectum. The mucosa of the large intestine is coated with barium and then the lumen is distended with air to produce the double contrast effect. In certain instances, a single contrast study using barium alone is used. If leakage from the colon is anticipated, e.g. following recent surgical anastomoses, the study is performed using a water-soluble contrast medium.

Preparation of the patient

The radiologist will provide detailed instructions to the patient concerning bowel cleansing, using hydration, cathartic pills and suppositories, and low residue diet. However, it is helpful if the referring clinician institutes a high fluid intake which is the single most important factor in achieving a clean colon. Also, it is important for the clinician to consider the patient's psyche and explain the nature of the examination, its importance and prepare the patient for some minor degree of discomfort during the procedure.

Importance of rectal examination

It is bad practice to refer a patient for barium enema without having at least performed a digital rectal examination and preferably proctoscopy or sigmoidoscope. There are two reasons at least for this recommendation. First, about one half of all large intestine cancers occur in the distal colon and rectum, often within range of the sigmoidoscope. Secondly, the barium enema does not exclude a lesion low in the rectum or anal canal, because the self-retaining balloon catheter obscures the region.

Indications for barium enema

1. Altered bowel habits

A patient who has established a regular pattern of bowel actions and becomes aware of a significant change, usually constipation, is a candidate for further examination. However, it is important to exclude agents which may produce a functional disturbance. These include drugs such as opiates and anticholinergics, a change in diet, particularly a lowered fluid intake, giving up smoking, or a change of life-style with suppression of the normal urge. In patients with a long history of irregularity the decision to investigate becomes more difficult.

2. Bleeding per rectum

The presence of bright blood mixed with the faeces is a strong indication for further investigation. Blood on the stool and splashed onto the toilet bowl is almost certainly due to haemorrhoids. The main colonic causes are carcinoma, diverticula, polyps, and forms of colitis. Melaena, or altered blood in the stool, usually arises from lesions above the colon, but occasionally from proximal colonic conditions such as carcinoma of the caecum.

3. Diarrhoea

Careful clinical examination is essential to narrow down the wide range of conditions causing this nonspecific symptom. The association of blood and mucus in the stool points to a large bowel organic origin and it should be remembered that episodes of diarrhoea may occur with obstructive lesions such as carcinoma of the left side of the colon. Patients with tumours low down in the rectum may also complain of diarrhoea and unsatisfied defaecation.

8.2 Carcinoma of the Colon

Carcinoma of the colon is common, affecting one in twenty-five Australians, but has a good prognosis if detected at an early stage. It is uncommon under the age of forty. The risk is increased three to fourfold if a first degree relative has had the condition.

Appearances on barium enema

1. Annular constricting ('Apple Core') (Fig. 8.1)

This type has features common to similar lesions elsewhere in the gut, e.g. oesophagus.

- A well-defined constant irregular stricture.
- An abrupt change from normal bowel to the stricture.
- Evidence of tissue proliferation ('shouldering').

2. Polypoid (Fig. 8.2)

Frequently, on the right side of the colon the tumour produces an intraluminal filling defect which does not produce obstruction until late in the disease, unless it intussuscepts or involves the terminal ileum. These patients often present with anaemia through chronic blood loss.

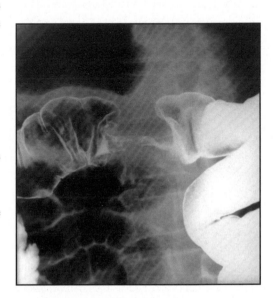

Fig. 8.1 Annular constricting ('apple core') carcinoma of transverse colon. Note the abrupt change from normal to abnormal calibre and the presence of tumour indenting the adjacent gas-distended bowel ('shouldering').

3. Carcinoma in ulcerative colitis
(Fig. 8.13)

Carcinoma frequently develops in longstanding ulcerative colitis and to a lesser extent in Crohn's colitis. The typical appearance may not be seen due to the general thickening of the bowel wall in the region. As a result, the annular constricting carcinoma may not show 'shouldering' but rather a tapered appearance, which can be confusing. Any persistent stricture in such a patient should be considered as carcinoma until proven otherwise.

4. Carcinoma and multiple polyps

Carcinomas may be multiple in the bowel or a carcinoma may be associated with benign polyps. A polyp larger than 1.5 cm in diameter, if sessile, is considered generally to be a carcinoma.

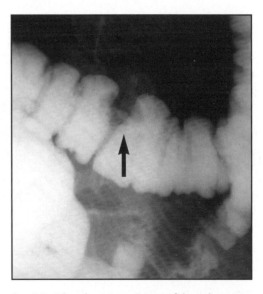

Fig. 8.2 Polypoid carcinoma (arrow) of the mid-transverse colon. Patient noticed bright blood in the faeces.

Demonstrating metastases

Local spread and spread to regional lymph nodes in the mesentery is assessed at operation. The tumours spread through the portal system to the liver and because the bulk of that organ precludes detailed examination at operation it is logical to perform CT to detect metastases as it has an accuracy of 85%. Some colonic liver metastases are calcified and visible on plain radiography.

8.3 Diverticular Disease

Radiological appearance

The appearance reflects the stage of the disease.

1. Uncomplicated diverticula
(Note: the plural is not 'i' or 'ae').

Diverticula form as protrusions of mucosa through the wall at points of penetration of the muscularis propria by the vasa recta. The three taeniae are disposed at 2, 6 and 10 o'clock around the lumen with the mesentery attaching at the 6 o'clock position. Diverticula do not arise between the two antimesenteric taeniae (i.e. 10 and 2 o'clock). Uncomplicated diverticula fill readily during barium enema and are easily recognized and the lumen of the colon is not reduced. This uncomplicated state is referred to generally as **diverticulosis**. Because the fundus of the diverticulum is closely related to the arterial branches in the wall, severe haemorrhage may occur, giving rise to problems in diagnosis of the site because diverticula are usually multiple.

2. Early diverticulitis

Diverticula in the sigmoid colon are prone to become infected. The first change is spasm of the bowel wall during filling with barium. The spasm prevents filling of the diverticula beyond the necks giving a serrated appearance of the bowel which is slightly reduced in luminal width (Fig. 8.3). A film made the next day may show the diverticula well filled with residual barium, giving a better appreciation of the extent of the condition.

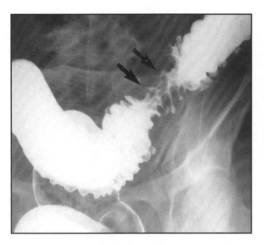

Fig. 8.3 Sigmoid diverticulitis. Relatively early changes. In the narrowed segment, due to spasm, only the necks of diverticula (arrows) have filled.

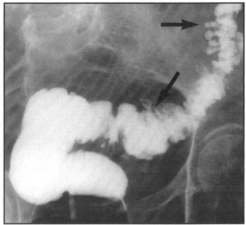

Fig. 8.4 Sigmoid diverticulitis. Some diverticula contain faecal filling defects (arrows). Thickened bowel wall with varying degrees of stenosis.

3. Chronic diverticulitis (Fig. 8.4)

The wall becomes considerably thickened, resulting in a long segment of narrowing, which usually tapers to the normal width and in most cases can be differentiated from the shorter very localized stenosis of carcinoma. The presence of diverticula along the extent of the narrowed segment indicates the nature of the disease and differentiation from carcinoma is usually not difficult.

4. Pericolic abscess and fistula formation

Fixity of a sigmoid loop with changes of chronic diverticulitis and an adjacent soft tissue opacity is consistent with the presence of a pericolic abscess. Adhesion to the bladder may result in a vesico-colic fistula with evidence of **pneumaturia**. CT is valuable in such cases as it virtually always shows some air in the bladder (Fig. 8.5). Rarely, air and barium may be seen in the bladder during barium enema (Fig. 8.6). Adhesion to the small bowel may

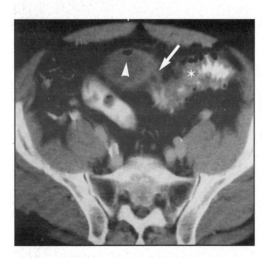

Fig. 8.5 Vesico-colic fistula due to diverticulitis. CT shows loop of sigmoid colon (*) with air-containing diverticula adherent to the thick-walled bladder (arrow). A bubble of gas is seen in the bladder (arrowhead). The patient presented with difficult-to-control urinary tract infection.

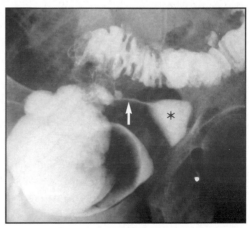

Fig. 8.6 Vesico-colic fistula complicating sigmoid diverticulitis. The barium-filled dependent portion of the bladder (*) and fistula (arrow) can be seen extending from the narrowed proximal sigmoid. The patient presented with pneumaturia as a symptom.

result in an **entero-colic fistula**, and with barium enema early filling of the small bowel, prior to the proximal colon, indicates the nature of the problem.

These patients present with severe diarrhoea as small bowel content is delivered directly to the distal colon.

8.4 Polyps

Polyps are seen in about 25% of all autopsies. Using double contrast techniques, polyps are frequently demonstrated radiologically.

Most polyps demonstrated by barium enema may be classified into:

1. Adenomatous
- Tubular.
- Villous.
2. Carcinomatous
3. Hamartomatous
- Peutz–Jegher syndrome.
- Juvenile.
4. Pseudopolyps
- e.g. in ulcerative colitis.

Patients with polyps may present with rectal bleeding, diarrhoea with mucus, or because the polyps have been found incidentally.

Appearance on barium enema

1. Adenomatous

Tubular adenoma

This is by far the commonest polyp. The appearance is of a smooth, hemispherical protrusion from the mucosal surface, usually measuring less than 1.5 cm in diameter (Fig. 8.7). The lesions may be multiple and evidence suggests they increase in frequency with age. Some tubular adenomas develop a stalk, particularly on the left side of the colon and have a characteristic appearance on barium enema (Fig. 8.8).

Villous adenoma

Villous adenoma is usually several centimetres across at its base and has a somewhat irregular surface due to its villous structure. The radiologist

usually reports such a finding as carcinoma and it is uncommon for the true nature of the lesion to be appreciated at radiological examination. These lesions have about a 43% chance of being malignant and often present because of diarrhoea with much mucus.

2. Carcinomatous (Fig. 8.2)

Particularly on the right side of the colon, carcinoma may appear polypoid rather than the more usual annular constricting 'apple core' appearance. It is generally accepted nowadays that most carcinomas develop from tubular adenomas (see below) and the likelihood of malignant change increases with the size of the polyp.

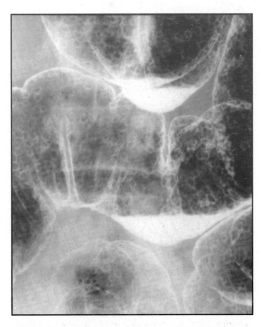

Fig. 8.7 Familial polyposis coli. Multiple small polyps throughout the gas-filled colon, all less than 1 cm in width.

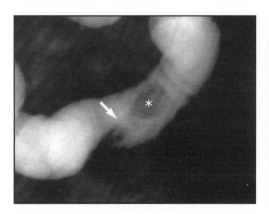

Fig. 8.8 Adenomatous polyp on a stalk. The single contrast barium enema clearly shows the round head of the polyp (*) and the stalk (arrow) extending down to the bowel wall, which is slightly enfolded.

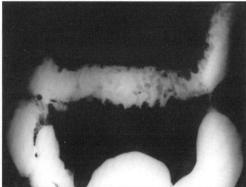

Fig. 8.9 Ulcerative colitis. Pseudopolyposis. The colon is markedly shortened and numerous filling defects are seen in the transverse colon due to oedematous residual mucosa.

3. Hamartomatous

Peutz–Jegher syndrome

The polyps contain smooth muscle and the small intestine is always involved when large bowel polyps are present. Radiologically, the appearance suggests a polypoid carcinoma because of the rather large size, but the smooth surface of the polyps may give a clue to diagnosis. Muco-cutaneous pigmentation is a feature.

Juvenile polyps

These polyps of early life contain connective tissue and distended ducts containing mucus. The condition is not pre-malignant.

4. Pseudo-polyps

In colitis, particularly ulcerative colitis, the mucosa between ulcerated areas becomes oedematous producing a polypoid appearance on barium enema. (Fig. 8.9)

Screening: colon adenoma-carcinoma sequence

Because colorectal carcinoma (CRC) is very common in Australia, affecting at least 6% of the population, it is important to recognize those at higher risk. To date, a satisfactory screening test which can be applied universally has not evolved. A family history of CRC in a parent or sibling increases the risk of CRC from 6% to 18%. The incidence of polyps and CRC increase in the older age groups, and in the 7th decade it is estimated that 70% of persons will have at least one tubular adenomatous polyp. Only about one in twenty polyps 5 mm in size is estimated to become malignant, and it may take years to do so. Certainly the size of a tubular adenoma increases the likelihood of CRC. For those less than 1 cm, the likelihood is 1%, from 1–2 cm 10%, and for polyps larger than 2 cm, 30% will be carcinomatous. In the absence of a reliable test for CRC, it is logical that those with a strong family history or known to have tubular adenomatous polyps, should undergo regular surveillance by barium enema or colonoscopy every two or three years. Recently **Virtual Colonoscopy** based on helical CT data has been shown to be equal to direct colonoscopy in detecting polyps larger than 1.2 cm (see Plate 1.1 in colour plates section).

Familial polyposis coli

Patients with this non-sex-linked Mendelian dominant hereditary abnormality (Fig. 8.7) present generally in the second decade of life due to rectal bleeding. The adenomatous polyps increase in size and number from birth and are not demonstrable before the age of about nine years. Most patients below this age with large bowel polyps have either juvenile polyposis or Peutz-Jegher syndrome. Radiology is not necessary to make the diagnosis as in 95% of these patients polyps can be seen on rectal examination. The barium enema demonstrates the extent of the involvement and the presence of already existing carcinomas. In most patients carcinoma is established before 30 years of age.

8.5 Colitis

Colitis has come to mean that a segment or the entire length of the large bowel is abnormal as opposed to a localized focal lesion. The suffix 'itis' is inappropriate as acute inflammation is not always present. Diarrhoea is usually a feature and frequently the presence of blood and mucus points to an organic abnormality in the large bowel.

Types:
- Ulcerative colitis.
- Granulomatous colitis, i.e. Crohn's disease.
- Ischaemic colitis.
- Radiation proctocolitis.
- Amoebic colitis.
- Pseudomembranous enterocolitis.

It is important to realize that the large bowel can respond to damaging agents only in a limited number of ways, e.g. ulceration, oedema, stricture. The macroscopic appearances produced by the various entities above may be similar, and hence, the radiological appearances may be difficult to differentiate. Despite this, there are features radiologically which help in most cases to make a diagnosis. The radiological appearances are described for the commonest conditions encountered.

Ulcerative colitis
Early diagnosis
Barium enema is not the way to confirm a provisional clinical diagnosis of ulcerative colitis.

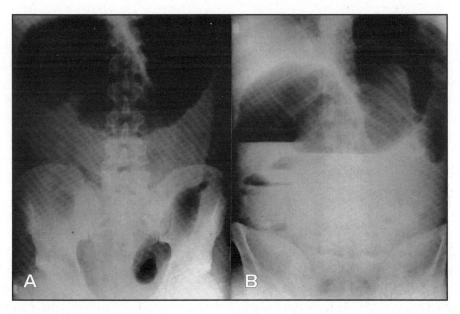

Fig. 8.10 Toxic megacolon. Acute fulminating ulcerative colitis. Supine (A) and erect (B) films show marked dilatation of large bowel which may be confused with a distal mechanical obstruction.

Ulcerative colitis is now considered always to involve the rectum and the diagnosis can be made by endoscopy and biopsy. Also, a barium enema examination may adversely affect the patient's condition and should be avoided until the condition is quiescent.

Plain films may demonstrate marked gaseous distension of the large bowel which is a feature of **toxic megacolon** (Fig. 8.10), the fulminating acute form of the disease which sometimes results in perforation.

Early changes seen on barium enema during remission are confined to the mucosa, which takes on a granular appearance (Fig. 8.11), and later ulceration, which does not penetrate the muscularis mucosae. These shallow ulcers are seen filled with barium on double-contrast films and occasionally the undermining of the ulcers give an apparent double edge to the barium-filled colon. Other early changes are a failure of the colon to empty well on after-evacuation films; a strange finding when diarrhoea is such a prominent symptom. Also, there may be an early loss of the haustral pattern.

Late diagnosis

The barium enema is valuable as it gives information concerning the degree and extent of the disease in the colon and also the presence of complications. The bowel preparation in these patients must be modified. Purgatives and suppositories should not be given to patients with a known diagnosis of ulcerative colitis. The bowel can be adequately prepared by increasing the fluid intake of the patient for at least two days prior to examination.

Advanced ulcerative colitis affecting the entire colon has a characteristic appearance, the so-called 'lead pipe colon' (Fig. 8.12). Haustral pattern is entirely absent and the margin of the colon relatively smooth as the mucosa is denuded as a result of ulceration. A striking feature is the marked narrowing and shortening of the entire large intestine.

Complications

1. Pseudopolyposis (Fig. 8.9)

The swellings of the mucosa between ulcers may be sufficient to cause confusion with familial polyposis coli, particularly as both conditions may present with diarrhoea. Rectal biopsy of a polyp rapidly differentiates the two conditions.

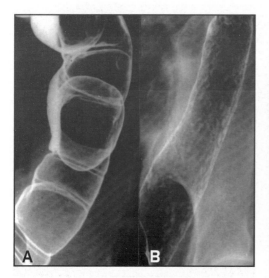

Fig. 8.11 Early mucosal changes of ulcerative colitis. Double-contrast enema shows the normal appearance of descending colon (A) compared with early ulcerative colitis (B). Note the lack of haustra and the irregularity of mucosa.

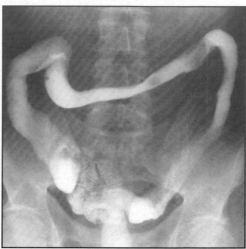

Fig. 8.12 End stage ulcerative colitis ('lead pipe appearance'). The large bowel is narrowed, shortened and lacks haustra.

2. Carcinoma

Because of the changes in the bowel wall with advanced ulcerative colitis, the classical changes of carcinoma, readily diagnosed in a normal colon, may not be present (Fig. 8.13). The carcinoma may have the appearance of a stricture with a gradual transition from the narrow neoplastic segment to the wider lumen. Ulcerative colitis patients have an increased risk of CRC, which occurs at an earlier age than in the general population. The risk is said to increase ten years after developing colitis and the risk increases at 10% for each ten years beyond.

3. Stricture

Because of the superficial nature of the mucosal ulceration focal strictures are uncommon, compared with Crohn's colitis. Because of the bizarre appearance of carcinoma in this condition any established stricture must be considered to be a carcinoma until proven otherwise by colonoscopy or operation.

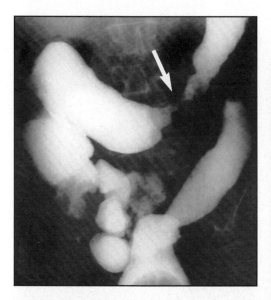

Fig. 8.13 Carcinoma complicating ulcerative colitis. In the transverse colon note the neoplastic narrowing (arrow) which is more tapered than the usual annular constricting tumour (compare Fig. 8.1). The entire colon is shortened and lacks haustration. The ileum is dilated.

Crohn's disease

Roughly 25% of patients with this disease of the bowel will have only small intestine involvement (see section 7.4), another 25% will have the disease limited to the colon and 45% will have both large and small gut affected. The remaining 5% have the disease in odd sites even as high as the upper gastro-intestinal tract. Perianal and perirectal inflammation has been reported in 36% of patients with this disease.

The features on barium enema may suggest the diagnosis (Fig. 8.14).

1. Segmental distribution

The rectum is not necessarily involved and there may be more than one segment affected with normal-appearing bowel between (skip lesions).

2. Strictures

Because the disease penetrates the coats of the bowel the lumen becomes reduced to a greater degree than seen in ulcerative colitis.

3. Mucosal changes

The deep penetrating ulcers give a spiculated ('rose thorn') appearance to the margins of the colon. The mucosal surface, seen best in the

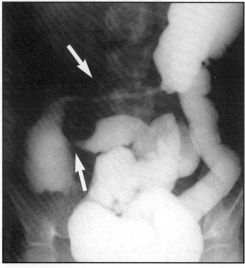

Fig. 8.14 Crohn's colitis. Extreme narrowing and shortening of the proximal transverse colon and terminal ileum (arrows) with relative sparing of the caecum ('skip lesions').

double-contrast enema, has a 'cobblestone' appearance due to the fissure-like ulcers in the swollen mucosa.

4. Small bowel involvement

The barium enema technique frequently outlines the terminal ileum. In Crohn's disease this may be narrowed (Fig. 7.8) whilst in ulcerative colitis the terminal ileum tends to dilate as the colon becomes increasingly abnormal (Fig. 8.13). CT is a useful adjunct in demonstrating the pathology of Crohn's disease.

5. Fistulae

As opposed to ulcerative colitis the penetrating nature of Crohn's disease may occasionally result in fistula formation with other organs, such as bladder, or even the skin. Anorectal fistulae are best shown by MRI, which displays well the fistulous track and relation to the pelvic floor.

Ischaemic colitis

Bowel ischaemia may produce widespread and fatal infarction or less severe segmental effects, which in the large bowel may be confused with other forms of colitis and in the small bowel may produce manifestations of malabsorption or symptoms consistent with intestinal angina.

In the large bowel, ischaemic colitis (Fig. 8.15) usually presents with the acute onset of abdominal colic and bloody diarrhoea.

Early changes on barium enema:

- An abnormal segment of colon is demonstrated, usually in the distal transverse colon or splenic flexure region, i.e. the watershed between superior and inferior mesenteric arteries.

- Mucosal swelling. Oedema and haemorrhage in the affected segment results in large mucosal swellings which bulge into the lumen (so called 'thumb printing'), markedly reducing the lumen.

- More severely affected patients may develop paralytic ileus at the onset of the condition with considerable gaseous distension of the bowel. Plain films in these cases may suggest the diagnosis by demonstrating increased

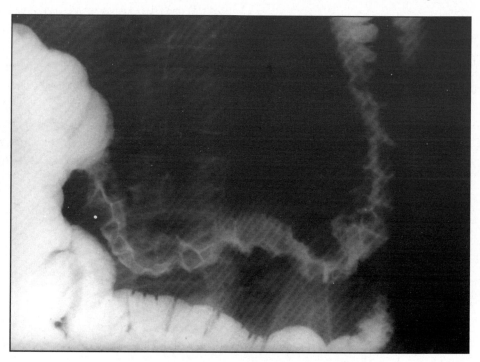

Fig. 8.15 Ischaemic colitis of the transverse colon. Mucosal swellings ('thumb printing') narrow the lumen.

bowel wall thickness. With the usual form of paralytic ileus, the intraluminal gas shadows lie close together, but with bowel wall thickening the lumina of adjacent loops appear somewhat separated.

- Air within the bowel wall. In more severe cases gas may track into the necrotic layers and be visible on plain films.

Late changes

In patients who survive, the ischaemic segment develops fibrous strictures with some areas of thinning so that within the generally stenosed length of bowel there may be several localized dilatations which have a rather characteristic appearance.

Conditions contributing to bowel ischaemia can be listed as follows:

1. Vascular disease
- Atherosclerosis.
- Thrombosis:
  - a. arterial.
  - b. venous.
- Embolus.
2. Poor perfusion
- Cardiac failure, e.g. irregular rhythms, left ventricular failure.
- Shunting:
  - a. shock.
  - b. mesenteric arteriovenous fistula, e.g. stab wound.

To produce organic changes within the bowel wall a number of these causes may be significant in any one patient. Ischaemia may also play a part in other forms of enterocolitis, e.g. pseudomembranous enterocolitis.

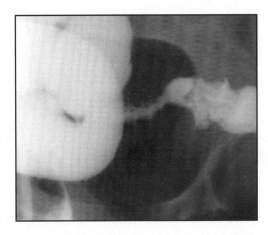

Fig. 8.16 Radiation colitis. A short segment of sigmoid colon is narrow but the transition to normal bowel is tapered without 'shouldering'. Radiotherapy was used to treat invasive uterine cancer.

Radiation colitis

Radiation therapy may be complicated by bowel wall changes due to obliterative arteritis. Most commonly seen in the sigmoid loop of women treated for pelvic malignant neoplasms.

It is important to emphasize again that the features described on barium enema for ulcerative colitis, Crohn's disease, ischaemic colitis and radiation colitis (Fig. 8.16) may prove helpful in suggesting the nature of the patient's problem. However, it should be remembered that other causes may produce similar appearances and in difficult cases evidence for these other causes, e.g. amoebiasis, should be sought clinically and by laboratory investigation.

Reference

See Chapter 6.

Biliary System

Although occasionally a distended gall bladder is palpable, in the majority of patients clinicians depend on diagnostic imaging to assess the status of the gall bladder and bile ducts. Patients with pathology in the biliary system may present clinically in various ways which can be listed.

- Dyspepsia and epigastric pain due to gallstones and chronic cholecystitis.
- Acute abdomen due to acute obstructive cholecystitis.
- Obstructive jaundice.
- Small bowel obstruction due to gallstone ileus.
- Postcholecystectomy syndrome.

9.1 Imaging Methods

Prior to considering the appropriate and cost-effective means of investigating such patients, the various techniques now available for imaging the biliary system should be known. In 1923 Graham and Cole, whilst conducting animal experiments on liver function by feeding iodine-containing compounds, found, by accident, that the gall bladder became opaque to x-rays. For decades oral cholecystography, known as Graham's test, served as the mainstay of biliary diagnosis. Today a range of imaging techniques is available.

Non-invasive methods

1. Plain radiography

Only about 15% of gallstones are opaque on plain x-ray films (Fig. 9.1) and about 80% on CT (Fig. 9.2). These methods are not considered cost-effective in most cases and the following techniques are preferred.

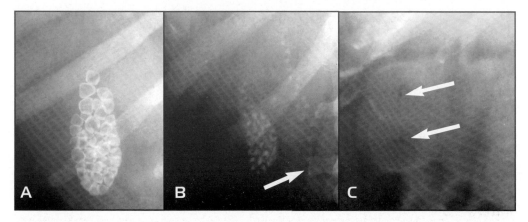

Fig. 9.1 Opaque gallstones. (A) Stones with calcified rims. (B) Opaque stones with lucent rims in gall bladder and CBD (arrow). (C) Two large stones with faintly calcified rims and tri-radiate gas shadows centrally (arrows).

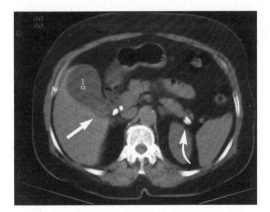

Fig. 9.2 CT showing a gallstone (arrow) in the neck of the gall bladder (1). The stone has a lucent centre and a moderately opaque rim. The calcification anterior to the left kidney (curved arrow) may be in the splenic artery; the opacity medial to the gallstone is of uncertain nature.

2. Ultrasound (US)

US is the preferred and usual way of demonstrating the gall bladder and bile ducts. The patient is fasted for 12 hours to relax the gall bladder, but no drugs or special preparation are required. US has the great advantage of allowing demonstration of other relevant organs in the upper abdomen. The distended gall bladder appears like other cystic structures in the body on US, with few if any echoes within the lumen, a slightly echogenic thin wall and increased transmission of sound to the tissues deep to the gall bladder shown as 'posterior enhancement'

(Fig. 9.3A). US also provides information concerning the common bile duct (CBD) (Fig. 9.3B). Normally the CBD should not exceed 4 or 5 mm in width although it can be slightly wider in patients following cholecystectomy. Adjacent structures are well seen, particularly the portal vein, lying posterior to the CBD and the head of the pancreas distally. By convention, longitudinal US images are viewed with the head of the patient to the left and the feet to the right, whilst transverse images are viewed as though looking from the feet upwards.

3. Oral cholecystography

Since Graham's discovery, special oral iodine containing contrast media, i.e. iopanoic acid, have been developed to outline the gall bladder. This medium is absorbed from the small bowel and behaves like bilirubin in the blood stream by associating with serum albumin. On reaching the liver, it is dissociated and passes into the bile, but it requires concentration in the gall bladder to become sufficiently opaque to be detected on radiographs (Fig. 9.4). On passing to the bowel again the medium is largely reabsorbed, so it is possible to reinforce the concentration of contrast medium in the gall bladder by repeated doses of the medium. On the evening before examination, the patient swallows several enteric-coated tablets

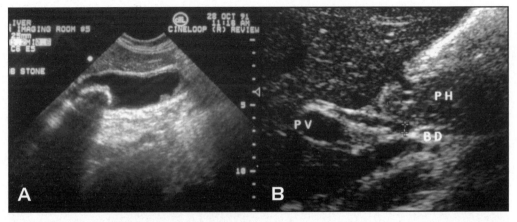

Fig. 9.3 (A) US showing a large gallstone in the gall bladder neck. Note the arc-shaped band of echoes from the front of the stone and the echo free band (acoustic shadowing) deep to the stone. (B) US of the common bile duct (BD). The duct lies anterior to the portal vein (PV). Pancreatic head (PH).

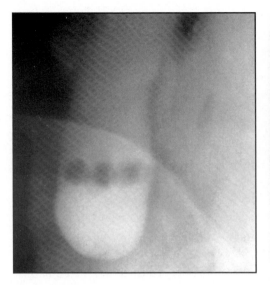

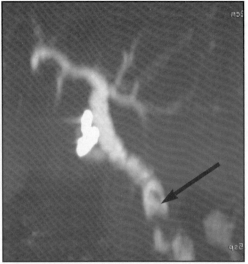

Fig. 9.4 Oral cholecystogram. The film made with the patient erect shows a group of non-opaque stones forming a level.

Fig. 9.5 Intravenous cholangiography. Helical CT shows a calculus in the distal end of the slightly dilated CBD (arrow). The gall bladder has been removed.

of the medium and fasts until the examination next morning, except for drinking water. The normal gall bladder will appear opaque on radiographs and gallstones are seen as lucent filling defects within the opacity. The ability of the gall bladder to contract after a fatty meal, i.e. chocolate, can be gauged. The CBD is not adequately demonstrated with this method.

4. Intravenous cholangiography

To demonstrate the bile ducts as well as the gall bladder with x-rays, a special intravenous contrast medium, i.e. iotroxate, was developed. Like the oral medium, it couples with serum albumin and passes through the liver into the bile. Unlike the oral medium, it is opaque without the need for concentration by the gall bladder, and the CBD is rendered opaque on the radiographs. Unlike the oral medium, once this material reaches the small bowel, it is not reabsorbed. With impaired liver function, this intravenous contrast medium passes out through the kidney and the biliary system is not outlined. Recently, intravenous cholangiography has been combined with helical CT to provide better detail of the CBD (Fig. 9.5).

5. Radionuclide cholangiography

After intravenous injection, technetium-labelled HIDA, or similar fat-soluble high molecular weight compound, is excreted through the liver into the bile, and its passage can be monitored with the gamma camera (Fig. 9.6). Failure of the biliary duct system to fill indicates impaired liver function. Presence of radionuclide in the CBD but not in the gall bladder is consistent with an obstructed cystic duct. Detail with this test is insufficient to demonstrate gallstones.

6. Magnetic Resonance Imaging (MRI)

Using special pulse sequence techniques MRI has the capability of multiplanar demonstration of the biliary tree without using contrast medium and will become more widely used in future. Currently, using a single breathhold technique, MRI is being promoted as a means of selecting cases for ERCP (see below and Fig. 9.7). MRI has the advantage over intravenous cholangiography of being equally effective in jaundiced and non-jaundiced patients. MRI can also show the pancreatic duct.

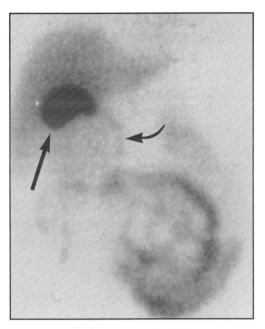

Fig. 9.6 Radionuclide cholangiogram. The liver, gall bladder (arrow), common bile duct (curved arrow) and small bowel are outlined following intravenous injection of technetium-labelled HIDA, a fat-soluble high molecular weight compound.

More invasive methods

1. Endoscopic retrograde cholangiopancreatography (ERCP)

After introducing an endoscope under heavy sedation through the oesophagus and stomach to the duodenum a fine catheter is passed through the ampulla of Vater into the common bile duct or pancreatic duct and contrast medium injected. The region of the ampulla is inspected and the method is particularly valuable for obstructions at the lower end of the common bile duct. If a gall-stone is obstructing, a therapeutic sphincterotomy may be performed for relief, and in some cases strictures may be balloon dilated (Fig. 9.8).

2. Percutaneous transhepatic cholangiography (PTC)

Using local anaesthesia and fluoroscopy or ultrasound, the radiologist passes a fine needle percutaneously from the lower lateral chest wall into the liver and aspirates bile from a dilated duct. A fine catheter is then inserted into the dilated biliary system and this allows contrast injections for more detailed diagnosis (Fig. 9.14A).

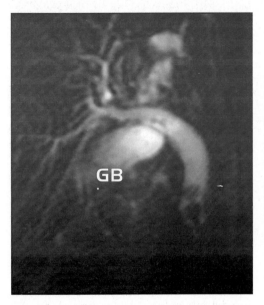

Fig. 9.7 MRI cholangiogram. The gall bladder (GB) and ducts are clearly shown with two calculi in the CBD.

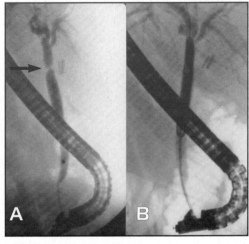

Fig. 9.8 Endoscopic retrograde cholangiopancreatography (ERCP). (A) The outlined CBD shows a postoperative stricture (arrow) with an adjacent surgical clip. (B) Transluminal balloon dilatation via the endoscope has successfully dilated the CBD narrowing.

9.2 Clinical Indications

1. Dyspepsia and epigastric pain

This common symptom complex may result from pathology in the gall bladder, stomach and duodenum or pancreas. If, after a period of empirical treatment, it is decided to investigate such a patient, upper abdominal ultrasound is recommended initially, but because US does not demonstrate the stomach or duodenum, a barium meal is also recommended (see section 6.4). Because US provides limited information concerning the pancreas, CT may be indicated (see section 10.12), particularly in those patients in whom US and the barium meal are normal. On US gallstones in a distended gall bladder are clearly demonstrated as mobile echogenic foci. Often gallstones completely reflect the sound waves producing an echo-free **acoustic shadow** (Fig. 9.3) deep to the stone. Such findings are virtually diagnostic of gallstones, but occasionally difficulty arises. In some patients with chronic cholecystitis, the gall bladder is markedly contracted around the gallstones, making identification of the gall bladder difficult. Also, a single small gallstone may impact in the neck of the gall bladder causing difficulties in diagnosis. In these cases, oral cholecystography may assist in clarifying the situation.

When the gall bladder opacifies during oral cholecystography, gallstones are usually easily identified as radiolucent filling defects. In an erect film, the gallstones tend to form a level in the bile (Fig. 9.4), which makes identification of even very small stones easier. If the cystic duct is obstructed the gall bladder will not opacify. However, this may also result from impairment of liver function, and, of course, if the patient failed to take the tablets on the previous evening! Carcinoma of the gall bladder is usually associated with gallstones and may be suspected if immobile filling defects encroach on the gall bladder lumen. If carcinoma is suspected, CT is performed.

2. Acute obstructive cholecystitis

Typically these patients are acutely tender over the gall bladder, with pain and fever, and virtually always have gallstones in the gall bladder with obstruction of the cystic duct. US is the investigation of choice to confirm the provisional clinical diagnosis. Gallstones can be demonstrated and local tenderness directly over the gall bladder confirmed. The acutely inflamed gall bladder wall may appear considerably thickened on US and complications such as pericholecystic abscess may be detected also (Fig. 9.9). Occasionally in such acutely ill patients, US reveals a dilated gall bladder with no obvious stones, yet consistent with a gallstone obstructing the cystic duct. In those cases HIDA radionuclide cholangiography is indicated (Fig. 9.10). Absence of gamma radiation from the gall bladder confirms the cystic duct obstruction.

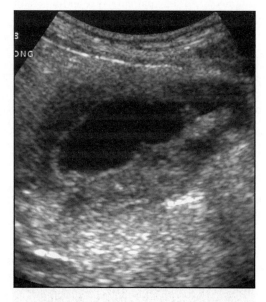

Fig. 9.9 Acute obstructive cholecystitis. The gall bladder is distended with a thick, echolucent wall (c.f. Fig. 9.3) consistent with inflammatory oedema. The calculus obstructing the cystic duct is not shown.

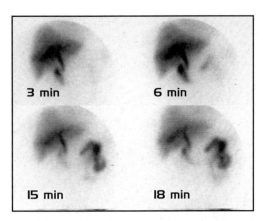

Fig. 9.10 HIDA radionuclide scan. Known gallstones with suspected acute cholecystitis. Interval scans show no filling of the gall bladder due to a blocked cystic duct, consistent with the diagnosis.

3. Jaundice

Whether jaundice is due to haemolytic or hepatotoxic causes, or biliary obstruction, can usually be made on clinical grounds and liver function tests. US is the primary imaging investigation and does not disturb the patient. **Because it is most important that biliary obstruction should not be missed, US should be employed in all patients presenting with jaundice.** The causes of obstructive jaundice most commonly encountered can be classified as follows:

In the lumen
- Gallstones.
- Hydatid cyst elements.
- Worms in some countries.

In the wall
- Cholangiocarcinoma.
- Strictures, including postoperative.

Outside the wall
- Carcinoma of head of pancreas.
- Metastases at porta hepatis.

In the duodenum
- Carcinoma of the ampulla of Vater.

In obstruction US demonstrates the dilated bile ducts and allows assessment of the level of obstruction and in many cases, the cause (Fig. 9.11). The normal CBD should not measure more than 5 mm in width. Gallstones can be detected in the gall bladder, but in the CBD, small stones less than 1 cm in width may not be demonstrated. If the obstruction is low down in the CBD, then the gall bladder, if present, will be dilated, whereas an obstructive lesion in the porta hepatis results in non-distension of the gall bladder. Masses in the pancreatic head, porta hepatis, or liver may be demonstrated. CT, in some cases, may be used to supplement the US findings (Fig. 9.12).

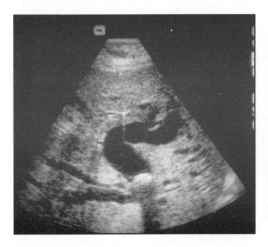

Fig. 9.11 Obstructive jaundice. US shows the 1.5 cm stone in the dilated CBD.

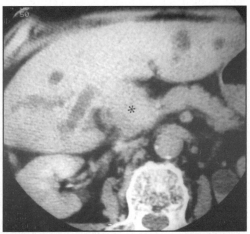

Fig. 9.12 Adenocarcinoma of the pancreatic head. CT clearly shows the neoplastic expansion of the pancreatic head (*). Note dilatation of intrahepatic bile ducts. Also see Fig. 10.24.

If the CBD is obstructed but the cause remains uncertain, further information may be obtained by ERCP (Figs 9.8 & 9.13). Sphincterotomy allows a stone to pass into the duodenum. If the obstruction is high up in the biliary tree, percutaneous transhepatic cholangiography (PTC) provides percutaneous drainage of bile and alleviation of the jaundice. Furthermore, it may be possible to biopsy an obstructing lesion by way of the drainage catheter, and for palliation a stent may be passed through the obstruction into the duodenum (Fig. 9.14). Rendering the patient free from jaundice, particularly when an inoperable tumour is present, may relieve considerable discomfort. In future, MRI will almost certainly be the next diagnostic test when US shows duct dilatation as it is non-invasive and requires no contrast medium (Fig. 9.8).

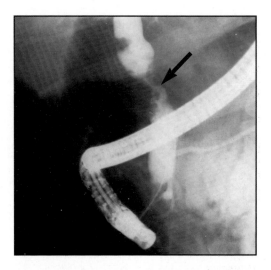

Fig. 9.13 Obstructive jaundice. Cholangiocarcinoma (arrow) shown by ERCP. The appearance of the lower end of CBD is due to sphincterotomy, not stone.

4. Gallstone ileus

Occasionally, as a result of acute obstructive cholecystitis, a fistula develops between the gall bladder and small bowel or duodenum allowing passage of gallstones into the gut. In some cases, a large gallstone may obstruct the distal small bowel, and if the stone is calcified it may be detected on a plain radiograph with associated changes of small bowel obstruction (see section 12.4). With such a fistula, plain films may show gas in the gall bladder and biliary ducts (Fig. 9.15).

5. Postcholecystectomy syndrome

Persisting symptoms, usually pain, following cholecystectomy may have various causes. First, because gallstones are very common, there may have been coexisting pathology elsewhere which was not relieved by the cholecystectomy. In particular, epigastric pain and dyspepsia may have its origins in lesions of the stomach, duodenum and pancreas. Also, a stone in the CBD may have been overlooked. Nowadays, laparoscopic

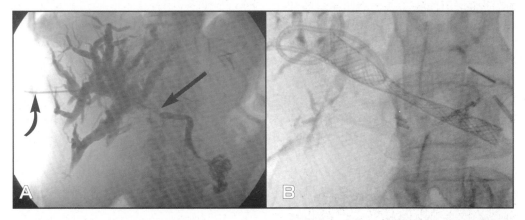

Fig. 9.14 Obstructive jaundice. Metastases at porta hepatis. (A) Percutaneous transhepatic cholangiography (PTC). The obstruction (arrow) and dilated ducts are outlined after needling (curved arrow). (B) Shows a stent, introduced percutaneously, passed through the lesion. Jaundice was relieved.

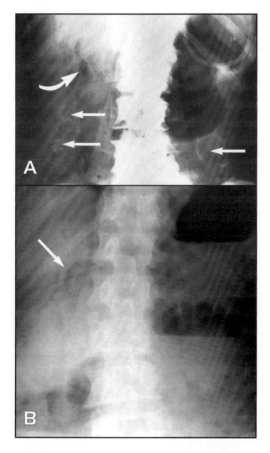

cholecystectomy is popular and this procedure does not allow for palpation of the CBD. Post-operative strictures may occur in the biliary duct system causing persisting pain, which is usually associated with jaundice. If too large a cystic duct remnant is left, it is thought that this may act as a focus of cholecystitis and continuing pain. Finally, the complex matter of biliary dyskinesia has been invoked as a possible cause of continuing pain. This refers to abnormal peristalsis and spasm involving the lower end of the CBD, a condition which may be alleviated with drugs. Ultrasound should be the first imaging investigation of these patients with postcholecystectomy symptoms, but ERCP, barium meal and upper abdominal CT may be indicated in particular cases.

Fig. 9.15 Gallstone ileus. (A) Several large gallstones with calcified rims (arrows) in the mid-abdomen. Gas in the gall bladder or CBD (curved arrow). (B) Erect film shows dilated stomach and an ileal loop, both with fluid levels. Suggestion of gas in the biliary system (arrow).

9.3 Imaging and Biliary Surgery

Surgeons require to know whether gall bladder stones are associated with stones in the CBD. If not, simple cholecystectomy is performed and the more extensive operation of duct exploration is avoided. With the availability of laparoscopic cholecystectomy, some surgeons arrange pre-operative intravenous cholangiography or, in some cases, ERCP to detect stones in the CBD, which may require open operation. Radiology may be used during and after operation to assist management.

Operative cholangiography

During operation, the surgeon injects contrast medium either directly into the CBD or by way of the cystic duct and a radiograph is obtained to demonstrate stones which may be present.

T-tube cholangiography

If the common bile duct is explored, and stones removed, it is usual to perform a radiograph about one week after injecting the percutaneously draining T-tube with contrast medium to check that no persisting calculus is present (Fig. 9.16).

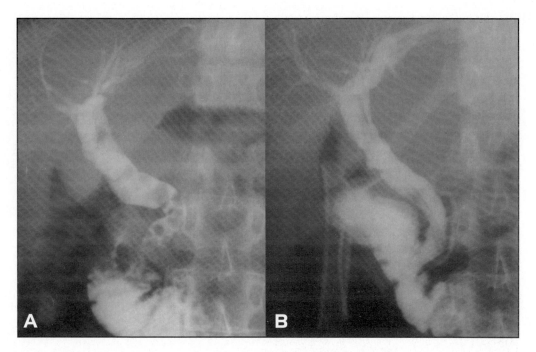

Fig. 9.16 (A) Operative cholangiogram performed by injecting the common duct. Previous cholecystectomy. Numerous calculi. (B) Post-operative T-tube cholangiogram showing no residual stones.

Reference

See Chapter 6.

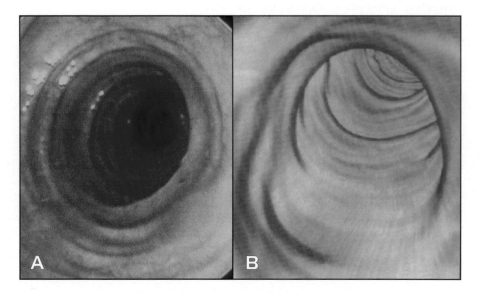

Plate 1.1 Virtual Colonoscopy
(A) Photograph taken during colonoscopy. (B) Photograph reconstructed at the same level from data obtained from helical CT after distending the bowel with air and administering an antispasmodic. Appearances are similar except that in (A) the colour of the mucosa is seen. The 3D reconstruction allows the entire colon to be viewed as through a colonoscope. Similar technology provides virtual bronchoscopy. (By courtesy of Dr. Joseph T. Ferrucci, Boston Medical Center.)

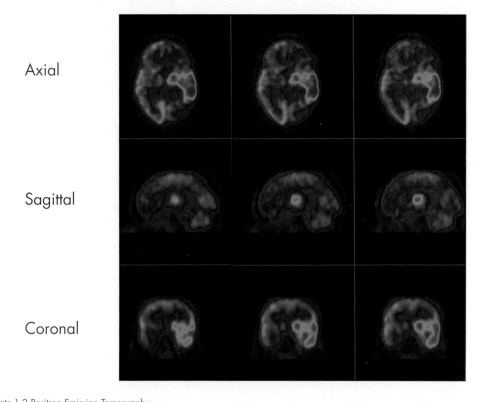

Plate 1.2 Positron Emission Tomography.
A left temporal glioma was resected 2 years previously followed by radiotherapy. Recent CT and MRI showed a persisting lesion but could not differentiate recurrent tumour from radiation damage. Following intravenous injection of glucose-labelled Flourine 18, a short-life radionuclide, the thin PET axial, sagittal and coronal sections display the metabolic activity as low (blue/green) or high (yellow/red). High metabolic activity in the lesion confirmed recurrent tumour.

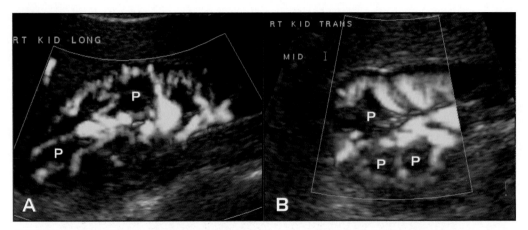

Plate 1.3 Power Doppler of normal kidney.
Based on the energy of moving blood, irrespective of velocity or direction, Power Doppler displays the renal vascularity in (A) longitudinal and (B) transverse sections. The relatively avascular pyramids (P) contrast with the vascular cortex.

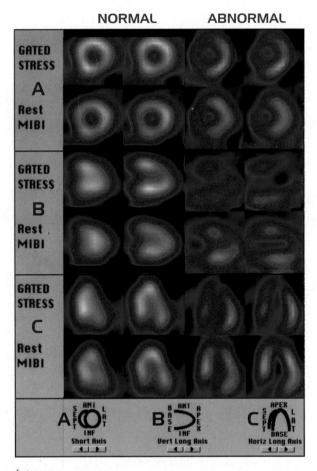

Plate 3.15 Myocardial perfusion scan.
Following intravenous injections of technetium-labelled sestambi SPECT (single photon emission computed tomography) sectional scans are obtained along the three cardiac axes during stress and then at rest. Perfusion ranges from poor (blue/green) to good (red/yellow). Shown, compared with a normal case, is an example of very poor perfusion of the septal and anterior left ventricular myocardium made worse by stress.

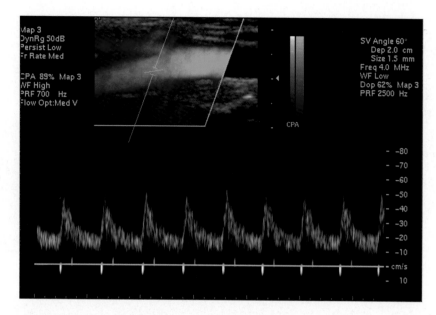

Plate 4.8 Carotid Bifurcation Duplex Doppler Ultrasound. Normal.
Colour flow Doppler (above) shows the internal carotid artery to have smooth margins and a homogeneous colour display consistent with laminar flow. The velocity graph (below) shows a clear window beneath the curve indicating no turbulence (compare Fig. 4.9C next page).

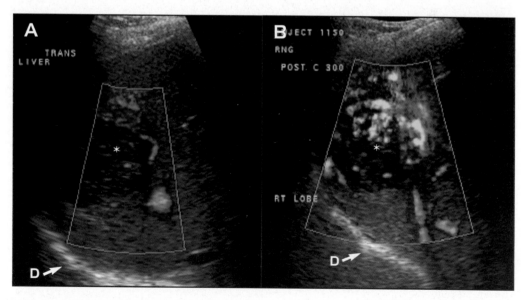

Plate 10.6 Hepatocellular carcinoma. Use of US contrast medium.
(A) longitudinal US section shows a rounded echolucent focus in the right lobe.(*). Power Doppler US suggests some vascularity in the lesion. (B) Power Doppler US after intravenous injection of US contrast agent (tiny gas-containing capsules) confirms the vascular nature of the neoplasm convincingly. (D) Diaphragm.

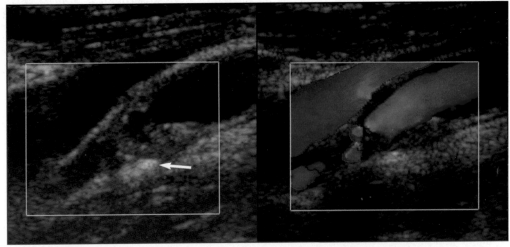

A - Greyscale   **B - Colour Flow Doppler (CFD)**

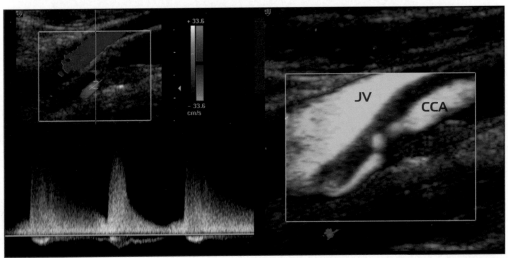

C - Duplex Doppler   **D - Power Doppler**

Plate 4.9 Carotid Bifurcation Ultrasound. Atherosclerotic stenosis.
Four techniques of displaying the severe stenosis are shown. (A) Greyscale US shows plaque narrowing the lumen of the internal carotid near the origin. The tiny calcified focus (arrow) is echogenic with an acoustic shadow. (B) Colour flow Doppler shows a range of colour at the stenosis consistent with turbulent flow. (C) Duplex Doppler shows the site of sampling (above) and the trace (below) showing spectral widening of the peak and filling-in of the window due to turbulence. (D) Power Doppler in which the colour display shows moving blood irrespective of velocity and direction. (CCA) Common Carotid Artery. (JV) Jugular Vein.

Liver, Pancreas and Spleen

The Liver

The liver is the largest abdominal organ. Despite this, it is difficult to examine clinically because of the overlying rib cage. Although the lower liver margin is often palpable, even assessing liver size is difficult because the upper extent is uncertain. Various imaging methods are available to display the state of the liver and it is important, at least for cost considerations, that the modality most appropriate to the clinical situation is selected.

10.1 Methods of Liver Imaging

Plain radiography of the liver may show calcifications most often due to colorectal carcinomatous metastases and occasionally hydatid cysts. However, plain radiography is most often non-contributory and not cost effective.

US generally is the most appropriate initial means of demonstrating the liver. The normal adult parenchyma has a uniform pattern, being equally echogenic with the spleen and more so than the kidney parenchyma. The diaphragm is easily recognized and the vascular and biliary branching within the liver clearly displayed as echo-free tubular structures. Doppler US techniques (see page

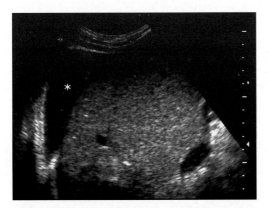

Fig. 10.1 US showing ascitic fluid (*) between normally echogenic liver and chest wall.

8) demonstrates fluid motion and clearly separates the blood vessels from the bile ducts. Ascites, particularly around the liver is well seen (Fig. 10.1).

CT provides fine detail of the liver parenchyma, which appears homogeneous. The blood vessels and bile ducts are seen as lower densities. Dynamic CT using a bolus of contrast medium clearly outlines systemic and portal vessels and differentiates them from the bile ducts. CT does not provide detailed information of the biliary tree because it is limited to transverse axial images.

Radionuclide scanning of the liver is occasionally indicated. The Kupffer cells lining the sinusoids, part of the reticulo-endothelial system, make up 25% of the cellular content of the liver and are scattered uniformly throughout. After an intravenous injection of technetium-labelled colloid particles the Kupffer cells, which take up the material, emit radiation, producing a uniform image on the gamma camera. Also, by using a blood pool radionuclide agent the vascularity of the liver and lesions within it can be demonstrated.

Magnetic resonance imaging (MRI) has had limited application in the abdomen because of problems with breathing and the longer exposure time required. Currently these problems are being overcome and the method shows considerable promise in particular clinical situations.

Hepatic angiography requires selective catheterization of the coeliac axis by way of percutaneous femoral artery puncture. The technique provides a detailed demonstration of the hepatic circulation and a dense 'hepatogram' during the capillary phase. The method allows for interventional therapeutic techniques such as tumour embolisation and cancerocidal drug infusion.

10.2 Clinical Indications for Liver Imaging

Liver imaging may be indicated in patients with:

- Diffuse Parenchymal disease.
- Focal liver lesions.
- Portal hypertension.
- Ascites.
- Jaundice (see section 9.2).
- Blunt abdominal trauma (see section 12.5).
- Liver transplantation.

10.3 Diffuse Parenchymal Liver Disease

In most cases of acute or chronic hepatitis, there is no clinical indication to image the liver. Histological diagnosis is obtained by liver biopsy. Cirrhosis, the end result of diffuse parenchymal disease resulting in fibrosis and scarring of the liver surface, can be shown by US or CT (Fig. 10.12A). The availability of US and CT has highlighted the frequency with which fatty infiltration of the liver occurs. It implies fatty accumulation in the hepatocytes and is seen in numerous conditions, particularly diabetes and alcohol abuse. On US the fatty areas appear echogenic whilst on CT fatty areas appear of lower density than normal parenchyma (Fig. 10.2). The condition, which may be patchy throughout the liver, for reasons unknown, has been shown to be reversible in alcoholics. Areas of fatty infiltration can be mistaken for focal masses on CT and US, but MRI, using fat suppression techniques, can differentiate these fatty areas. The dense liver in haemochromatosis, due to iron deposition, can be demonstrated with CT and is also clearly shown by MRI.

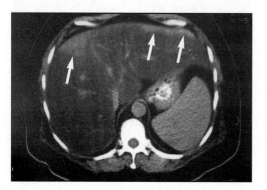

Fig. 10.2 Diffuse fatty infiltration of the liver. Most of the liver is considerably less dense than the spleen and the hepatic blood vessels and ducts can be seen as relatively dense in this non-contrast study. Peripheral areas of normal liver echogenicity remain (arrows).

10.4 Focal Liver Masses

Most masses encountered are included in the following list:

Neoplasms

   Benign:

- Cavernous haemangioma.
- Focal nodular hyperplasia (FNH).
- Liver cell adenoma.

   Malignant:

- Metastases.
- Hepatocellular carcinoma (HCC).
- Cholangiocarcinoma.

Cysts

- Simple unilocular.
- Polycystic liver disease.
- Hydatid (Fig. 10.3).

Abscesses

- Pyogenic.
- Amoebic.

US is very sensitive in detecting focal liver masses and is the recommended method (Fig. 10.4), except when monitoring cancer patients for liver metastases when CT or MRI provides serial images which are more easily compared (Fig. 10.5). The recent development of **Power Doppler US,** which displays moving blood (see section 1.2), allows assessment of the vascularity of suspected focal lesions (Plate 10.6 in colour plates section).

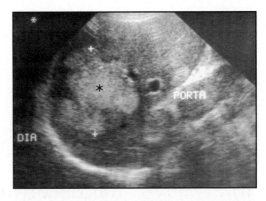

Fig. 10.4 Hepatocellular carcinoma. The large echogenic tumour (*) is seen centrally within the right lobe of the liver on US. The curved echogenic band is due to the diaphragm (DIA).

The introduction of US and CT has drawn attention to several benign hepatic neoplasms which may be confused with more serious abnormalities. **Cavernous haemangioma** is quite common, occurring in about 7% of autopsies. The lesion is usually less than 5 cm across and hyperechoic on US (Fig. 10.7). With CT the tumour appears less dense than surrounding liver and the diagnosis is confirmed by delayed dynamic CT when the contrast-filled vascular spaces render the lesion isodense with the surrounding parenchyma (Fig. 10.8). The same can be demonstrated using radionuclide scanning (Fig. 10.9).

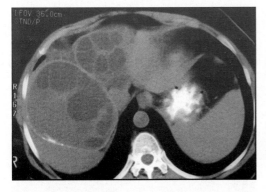

Fig. 10.3 Hydatid cysts. CT clearly shows two large cysts within the liver, one with calcification within the wall and both containing numerous daughter cysts.

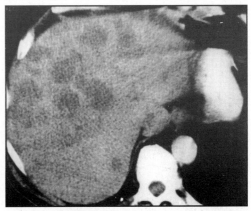

Fig. 10.5 Multiple liver metastases from colon cancer. The rounded metastases are relatively lucent compared with the parenchyma on CT following intravenous contrast enhancement.

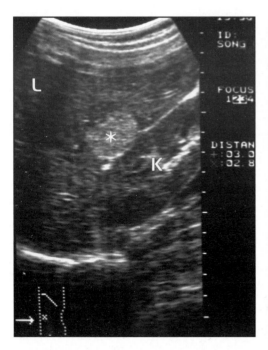

Fig. 10.7 (above) Cavernous haemangioma. The typical, but non-specific echogenic lesion (*) in the right lobe of liver (L) overlies the kidney (K) in this sagittal section.

Fig. 10.8 (right) Cavernous haemangioma confirmed by contrast-enhanced CT. (A) Soon after IV contrast injection the lucent lesion (*) is unchanged. (B) 30 seconds later filling in by peripheral blood vessels begins. (C) 10 minutes later the lesion is no longer visible confirming the diagnosis.

Fig. 10.9 (below) Cavernous haemangioma confirmed with radionuclide. The series of scans shows progressive accumulation of the isotope completely filling in the initial defect (arrow). The lesion was first detected on US.

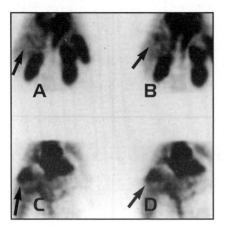

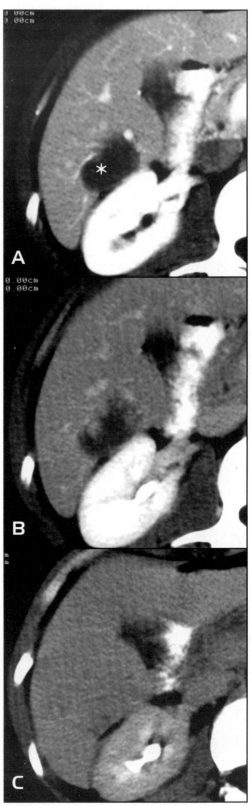

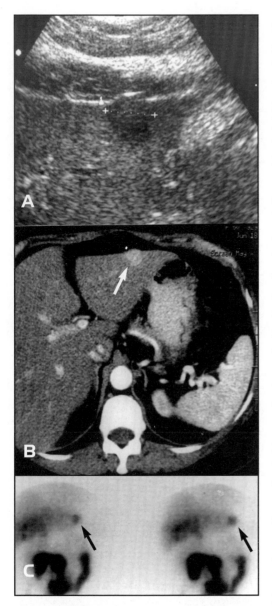

Fig. 10.10 Focal nodular hyperplasia (FNH) in a 30 year old female. (A) The rounded lesion is slightly hypoechoic on US. (B) Dynamic contrast CT shows the lesion to be vascular becoming opaque (arrow). (C) Radionuclide scan with technetium-labelled sulphur colloid shows uptake in the nodule consistent with it containing Kupffer cells and the diagnosis (arrow).

Focal nodular hyperplasia (FNH) is an unusual focal tumour, of unknown aetiology, that is asymptomatic and usually is discovered incidentally close to the free edge of the liver and usually in women younger than 40 years of age.

The well-circumscribed mass is composed of normal hepatic elements and the incidence has been related to the use of oral contraceptives. On US the texture is similar to that of liver parenchyma although often slightly hypoechoic. Because FNH contains Kupffer cells it takes up the radionuclide, like normal liver distinguishing FNH from the other benign tumours (Fig. 10.10).

Liver cell adenoma is relatively rare and consists of hepatocytes but no Kupffer cells or biliary elements and is well encapsulated. The appearance on US may be similar to FNH and these tumours have also been related to the use of oral contraceptives. The lesion is very vascular and spontaneous haemorrhage with rapid increase in size may occur, or, if near the surface, intraperitoneal bleeding may lead to an abdominal emergency. It is considered pre-malignant.

The liver is the commonest site for blood borne **metastases**, slightly more so than the lung. They are mostly multiple and have nonspecific appearances on US and CT, giving no hint of the primary site. Metastases are usually less dense on CT (Fig. 10.5) than the surrounding liver. Many enhance following intravenous contrast medium. Some are calcified, particularly colorectal metastases. On US the appearances are variable.

Hepatocellular carcinoma (HCC) usually occurs in cirrhotic livers. The US and CT appearances are nonspecific (Fig. 10.4) but the presence of cirrhosis and a heterogeneous single mass within the liver is strongly suggestive of HCC, particularly if evidence of portal venous invasion is demonstrated. Cholangiocarcinoma in the majority of cases involves the biliary system below the porta hepatis (Fig. 9.15) but may extend into the liver where it has a nonspecific appearance, although usually associated with bile duct dilatation.

10.5 Portal Hypertension

Portal hypertension, or increase in portal venous pressure above the norm of about 20 cm of water is due to obstruction to the portal venous system at various levels:

- Suprahepatic: Due to obstruction of hepatic veins (Budd–Chiari syndrome) by thrombosis, a congenital web, or adjacent tumours or abscesses. Constrictive pericarditis and tricuspid incompetence may also increase the pressure in hepatic veins.
- Intrahepatic: Due to cirrhosis in most cases.
- Infrahepatic: Due to thrombosis in the portal vein, or its branches, resulting from pancreatitis, or other infective or neoplastic processes. Infrahepatic obstruction, due to thrombosis, not infrequently complicates intrahepatic obstruction, due to cirrhosis.

Portal hypertension leads to the opening up of portal-systemic venous collateral pathways, particularly in the lower oesophagus, between the spleen and left kidney, and in the rectum. Patients with portal hypertension often present with gastrointestinal bleeding from oesophageal varices (see Chapter 6). Other clinical manifestations depend on the level and severity of portal obstruction. Some patients present with unexplained splenomegaly and others with hepatomegaly, depressed liver function or ascites.

Displaying the portal system

Various techniques are available now to demonstrate the status of the portal venous circulation, with minimal disturbance to the patient.

1. Ultrasound

US is the preferred method for assessing patients with suspected portal hypertension. The portal vein can be imaged in virtually all cases as it approaches the liver, but the splenic vein and tributaries may be obscured by bowel gas. US is based on the average velocity of sound in the soft tissues and the transmission through gas-filled bowel is quite different, severely degrading the image. The hepatic veins and the upper inferior vena cava are well seen, so that suprahepatic obstruction may be demonstrated (Fig. 10.11). Colour Doppler US clearly demonstrates flow in the veins and an early sign of portal hypertension is the opening up of the vein in the ligamentum teres, i.e. the peri-umbilical vein, with flow of blood towards the umbilicus (Fig. 10.12). Large portal-systemic collateral veins, particularly the coronary vein, joining the portal and oesophageal veins (Fig. 10.13) may be shown by US and the direction of flow by Doppler. Ascites is well seen and the biliary system also. The size of the liver can be assessed and the presence of cirrhosis suggested, although liver biopsy is required for a better assessment.

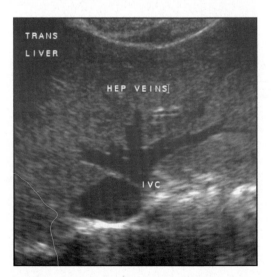

Fig. 10.11 Cardiac failure. US showing distended inferior vena cava (IVC) and the three major hepatic veins.

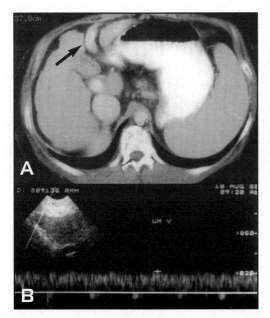

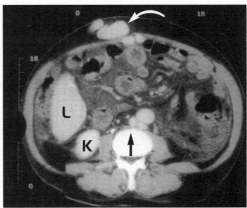

Fig. 10.14 Dynamic CT in portal hypertension. A rapid series of scans during a bolus injection of contrast shows numerous collateral vessels (arrow) in the retroperitoneum and a large venous connection at the umbilicus (caput medusa) (curved arrow). Ascites separates the bowel loops. L=Liver. K=upper pole of right kidney.

Fig. 10.12 Portal hypertension. (A) CT following contrast injection shows the small irregular cirrhotic liver and a large patent peri-umbilical vein (arrow). (B) Duplex Doppler US confirms patency of the peri-umbilical vein in another patient by showing a venous flow graph directed towards the probe and the umbilicus anteriorly.

2. Dynamic CT

If a series of body sections is made through the region of the portal vein whilst a bolus of contrast medium is injected good opacification is obtained within the portal system. The spleen can be assessed and the retroperitoneal tissues with portal-systemic collaterals also (Fig. 10.14).

3. Magnetic resonance imaging (MRI)

Using intravenous gadolinium contrast, MRI has evolved to a point where the abdominal arteries and veins can be demonstrated in a single breath-hold.

4. Angiography

The availability of less invasive methods has led to catheter angiography being reserved for special cases.

5. Transhepatic portal venography

After needling a portal vein radicle percutaneously through the liver a fine catheter is introduced and passed retrogradely down into the portal system. This technique provides excellent portal venograms and allows direct pressure measurements, but is reserved for special situations.

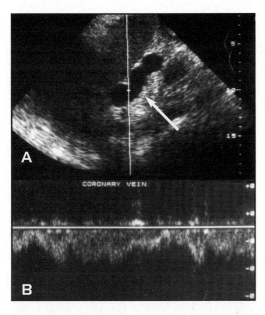

Fig. 10.13 Cirrhosis. Portal hypertension. Duplex Doppler US. (A) A large coronary vein (arrow) is shown clearly. (B) Doppler trace shows the flow to be away from the probe, i.e. below the baseline, consistent with a collateral circulation to the oesophageal venous plexus.

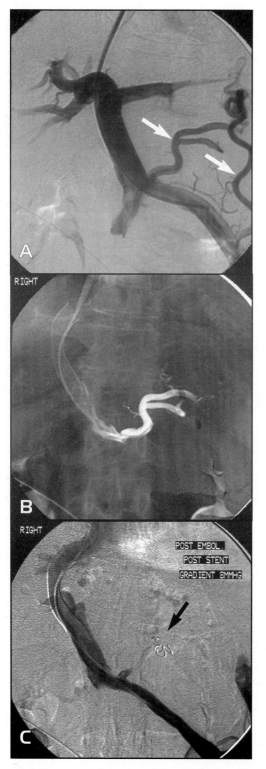

Interventional radiology

Radiological methods are used to assist in the management of severe portal hypertension. A catheter introduced at transhepatic portal venography can be directed into the collateral vein feeding the oesophagus and the oesophageal varices may be embolised. However, this approach is no longer popular as it does not reduce the hypertension. **Transjugular intrahepatic portosystemic shunting** (TIPS) is a percutaneous technique for directly reducing the portal venous pressure. A catheter is passed percutaneously into the jugular vein and directed through the heart into the hepatic veins and then by passing a long needle through the catheter a communication is made with a portal vein branch. The catheter is then advanced into the portal vein and the communication is maintained by introducing a metallic stent (Fig. 10.15).

Fig. 10.15 Transjugular intrahepatic portosystemic shunt (TIPS) in cirrhosis and portal hypertension. (A) Portal venogram through catheter introduced from the neck and by needle from the hepatic to the portal venous system. Collaterals to oesophagus (arrows). (B) Portosystemic stent in place but collaterals still patent (C). Final result after embolising collaterals with coils (arrow).

10.6 Ascites

Accumulation of fluid in the peritoneal cavity is usually due to one of the following:

1. Cirrhosis and liver failure.
2. Carcinomatous peritoneal metastases.
3. Transudates from heart or kidney failure.
4. TB peritonitis.
5. Leakage of bile or bleeding from intra-abdominal organs.

By the time a patient presents with abdominal distension due to ascites the cause will usually be apparent from the clinical history and examination. Because gas-filled loops of bowel move centrally in the presence of a large ascites, abdominal percussion clinically demonstrating flank dullness will usually differentiate ascites from a large abdominal tumour, i.e. an ovarian cyst. Cytology and bacteriology of the aspirated ascitic fluid will usually clarify the diagnosis. When the diagnosis is uncertain CT should be performed prior to aspiration. CT, like US (Fig. 10.1), does not differentiate the type of fluid but indicates the preferred site of aspiration and frequently provides evidence of the underlying cause, particularly if malignant neoplasm is present. In malignant ascites matting together of bowel loops and the omentum is seen on CT (Fig. 10.16) and the ovaries are well demonstrated, a common site of the primary in such cases. Non-neoplastic ascites tends to spare the

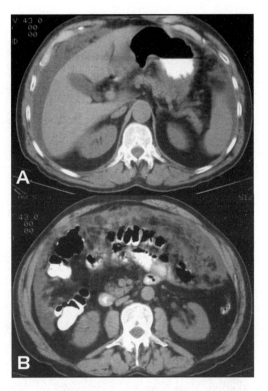

Fig. 10.16 Ovarian carcinoma. Malignant ascites. (A) CT shows ascitic fluid around the liver and spleen. (B) Typical matting of the omentum, bowel loops and the abdominal wall due to metastases.

lesser sac, which is usually involved if the cause is peritoneal seeding by tumour. Evidence of portal hypertension consistent with liver failure is also well shown. If more detailed information concerning the intrahepatic circulation is required then Doppler US may be indicated.

10.7 Jaundice   See page 152

10.8 Liver Trauma   See section 12.7

10.9 Liver Transplantation

In the immediate post-operative period problems may arise in respect to the integrity of anastomoses of bile ducts and vessels. US is the recommended method of monitoring such patients, particularly as it is readily performed at the bedside.

The Pancreas

Unlike the liver the pancreas lies almost entirely in the retroperitoneal space. Prior to the present decade the pancreas defied demonstration by available radiological methods.

10.10 Methods of Pancreatic Imaging

Apart from calcifications resulting from pancreatitis and demonstrable on plain films, and widening of the duodenal loop shown on barium studies, suggestive of pancreatic head cancer, the pathological anatomy of the pancreas remained a mystery short of exploratory laparotomy. Nowadays the duct system can be shown by ERCP (Fig. 10.17), or more recently by MRCP (magnetic resonance cholangio pancreatography) (Fig. 10.23), and the organ itself by CT or US, if no bowel gas intervenes. Unlike the liver, the pancreas does not have a single arterial supply but branches arise from the gastroduodenal and splenic arteries. For detailed vascular studies selective arteriography is used by guiding a fine catheter into the appropriate arterial branch. Detection of occult functioning islet cell tumours may be difficult and occasionally transhepatic portal venous catheterization and sampling of the draining pancreatic venous blood may assist in localization. In addition radiologists can perform fine needle biopsy of suspicious areas within the pancreas, guided by US or CT.

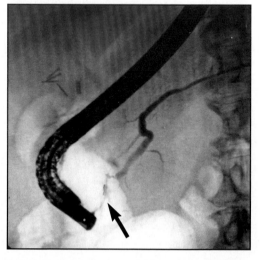

Fig. 10.17 ERCP with injection of the main pancreatic duct (arrow) which is seen to taper as it passes across the midline and with fine lateral branches to the parenchyma.

Indications for imaging the pancreas

- Acute pancreatitis.
- Chronic pancreatitis.
- Suspected pancreatic tumour.

10.11 Acute Pancreatitis

Patients with acute pancreatitis present with acute upper abdominal symptoms, particularly pain. In severe cases the patient may have acute circulatory failure whilst in milder cases there is less generalized disturbance.

The erect chest film

It is important to exclude the possibility of a perforated peptic ulcer, by obtaining an erect chest film (not erect abdomen). This view shows free gas beneath the diaphragm well (Fig. 12.2), consistent with a perforation. In acute pancreatitis this view may show a small left sided pleural effusion, consistent with the inflammatory process involving the lesser sac.

Complications of acute pancreatitis

Until recently the terminology applied to the complications was confused, but recently the following nomenclature has been accepted internationally:

Early:

- Acute fluid collections.
- Pancreatic necrosis.

Later:

- Pseudocysts.
- Pancreatic abscess.

Acute fluid collections occur in 30–50% of cases and more than half regress spontaneously (Fig. 10.18). The nature of the fluid on CT is not clear but it may contain bacteria. The collections lack a clearly-defined wall and are well shown by CT as lying in the peri-pancreatic soft tissues or in adjacent peritoneal spaces. Some acute fluid collections will go on to form pseudocysts or abscesses.

Pancreatic necrosis may be diffuse or focal and is usually associated with severe manifestations of the disease. Using contrast-enhanced CT the diagnosis of necrosis is made when areas of pancreas are shown to be nonperfused. The presence of necrosis,

particularly if infection is superadded, significantly worsens the prognosis (Fig. 10.19).

Pseudocysts contain pancreatic fluids surrounded by a well-formed wall without an epithelium. They rarely develop in less than four weeks from the acute episode and are well seen on CT (Fig. 10.20). Pseudocysts may track extensively in the upper abdomen and even into the mediastinum. A pseudocyst may resolve or continue to expand, requiring surgery, usually anastomosis, i.e. 'marsupialisation', to the bowel. Some respond to percutaneous aspiration.

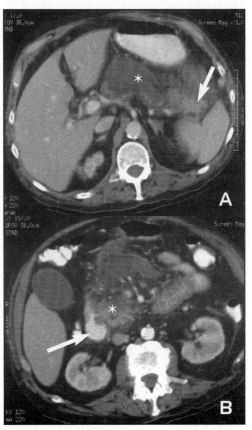

Fig. 10.19 Acute pancreatitis with necrosis. (A) Dynamic CT shows enhancement of the tail of the pancreas (arrow) but not the body (*), consistent with necrosis. (B) A section 2 cm lower shows a swollen pancreatic head (*) indenting the contrast-filled duodenum (arrow) and heterogenous opacity of the adjacent pancreatic tissue consistent with areas of necrosis.

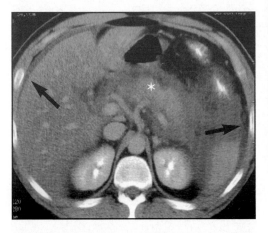

Fig. 10.18 Acute pancreatitis. CT following contrast shows the enhanced pancreas (*) surrounded by non-enhancing areas consistent with oedematous inflammatory tissue. Note the small amount of ascites over the liver and spleen (arrows).

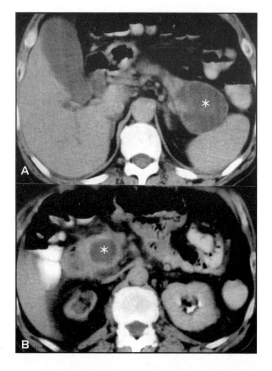

Pancreatic abscess may result from bacterial contamination of a pseudocyst or occasionally following pancreatic trauma. Usually indistinguishable from pseudocyst on CT pancreatic abscess may be suspected from the clinical manifestations. The diagnosis may be confirmed by needle puncture guided by US.

Once the diagnosis of acute pancreatitis is made in mild cases there is no imperative for early detailed imaging. In severe cases CT is indicated to assess pancreatic necrosis. Later CT or US are suitable for detecting pseudocyst formation.

Fig. 10.20 Pancreatic pseudocysts. CT shows two well defined cysts (*) in the tail (A) and the pancreatic head (B). Several weeks after acute pancreatitis. Note the shrunken right kidney.

10.12 Chronic Pancreatitis

Patients usually present with upper abdominal pain and digestive disturbances. In this regard differentiation from biliary and gastroduodenal pathology may be difficult. In this condition the pancreas undergoes continuing degeneration and classically the triad of calcification on plain radiographs, steatorrhea and diabetes is diagnostic. However these severe manifestations are seen in less than 30%. In most patients presenting with upper abdominal pain and dyspepsia, it is wise to first exclude pathology in the biliary system using US and the gastroduodenal region by barium meal. If negative the pancreas then may require examination and CT is recommended. However, in patients with steatorrhea, CT should be the initial imaging examination.

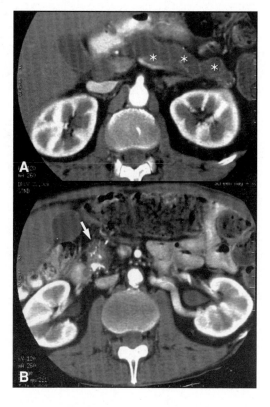

Fig. 10.21 Chronic pancreatitis. Post contrast CT. (A) The pancreatic duct (*) in the body and tail is grossly dilated with only a shell of pancreatic tissue. (B) The pancreatic head is small and contains numerous calcifications (arrow).

CT demonstrates the size of the pancreas and the presence of calcification and may, in some instances, demonstrate the pancreatic duct (Fig. 10.21). The definitive diagnosis of chronic pancreatitis is made by ERCP, but this is more invasive than CT, and may not be required in many cases. The pancreatic duct in this condition is generally dilated and strictures commonly occur (Fig. 10.22). Calcifications may be seen within the pancreatic substance or within the ducts. Magnetic resonance cholangio-pancreatography (MRCP) has the potential to replace ERCP as the primary modality to demonstrate the pancreatic duct. Non-invasive, it shows the duct both proximal and distal to an obstruction (Fig. 10.23) and does not require contrast. Pancreatic duct obstruction may require surgery or interventional radiological techniques for correction.

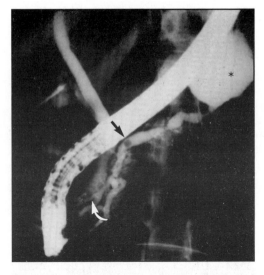

Fig. 10.22 Chronic pancreatitis. ERCP shows irregularity of the main pancreatic duct with stenoses and filling of a cystic space within the pancreas (*). The small radiolucency within the duct is probably an air bubble (arrow). Note retrograde filling of the accessory pancreatic duct (curved arrow).

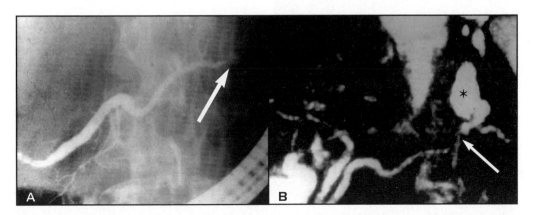

Fig. 10.23 Recurrent pancreatitis. (A) ERCP shows the slightly irregular duct obstructed (arrow). (B) Magnetic resonance cholangio-pancreatography (MRCP) shows the entire duct including the portion in the pancreatic tail proximal to the obstruction (arrow). A fistulous track (*) extends upwards towards the left hemidiaphragm. (By courtesy of Dr. Joseph T Ferrucci, Boston Medical Centre.)

10.13 Pancreatic Tumours

Most primary tumours of the pancreas are of the following types:

- Ductal adenocarcinoma.
- Mucinous macrocystic adenoma or carcinoma.
- Serous microcystic adenoma.
- Islet cell tumours.

Adenocarcinoma

This is the commonest tumour (90%) and is usually a solid mass which tends to metastasise to the liver and lymph nodes and has a poor prognosis. The pancreatic duct is frequently obstructed by such a tumour and, as a result, the tail of the pancreas may atrophy. Tumours in the pancreatic head frequently involve the common bile duct resulting in jaundice (Fig. 10.24).

Diagnosis can now be made in most cases by combining CT, ERCP and percutaneous fine needle biopsy. CT demonstrates the size and shape of the pancreas very well but usually does not allow differentiation between neoplastic tissue and normal pancreatic parenchyma with sufficient degree of confidence. CT may show extension of tumour beyond the pancreas with encasing of adjacent blood vessels (Fig. 10.25).

ERCP or MRCP outlining the pancreatic duct will demonstrate any local obstruction. If a localized pancreatic swelling is seen on CT or US

the diagnosis of carcinoma can be confirmed by percutaneous fine needle biopsy.

Cystic tumours

The two cystic tumours are uncommon and well demonstrated by CT. The macrocystic tumour has a high malignant potential and consists of moderately large multilocular cysts, containing mucinous material, and arises most frequently in the body or the tail of the pancreas (Fig. 10.26). It may be confused with a pseudocyst. The microcystic adenoma is often quite large and is benign, consisting of many very small cysts containing serous fluid.

Islet cell tumours

These tumours are small, usually about 1 or 2 cm in size, and many are functional, producing hormones, and associated with particular clinical syndromes. The indication for searching for such a tumour is entirely dependent on the clinical indications. Insulinomas are associated with

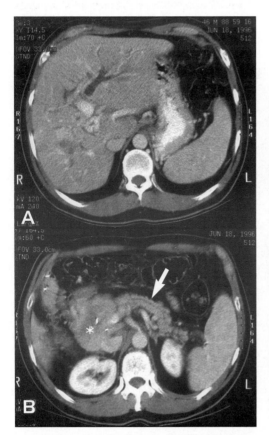

Fig. 10.24 Obstructive jaundice. Carcinoma of pancreatic head. (A) Radiolucent dilated intrahepatic bile ducts contrast with the blood vessels. (B) An heterogeneous mass (*) in the pancreatic head. Remainder of pancreas appears atrophic with the duct slightly dilated (arrow).

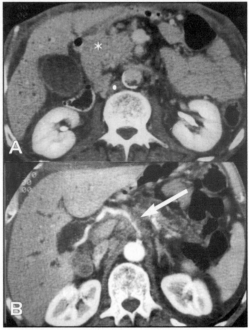

Fig. 10.25 Pancreatic adenocarcinoma with local spread. (A) An irregular mass (*) is seen in the neck of the pancreas. (B) Dynamic CT shows irregularity of the lumen of the hepatic artery arising from the coeliac axis with surrounding neoplastic tissue (arrow).

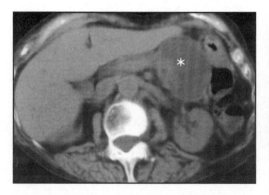

Fig. 10.26 Macrocytic carcinoma of pancreas. CT shows the largely cystic tumour (*) in the pancreatic tail with some solid tissue medially.

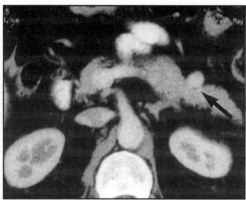

Fig. 10.27 Islet cell tumour. CT following IV contrast clearly shows the small rounded tumour near the tail of the pancreas which enhances strongly (arrow).

hypoglycaemia and tend to affect older people. Gastrinomas secrete large amounts of gastrin, which induces high acidity in the stomach with the development of peptic ulcers in the stomach and the duodenum, i.e. Zollinger–Ellison syndrome. Both tumours may be part of a Multiple Endocrine syndrome.

Islet cell tumours are difficult to demonstrate. CT, with contrast enhancement, may show a tumour within the pancreas (Fig. 10.27) and selective arteriography may demonstrate a localized pathological circulation. In some cases percutaneous transhepatic portal vein catheterization is performed to obtain blood samples from parts of the pancreas to localize the tumour more accurately. Recently intra-operative ultrasound, with pancreatic palpation, has been found to demonstrate the vast majority of insulinomas.

The Spleen

The spleen is visualised in most abdominal radiological examinations, but it is unusual clinically to require imaging of the spleen alone. Significant splenic enlargement is usually easily detected by clinical examination.

10.14   Imaging the Spleen

The spleen is seen on plain abdominal radiography, US, CT, MRI and radionuclide studies with agents targeting the reticulo-endothelial system. For specific clinical problems related to the spleen CT is the recommended initial investigation. On CT the spleen is of homogeneous density, slightly less dense than the liver and more than the kidney parenchyma. Accessory spleens are not uncommon and usually located close to the splenic hilum. Sometimes a localized nodule from the lower margin may be confused with a tumour arising from the upper pole of the left kidney.

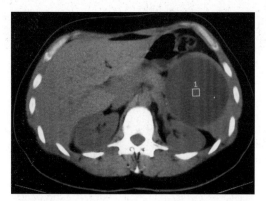

Fig. 10.28 Splenic epidermoid cyst. CT shows the cyst (1) of fluid density (less than 20 Hounsfield units) without evidence of a wall.

Indications for imaging the spleen

- Blunt abdominal trauma – see section 12.9.
- Splenomegaly.

Causes of splenomegaly

- Lymphoma and leukaemia.
- Portal hypertension (see section 8.3).
- Cysts (parasitic / non-parasitic).
- Carcinomatous metastases.

In lymphoma and leukaemia, the spleen, although enlarged, usually has a homogeneous texture on CT. Sometimes the abnormal tissue is nodular and is seen in contrast to the normal splenic tissue. The presence of abdominal lymphadenopathy strengthens the likelihood of the diagnosis. Hydatid cysts may occur in the spleen. Cysts may also result from trauma and haemorrhage. Epidermoid cyst (Fig. 10.28), containing cholesterol crystals, is occasionally encountered, particularly in young females. Of interest is the finding that such fluid, unlike cysts generally, may be quite echogenic on US. Primary splenic tumours are rare but occasionally malignant metastases may be recognized as low density focal lesions within the splenic parenchyma. Infarcts may also be demonstrated as wedge-shaped areas of decreased attenuation extending to the capsule of the spleen, and not enhancing after administration of intravenous contrast medium.

Reference

See Chapter 6.

Although enlarged kidneys become palpable, and the distended bladder also, the detection of most urinary tract abnormalities requires special investigation. Whilst endoscopy of the bladder and urethra is valuable in particular cases, radiology is required in most patients with urinary tract problems. A wide range of techniques is used in urinary tract radiology and it is important that the appropriate examination is requested for the particular clinical problem.

11.1 Intravenous Urogram (IVU)

In patients with normal, or slightly impaired, renal function the IVU is an excellent means of imaging the entire urinary tract and it is the first imaging investigation in many cases. When renal function is significantly impaired (serum creatinine above 0.5 mmol/litre) the intravenous contrast excretion is inadequate and other methods, e.g. plain radiography, US and CT, are used.

Preparation of the patient for IVU, which always includes plain radiography, need not be rigorous. Food and fluid restriction is not required but a mild purgative is valuable to clear the urinary tract of overlying faeces and gas.

Various phases of contrast excretion are filmed in urography following intravenous injection of the water-soluble iodine-containing contrast medium (Fig. 11.1). **Plain films** are made prior to injection, particularly to demonstrate opaque calculi. A film soon after injection records the **nephrogram**, i.e. parenchymal opacification due to contrast in the blood vessels and nephrons. Later the pelvi-calyceal system is outlined, i.e. the

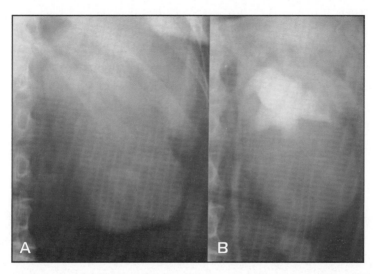

Fig. 11.1 Intravenous urogram (IVU). Renal cell carcinoma. (A) Nephrogram at conclusion of injection. (B) Pyelogram confirms a mass in the lower pole of uncertain nature, probably either cyst or neoplasm. US is indicated.

pyelogram phase, and this is enhanced by using an ureteric compression belt. To outline the ureters a film is made immediately after the belt is released. Views of the bladder and an '**after micturition**' film conclude the procedure.

Reactions to the contrast medium are relatively common but are usually mild, consisting of urticaria, transient nausea, and sometimes vomiting. Rarely, serious cardiovascular collapse may occur soon after injection and the mortality from such a complication is about 1 in 250,000. Although a very occasional happening, staff in radiology departments are trained and prepared to deal with such an occurrence.

The role of imaging techniques in diagnosis in the urinary tract will be considered according to the main presenting clinical feature.

11.2 Haematuria

The presence of blood in the urine, whether macroscopic or microscopic, is abnormal and a cause should always be sought. Haematuria is a non-specific symptom with many causes, but the majority fall into the following categories.

1. Anticoagulant therapy

The use of anticoagulants is widespread and should be excluded by questioning to avoid unnecessary investigation. However, it should be remembered that occasionally, the presence of a focal lesion such as a tumour first becomes apparent on administering these drugs, which provoke the bleeding.

2. Diffuse renal parenchymal disease

The various forms of nephritis may present with haematuria. Clinical findings and urinalysis are usually diagnostic. Apart from casts the red blood cells in the urine may appear slightly damaged or crenated if they have passed through the glomeruli and tubules.

3. Tumours

Painless haematuria is the commonest presenting symptom in renal cell carcinoma and transitional cell tumours of the kidney, ureter and bladder. However, Wilm's tumour in children rarely presents with haematuria.

4. Urinary calculi

Stones in the urinary tract may occasionally present because of bleeding resulting from irritation and ulceration of the mucosal surface.

5. Urinary tract infections

Only occasionally is bleeding a prominent feature with urinary infection and the diagnosis is usually revealed by urinalysis.

6. Benign prostotamegaly

Not infrequently patients with bladder neck obstruction first present because of haematuria, which may be quite heavy. It is generally attributed to venous bleeding, perhaps associated with straining, but the exact mechanism remains uncertain.

Painful haematuria is more frequently associated with calculus whilst painless favours neoplasm. It should be remembered that occasionally tumours in the upper urinary tract may be associated with quite severe clot colic. Bleeding from the upper urinary tract may be distinguished from that from the bladder and urethra as the urine, when passed, is more uniformly blood stained.

Lower tract bleeding is usually more prominent at the beginning or end of micturition.

Intravenous urography, which always includes plain film radiography, is the first imaging investigation for haematuria except in those who have a clear-cut diagnosis of diffuse renal parenchymal disease, e.g. acute glomerulo-nephritis. The IVU is a sensitive means of revealing focal abnormalities within the drainage system and some lesions within the kidneys. The abnormalities, however, are often non-specific and further investigations are required to establish an absolute diagnosis on which to plan treatment.

Haematuria – no cause found on IVU

It is most important to realize that, particularly in older patients with haematuria, investigation should not cease if a normal IVU is obtained. The commonest cause of haematuria is a bladder tumour and they can be missed, if small, on an IVU. Cystoscopy should be performed. Also, the IVU may not detect small tumours within the renal parenchyma, and CT, which is a more sensitive method of demonstrating such lesions, should be requested if the IVU is normal. If diffuse parenchymal disease of the kidneys is suspected a renal biopsy may be indicated.

If all investigations prove negative it is important that haematuria patients should not be lost to follow-up. In particular cystoscopy should be repeated at the time of further bleeding and ureteric specimens of urine obtained to determine whether the bleeding is unilateral.

11.3 Renal Masses

A renal mass (Fig. 11.1B), often referred to as a space-occupying lesion, may produce symptoms, frequently haematuria, or may be detected incidentally when CT or US is performed for another purpose. In fact, because of the frequency of cross-sectional imaging and the inclusion of the kidneys within the field of examination incidental detection of renal space lesions is the most frequent presentation. Before listing the more commonly encountered renal masses the significance of simple or solitary cysts of the kidney will be emphasized, as the strategy of investigating a renal mass is largely concerned with separating the simple cyst from a range of usually solid masses, which on occasions may be semisolid or even cystic.

Simple cysts

Simple cysts are extremely common and most of the elderly, at autopsy, are shown to have one or more. The frequency increases with age but cysts are relatively common also in younger adults and occasionally in children. The size varies from 1cm or less to greater than 10 cm in diameter. The majority are only 1 or 2 cm across with larger sizes seen less frequently.

Simple cysts contain straw-coloured fluid and have a very thin lining of flattened cells with no cleavage plane from the interstitial tissue. For practical purposes malignant change in the lining cells does not occur. For this reason conservative management is justified for all but the few large cysts which may be compromising the surrounding renal tissue. Multicystic kidneys will be discussed separately (see section 11.4).

It is important that strict criteria are used for diagnosing simple cyst. Failing to recognize a malignant tumour, particularly a renal cell carcinoma, which may be largely cystic on occasions, may seriously alter the outcome for the patient. Simple cyst diagnosis depends on US or CT.

Ultrasonography (US)

US is a valuable and readily available means of separating simple cysts from solid tumours by demonstrating the anatomical and sonographic features of the mass (Fig. 11.2).

Anatomical features

1. Cysts tend to be spherical.
2. Cysts have no demonstrable wall thickness.

Sonographic features

1. An absence or paucity of echoes within the cyst.
2. Enhancement of echoes from tissue beyond the cyst. This is due to the better transmission of sound through the cyst fluid compared with the soft tissue on each side of the lesion which attenuates the sound.

Computed tomography (CT)

The anatomical features are the same as for US (Fig. 11.3) and it is particularly important that no demonstrable wall should be seen on the cyst (Fig. 11.4). CT allows the density of the fluid content to be measured and this should not exceed 25 HU (Hounsfield units).

Renal cyst puncture

Fine needle cyst puncture is relatively simply performed under radiological control, and occasionally this is required for diagnosis. In the few patients in which a large cyst interferes with renal function cyst puncture with the introduction of absolute alcohol may lead to resolution of the lesion.

Diagnostic protocol

If a mass lesion is first detected on IVU or nuclear scan, US is indicated to determine whether the lesion is a simple cyst or not. On IVU both cystic and solid lesions have similar density and cannot be separated unless calcification is seen in the mass. With nuclear scanning both cystic and solid lesions fail to take up the isotope. A diagnosis of simple cyst is made if the US criteria are fulfilled, but if any doubt exists (Fig. 11.4) or the lesion is clearly not a simple cyst then CT is performed. This protocol, frequently referred to as an **algorithm**, is now well established.

The following short list includes most of the focal mass lesions encountered.

Cysts

- Simple Cyst – *extremely common.*
- Hydatid – *very uncommon.*

Tumours – malignant

- Renal cell carcinoma (RCC).
- Transitional cell carcinoma (TCC).
- Wilm's tumour (Nephroblastoma).

  Occurs between the ages of one to five years with a peak at three years of age.

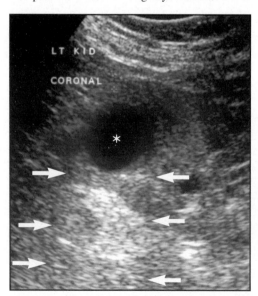

Fig. 11.2 Simple cyst in left kidney. The lesion (*) is echolucent, rounded, and without evidence of a wall. Note the band of increased echogenicity (between arrows) deep to the cyst (posterior wall enhancement), compared with tissue on either side.

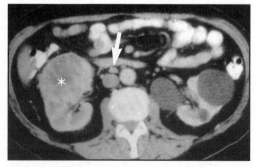

Fig. 11.3 Contrast-enhanced CT showing three cysts in the left kidney. The density of the cysts, which have no visible wall, was less than 20 Hounsfield units and they did not enhance with contrast. Note the mass in the right kidney due to a renal cell carcinoma (*) which has enhanced, and a metastatic lymph node (arrow) anterior to the IVC.

- Lymphoma – occasionally primary.
- Metastases.

Tumours – benign

- Angiomyolipoma.

Abscess – *uncommon*

Renal cell carcinoma (RCC)

RCC is an immunologically dependent tumour and cases have been recorded occasionally of multiple pulmonary metastases regressing after removal of the primary tumour. Although malignant the prognosis with treatment is relatively good (cf. lung). When confined to the renal capsule the five year survival is about 70%, falling to about 55% if the tumour extends into the perirenal fascial space. If the renal vein is involved, as frequently occurs, the survival falls to about 40%. If nodes are involved the prognosis at five years is about 20% and with distant metastases or penetration of the perirenal fascia only 5%.

In recent years more information is available on the behaviour of small RCCs which have been

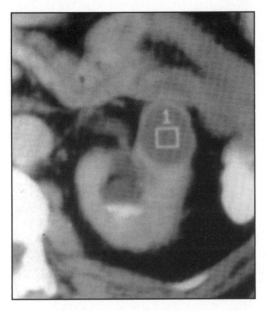

Fig. 11.4 Cystic renal cell carcinoma. Although rounded and fluid-containing (15 Hounsfield units) the presence of a definite wall indicates the diagnosis (cf. Fig. 11.4).

found incidentally (Fig. 11.5). Although very occasionally an RCC less than 3 cm in diameter may metastasise, the vast majority of tumours less than 3 cm in diameter have an excellent prognosis following surgery and it seems that partial nephrectomy in such cases is adequate. Clearly the radiologist has an important responsibility in detecting these small tumours and clearly differentiating them from simple cysts. Another problem in diagnosis is that very occasionally RCC may develop as a cystic lesion containing straw-coloured fluid (Fig. 11.4), but, in such cases, both on US and CT the presence of a wall to the cystic lesion should indicate the true nature of the abnormality.

CT appearance of RCC (Figs 11.6, 11.3)

Prior to injecting intravenous contrast an RCC appears less dense, at least in part, than the normal renal tissue. Following contrast heterogeneous enhancement of the lesion is expected. CT also shows involvement of renal veins, the state of the adjacent lymph nodes and the presence of metastases in adjacent sites. The CT appearance is non-specific and similar findings may be seen with other solid renal tumours including lymphoma and metastasis. The clinical picture assists in differentiating these conditions. If the findings strongly favour RCC radical nephrectomy, i.e. removing the kidney and the perirenal tissues, is performed, except for tumours less than 3 cm. If any doubt exists renal biopsy may be performed or surgical exploration of the kidney to determine the appropriate management.

Wilm's tumour

The commonest solid renal mass in childhood, the appearance may range from the benign renal blastema (Wilm's tumour in-situ) to a sarcomatous aggressive form. With a peak age of three years haematuria is not usually macroscopic and children present because of a palpable mass or, occasionally, anorexia, anaemia or hypertension. US usually

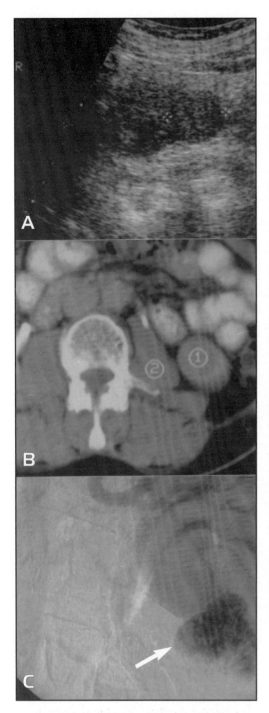

Fig. 11.5 Small renal carcinoma detected incidentally. (A) US shows 2.78 cm echogenic mass in lower pole of left kidney. (B) CT shows the homogeneous mass (1) of soft tissue density. (C) Arteriogram, showing tumour vascularity (arrow).

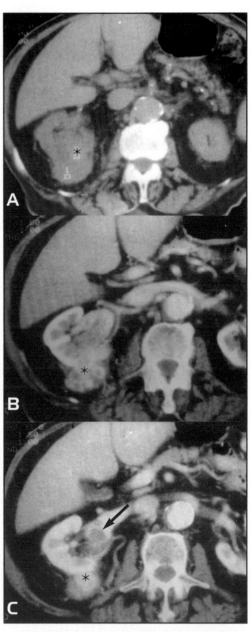

Fig. 11.6 Renal cell carcinoma. (A) Non-enhanced CT shows irregular mass on right kidney(*). (B) Dynamic contrast enhanced CT. The arterial phase shows patchy enhancement of the tumour. (C) A later phase of the same study, but at a slightly higher level shows filling of renal veins. A filling defect is seen in the right renal vein indicating extension of the tumour (arrow).

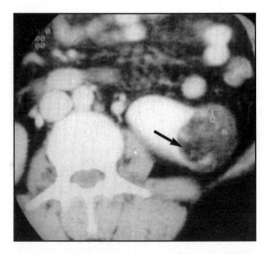

Fig. 11.7 Angiomyolipoma. Dynamic contrast-enhanced CT scan. In this late phase patchy enhancement of the tumour in the left kidney is seen but areas of persisting low density (black) consistent with fat provide the diagnosis (arrow).

confirms the diagnosis showing a heterogeneous mass which may extend to the vein and IVC.

Neuroblastoma, which affects the same age group, can be shown by US to lie outside the kidney.

Transitional cell carcinoma (TCC) *(see section 11.6)*

Angiomyolipoma

This hamartomatous tumour may occur in patients with tuberose sclerosis or as an isolated lesion. Haematuria is common and radiologically the tumour is evident by the presence of fat within it. This may be seen in some cases during IVU and confirmed on CT where fat has a very low density (-70 HU) (Fig. 11.7). The lesion is benign but resection may be required to control bleeding. Tuberose sclerosis patients may have periventricular brain calcifications, 'honeycomb' lungs or bone lesions.

11.4 Multicystic Kidneys

Apart from simple cysts (see section 11.3) which may be multiple, multicystic renal disease has been described in a wide range of conditions. The multiple cysts are readily detected by US, CT, MRI and if the cysts are large by IVU.

Polycystic kidneys

This term is used to include two genetically determined conditions, **autosomal dominant polycystic kidney disease (ADPKD)** and **autosomal recessive polycystic kidney disease (ARPKD)**. ADPKD is the commonest hereditary renal disorder and is usually detected in middle age or earlier and generally ends in renal failure after many years. Loin pain, haematuria, hypertension, or a family history may lead to detection and the kidneys may be palpable clinically. Berry aneurysms are more common in ADPKD and subarachnoid haemorrhage may be the presenting event. Before renal function is affected an IVU

may be performed and usually distortion of the calyces and bilateral renal enlargement point to the diagnosis (Fig. 11.8). Occasionally the cysts may be quite small and the calyces relatively undisturbed. The cysts are clearly identified by ultrasound, CT or MRI and cysts may be present in the liver, pancreas and spleen also (Fig. 11.9). Liver failure does not occur, but surface lesions may cause peritoneal pain.

ARPKD is uncommon and usually affects neonates. The enlarged kidneys, due to cystic collecting tubules, are associated with periportal fibrosis and it is usually liver failure which predominates, resulting in a poor prognosis.

Acquired cystic kidney disease

This title is reserved for long-term dialysis patients who frequently develop multiple cysts throughout the renal parenchyma. The kidneys are usually much smaller than in the terminal stages of polycystic kidney disease. RCC develops in 7%.

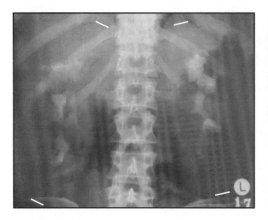

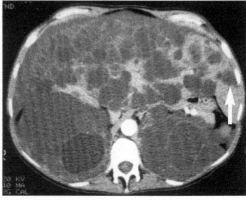

Fig. 11.8 Polycystic kidneys (ADPKD). IVU. The large kidneys (poles marked) function moderately well. The degree of pyelographic distortion is minor yet CT showed extensive cystic changes bilaterally.

Fig. 11.9 Advanced polycystic kidneys (ADPKD). Gross enlargement of kidneys and liver with cysts also in the spleen (arrow).

Medullary sponge kidney (MSK)

MSK is a developmental condition affecting the collecting ducts in the medullary pyramids. Small cystic spaces communicating with the duct system are usually evident on IVU. The condition may affect a single pyramid or be more widespread in one or both kidneys. Tiny calculi may develop within the cystic spaces and frequently migrate to the ureter, causing colic.

These calculi may be seen in the pyramids on plain films and following intravenous contrast numerous small cystic spaces, including those with calculi, become opaque (Fig. 11.10). Apart from episodes of colic the prognosis in MSK is good. On IVU the appearance needs to be distinguished from renal papillary necrosis.

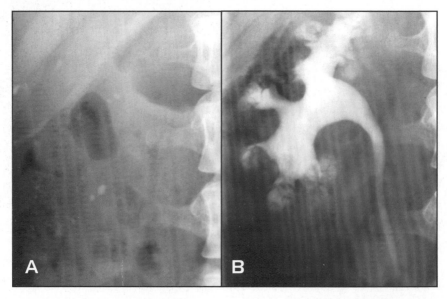

Fig. 11.10 Medullary sponge kidney (MSK). (A) Plain film: numerous round calculi within small cystic spaces in the medullary pyramids. (B) IVU outlines numerous cysts in the pyramids and also linear opacities due to dilated collecting ducts.

11.5 Ureteric Obstruction

Ureteric colic is disturbing for the patient and is usually recognized clinically because of referred pain in the loin and groin, corresponding to the lower thoracic and lumbar dermatomes. Lower ureteric obstruction may produce referred pain in the scrotum consistent with the first lumbar dermatome. Ureteric colic points to a degree of ureteric obstruction but is nonspecific.

Causes of unilateral ureteric obstruction

a. Mechanical

In the lumen
- Stone, blood clot, sloughed papilla.

In the wall
- Transitional cell tumour, stricture, e.g. TB.

Outside the wall
- Metastatic carcinoma, lymphoma.
- Primary cervical uterine carcinoma.
- Retroperitoneal fibrosis.

In the bladder
- Carcinoma. Ureterocoele.

b. Functional

Due to altered peristalsis
- Pregnancy – physiological.
- Pelvi-ureteric junction obstruction – common (Fig. 11.11).
- Vesico-ureteric junction obstruction (primary obstructive megaureter) – uncommon.

Urinary calculi

Calculus is by far the commonest cause of acute ureteric colic. Some are opaque on plain radiography.

1. Calcium oxalate – opaque.

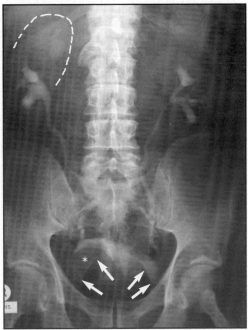

Fig. 11.12 Double right ureter and large ureterocoele. The ureter draining the upper portion of the kidney typically has an ectopic orifice in the bladder, or sometimes extravesical, and may develop an ureterocoele, as in this case (*). Back pressure has lead to loss of function in the upper pole (marked with a white line). The lower ureter, in this case, drains normally to the trigone but may show changes of vesico-ureteric reflux. Gas distends the rectum (arrows).

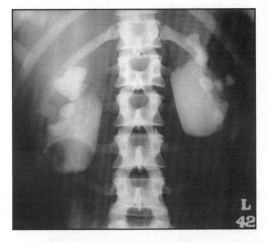

Fig. 11.11   Bilateral pelvic-ureteric junction obstruction. Moderate dilatation (clubbing) of calyces on the right with reduced renal parenchyma is consistent with moderate back pressure renal atrophy.

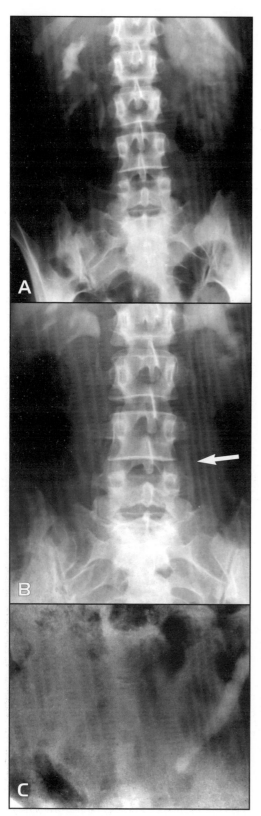

2. Ammonium-magnesium-calcium phosphate (i.e. triple phosphate or 'infection' stone or struvite) – opaque.
3. Uric acid – non-opaque.
4. Cystine – moderately opaque if large. Smaller stones non-opaque.

   Note: All of these stones are opaque on CT.

The majority of calculi in the ureter cause only partial obstruction and 85% of those less than 6 mm in size will pass spontaneously.

Double ureter and ureterocoele

A ureterocoele is a dilatation of the submucosal portion of the ureter as it passes through the bladder wall. There may be a 'pin-hole' ureteric orifice and some degree of ureteric obstruction. Ureterocoele is commonly seen when double ureters extend to the bladder (Fig. 11.12). In such cases the ureter from the lower part of the kidney drains to the normal site but the ureter from the upper renal pole has an ectopic orifice, usually along a line from the trigone to the posterior urethra. It is the ectopic ureter which often has a ureterocoele leading to non-function of the upper part of the kidney.

Acute renal colic

Emergency intravenous urogram

The IVU remains the preferred means of investigation. US to demonstrate ureteric dilatation combined with plain radiography to detect opaque stones has proponents. More recently helical CT has its proponents but is expensive and not always readily available.

Plain radiography of the urinary tract should be performed to detect the presence of opaque calculi but, in fact, only one third of calculi are

Fig. 11.13 Acute left ureteric obstruction by calculus. Limited IVU. (A) Five minutes after IV contrast injection the left kidney is enlarged with a persisting nephrogram. (B) 20 minutes later the dilated left ureter extends to the pelvis (arrow). (C) A view after micturition shows obstruction at the vesico-ureteric junction. Review of the plain film showed a tiny opaque calculus which passed two days later.

clearly identified on plain films made under these circumstances. About 20% of calculi are nonopaque but even opaque ureteric stones may be missed because they are very small and frequently obscured by overlying bowel content. In the bony pelvis, ureteric calculi, which are usually irregularly ovoid, differ from **phleboliths**, small calcified venous thrombi which are round, often with a lucent centre. The limited IVU during colic is valuable as it documents objectively the presence and level of ureteric obstruction and often the cause. Most ureteric calculi pass spontaneously. If the investigation is delayed until the symptoms subside after passage of the stone, then some doubt may exist, in the presence of a normal urogram, as to whether ureteric obstruction was the cause of the symptom.

Urographic evidence of acute ureteric obstruction (Fig. 11.13)

1. Delayed appearance of the pyelogram.
2. Dense persisting nephrogram.
3. Renal enlargement on the side of obstruction.
4. Dilatation of the upper urinary tract.
5. Evidence of the obstructing lesion.

As contrast gradually enters the drainage system delayed films will show the degree of upper ureteric dilatation, the level of the obstruction, and often the cause of the obstruction.

Follow-up studies

When the radiologist detects the signs of ureteric obstruction it is usual to give a further injection of contrast medium and to wait some time, even several hours, before making a further radiograph. A film made then, in the prone position may demonstrate the dilated ureter down to the obstructing lesion.

In high degrees of ureteric obstruction there may be virtually no opacification of the upper ureter. In these cases, dilatation of the upper ureter can be confirmed using US and the ureter above the obstruction can be outlined easily using the technique of **percutaneous antegrade pyelography**. Alternatively, cystoscopy and retrograde pyelography can be performed, but requires a general anaesthetic in males.

Percutaneous antegrade pyelography

Under local anaesthetic, a fine gauge needle is introduced into the pelvis of the ureter under US control with the patient lying prone. The pressure can be recorded and samples of urine taken for study. Using the image intensifier, contrast medium can then be introduced to outline the dilated obstructed system (Fig. 11.14A).

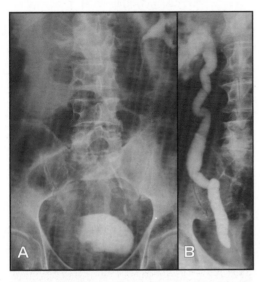

Fig. 11.14 Bladder transitional carcinoma obstructing right ureter. (A) Filling defect in bladder and non-functioning right kidney. (B) Percutaneous antegrade pyelogram shows obstruction at the bladder and no tumours in the right upper tract.

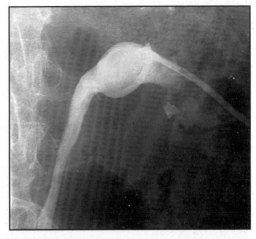

Fig. 11.15 Percutaneous nephrostomy. Pigtail catheter drainage.

Following such a 'skinny needle' pyelogram the radiologist, after consultation with the clinician, may be requested to perform percutaneous temporary nephrostomy, particularly if the ureteric obstruction is of high degree.

Percutaneous nephrostomy

Under radiological control, a needle catheter system is introduced in the loin through the renal substance into the dilated upper ureter. The fine catheter then provides urinary diversion until such time as definitive action is taken to overcome the obstruction (Fig. 11.15).

Causes of bilateral ureteric obstruction

a. Mechanical

Bladder outlet obstruction

- Prostate: hypertrophy or carcinoma.
- Urethral stricture.
- Posterior urethral valves.

Bilateral ureteric obstruction

- Procidentia (uterine prolapse).
- Cervical uterine carcinoma.
- Retroperitoneal fibrosis, lymphoma or metastasis.
- Aortic aneurysm (rare).

b. Functional

- Pregnancy.
- Bilateral pelvic-ureteric junction obstruction.

With incomplete bilateral obstruction and insignificant impairment of function the urinary tract may be outlined by IVU. With impaired renal function, and elevated serum creatinine levels, US is indicated and demonstrates dilated upper tracts and may indicate the level and cause of obstruction. Antegrade pyelography, CT and occasionally retrograde pyelography may be required. Bladder neck obstruction is discussed in section 11.9.

11.6 Non-Opaque Filling Defects

Urography may reveal a non-opaque filling defect consistent with an intraluminal mass within the pelvicalyceal system, the ureter, or the bladder. A filling defect may be due to:

- Transitional cell tumour.
- Non-opaque stone.
- Blood clot.
- A sloughed papilla.
- Occasionally a foreign body.

Upper urinary tract filling defects

When a non-opaque filling defect is seen in a kidney on IVU it may be difficult to determine the cause (Fig. 11.16). The next investigation is CT. All mineraloid calculi, even those non-opaque on IVU, are opaque on CT. Also, CT may reveal the full extent of a TCC, which, on occasions, may

extend well out into the renal parenchyma, simulating an RCC. Although TCC is of relatively

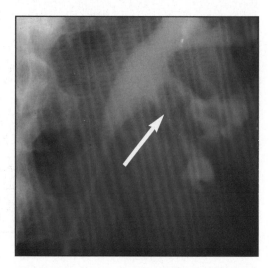

Fig. 11.16 Haematuria. Transitional carcinoma in lower major calyx (arrow). The non-opaque filling defect could also be due to blood clot or non-opaque calculus or sloughed papilla.

low vascularity, dynamic CT following contrast injection may show tumour enhancement. Sloughed papillae may be shown to lie freely in the drainage system on CT and do not enhance following contrast injection. Blood clot tends to break up over time and a repeat examination some days later may show a totally different appearance. The diagnosis of TCC may be confirmed in some cases by urinary cytology, preferably in a specimen obtained from a retrograde catheter.

Lower urinary tract filling defects

Bladder tumours are the commonest cause of haematuria and small tumours may not be seen within the contrast-filled bladder on IVU. Also, overlying bowel gas shadows may cause confusion with larger bladder tumours. For these reasons most patients presenting with macroscopic haematuria should undergo cystoscopy irrespective of the findings on IVU.

Cystoscopy is an effective means of diagnosing and in many cases treating less invasive bladder tumours. The urogram is valuable in demonstrating the presence of ureteric obstruction, a relatively common complication of invasive bladder tumours. Also, it may indicate whether the tumour is pedunculated or sessile (Fig. 11.17). The IVU may reveal the presence of a tumour within a bladder diverticulum, a circumstance which may escape detection at cystoscopy.

The grading of bladder tumours, particularly the extent of local invasion of the bladder wall, remains inaccurate despite the development of the newer imaging methods of CT and MRI. CT and MRI do provide some information concerning the pelvic and abdominal lymph nodes. CT can detect enlarged lymph nodes but involved nodes which are not enlarged will not be detected by this method. Recent studies suggest that MRI may be more effective.

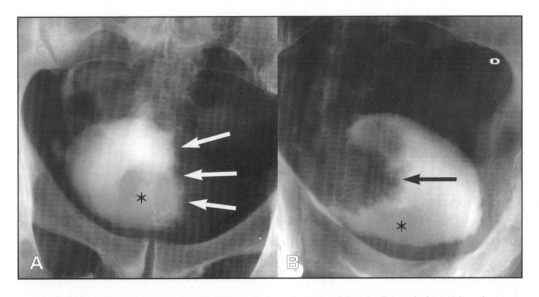

Fig. 11.17 Transitional cell carcinoma of the bladder on IVU (arrows). (A) Sessile. (B) Papillary. In both, an enlarged prostate causes a filling defect in the bladder base (*).

11.7 Urinary Tract Infections

Cystitis is extremely common and infection involving the upper urinary tract, usually referred to as **acute pyelonephritis**, frequently occurs. The diagnosis is made clinically and from urinalysis. Numerous polymorphs, within casts if pyelonephritis is present, are seen in the urine and culture on blood agar plates grows most organisms, particularly E.coli but not M.tuberculosis. Urinary tract infections may be categorized as follows.

1. Ascending infection

Very common in women of all ages, but less common in men. The organisms, usually E.coli, ascend from the perineum to produce cystitis and less frequently upper urinary tract infection. It is now known that the risk of significant structural damage to the kidneys mainly exists in the early years of life, although the results of that damage may not become clinically apparent until adulthood. The resultant pathological changes of focal scarring have been recognized for years and called chronic atrophic pyelonephritis. Nowadays, with a better understanding of the pathogenesis, a more appropriate title is **reflux nephropathy.**

2. Blood-borne infection

Relatively uncommon compared with ascending infection. Blood-borne organisms, e.g. staphylococcus or streptococcus, may result in a perirenal or intrarenal abscess. Diabetics are prone to this form of infection. Tuberculosis is also blood borne.

3. Tuberculosis

Tuberculosis is suspected when blood agar cultures fail to grow an organism in a case of pyuria. This so-called '**sterile pyuria**' is typical of TB and calls for special staining and plating on Lowenstein's medium.

4. Infection with a pre-disposing cause

Certain conditions in the urinary tract increase the likelihood of infection developing secondarily. These include:

- Stasis, e.g. pelvi-ureteric junction obstruction, bladder neck obstruction, vesico-ureteric reflux.
- Calculus.
- Diabetes.
- Papillary necrosis.

Reflux nephropathy

Before considering the indications for radiology in the management of urinary tract infection, it is crucial to understand the present state of knowledge in respect to vesico-ureteric reflux, ascending urinary infection, and the likelihood of developing renal damage. The present state of knowledge can be summarized as follows:

1. Some degree of **vesico-ureteric reflux (VUR)** is very common in children. With **high pressure reflux** during micturition the upper urinary tract distends significantly and this is distinct from **low pressure reflux** in which no upper tract distension occurs. From about the age of 7 years the frequency and severity of reflux diminishes in the vast majority of young people and high pressure reflux persisting into adulthood is very uncommon.

2. VUR results from the relatively short intramural course of the lower end of the ureter. Changes during growth result in correction of the problem in most people.

3. In very young children, below the age of about 5 years, with high pressure reflux, urine may be forced into the nephrons through incompetent collecting duct orifices on the papillae. This condition is referred to as

intrarenal reflux and more commonly occurs in the upper and lower poles due to the particular anatomy of the papillae in those regions.

4. Repeated intrarenal reflux, particularly of infected urine leads to focal scarring in those portions of the kidneys.

5. Even in the absence of scarring, unilateral high pressure reflux may lead to retarded growth of the kidney on that side, resulting, in adult life, in a considerable discrepancy in size of the two kidneys, although retaining a normal anatomical configuration, the so-called **hypoplastic kidney**.

6. Low pressure reflux, without distension of the upper urinary tract during micturition, may contribute to the recurrence of upper urinary tract infection in patients with cystitis but does not pose a significant risk to the integrity of the renal parenchyma.

Imaging investigations in urinary tract infection

1. Children

Urinary tract infection may be occult in the very young and it is important to detect it. Baseline investigation is regarded as important in infants and young children after a documented initial episode, because of the potential renal parenchymal damage.

Micturating cysto-urethrogram (MCU)

MCU is used to demonstrate the degree and severity of VUR, and in patients with high pressure reflux to detect intrarenal influx which indicates a risk to the kidney of developing scarring (Fig. 11.18). Children with high pressure reflux generally are prescribed urinary antiseptic therapy for several years until such time as reflux wanes. Further assessment of the degree of VUR, if required, is made using radionuclide MCU which reduces the radiation dosage very significantly.

Radionuclide renography

The status of the renal parenchyma is assessed most conveniently in children using radionuclide imaging with an agent which is taken up and persists in the renal parenchyma for some time (Fig. 11.19). Such an agent is Technetium-labelled DMSA (Di-mercapto-succinic acid). A defect in the scan indicates an area of parenchymal involvement, which may return to normal, but if persistent is consistent with a scar.

2. Adults

Acute urinary tract infection in adults, much more common in women, is usually caused by E.coli. Cystitis usually does not require radiological investigation. Acute pyelonephritis, due to ascending infection, but usually without VUR in adults, does justify imaging of the urinary tract, particularly if episodes are repeated.

IVU

This provides a good overview in adults, providing information concerning the presence of conditions which predispose to urinary tract

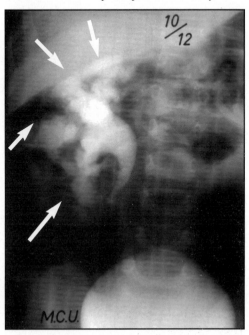

Fig. 11.18 Micturating cysto-urethrogram (MCU) in 10 month old child. High pressure right-sided vesico-ureteric reflux with intrarenal reflux (arrows).

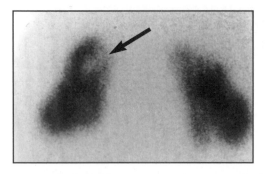

Fig. 11.19 Renal radionuclide scan in three year old child. Technetium-labelled DMSA is taken up by renal parenchyma. Defect in R upper pole (arrow) consistent with intrarenal reflux and potential scarring. High pressure VU reflux on MCU.

infection, i.e. stones and stasis, and also information concerning the state of the kidneys and whether focal renal scarring is present, as a legacy of childhood infections (Fig. 11.20). Also the 'after micturition' film, made immediately after emptying the bladder, provides an assessment of residual urine.

MCU

If the 'after micturition' film shows a moderate residue in the bladder then a MCU may be justified as VUR may have persisted into adult life and be the cause of the residuum. The same information can be obtained clinically by the patient voiding a second time a minute or so after the first micturition.

Note: It is important to remember that in women particularly a significant amount of radiation is received by the ovaries during IVU. Criticism has been levelled at the injudicious use of the IVU in urinary tract infection patients. It is unusual for a further IVU to be necessary should further episodes of pyelonephritis develop.

Urogenital tuberculosis

The postprimary dissemination of mycobacteria may result in foci in the urogenital tract in similar fashion to the development of lesions in the meninges, bone, joints, and adrenals. Urogenital TB is seen occasionally in Australia. Only about 10% have active pulmonary tuberculous lesions on chest x-ray. The initial granuloma occurs in the cortex and from that site spread may occur throughout the parenchyma or more frequently along the urinary tract. Lesions occur in the renal papillae and may caseate and ulcerate, communicating with the calyces. Spread along the ureter to the bladder may occur and cystitis may be the presenting symptom. In the male TB

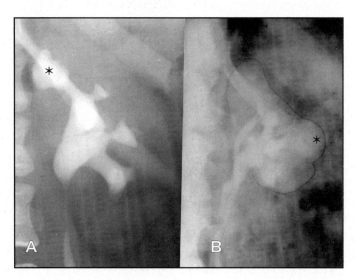

Fig. 11.20 Reflux nephropathy. (A) The upper calyx is dilated and clubbed with gross loss of overlying renal parenchyma (*). (B) A more severe case with gross scarring over the lower pole and the left mid zone. The renal outline has been marked. Note the hypertrophied parenchyma over unaffected calyces (*).

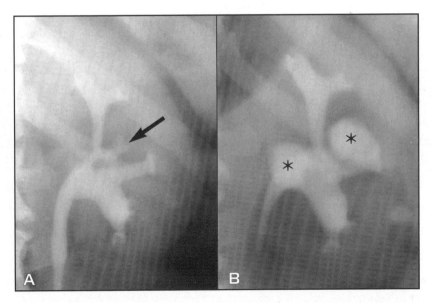

Fig. 11.21 Renal tuberculous ulceration. (A) Initial IVU showing ill-defined calyx (arrow). (B) One year following anti-tuberculous therapy two smooth-walled clubbed calyces (*) have resulted from sloughing of the caseous papillae. Urine became negative for mycobacteria.

lesions may be seen in the epididymis, vas, seminal vesicles, and prostate which may be the result of direct seeding or secondary to urinary tract involvement. In females, TB salpingitis and endometritis may cause infertility.

Radiological appearances

A broad spectrum of appearances may be seen radiologically resulting from various

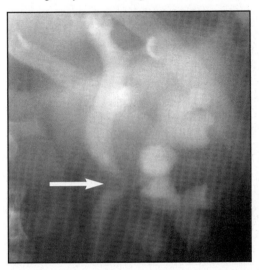

Fig. 11.22 Renal tuberculosis. Severe stricturing of the renal pelvis (arrow).

combinations of the following pathological features of the disease.

a.   Papillary ulceration

The initial lesion in the papilla may be difficult to detect until ulceration has occurred resulting in irregularity and loss of the normal papillary impression. Further ulceration results in cavity formation (Fig. 11.21).

b.   Stricturing

Stenotic lesions involving the pelvicalyceal system, ureter, or bladder are typical of TB and any urinary stricture should raise the possibility of the disease (Fig. 11.22). Focal strictures in the calyces or in the ureter may result in total obstruction, closing off the affected portions of the urinary tract, where the tuberculous process may continue but with the urine remaining sterile in some patients. Total destruction of the renal substance above a closed-off ureter is referred to as an **'autonephrectomy'**. Usually the destroyed renal substance is calcified. Because of the tendency to stricture formation it is important following a course of therapy for renal tuberculosis that radiology be performed some months after the urine becomes sterile to check on whether ureteric stenosis has developed, because subsequent back pressure atrophy of the kidney could occur.

c.   Calcification

Caseous TB lesions frequently calcify and such lesions may be detected on plain radiography (Fig. 11.23). Most often this calcification is seen in the kidney, but also occasionally in the prostate, seminal vesicle, vas and epididymis.

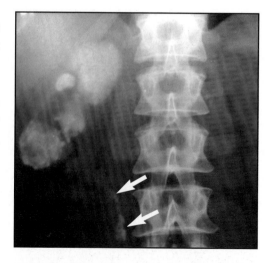

Fig. 11.23   Tuberculous auto-nephrectomy. The renal parenchyma is replaced by calcified caseous tissue. Calcified foci in the ureter (arrows).

11.8 Renal Papillary Necrosis

The renal papilla is the tip of the medullary pyramid, which is seen on urography as a conical filling defect indenting a minor calyx. In certain pathological states the papillae may become necrotic and the tissue may slough to a varying degree. The basis of the lesion is considered to be ischaemic necrosis and related to the particular intrarenal arterial anatomy which results in the papillae having a rather tenuous blood supply through the vasa recta which descend through the pyramid from the cortico-medullary junction. Prior to the 1950s renal papillary necrosis (RPN) was seen only occasionally and usually as a complication of diabetes or acute ureteral obstruction with infection. About this time many cases of RPN resulting from analgesic nephropathy

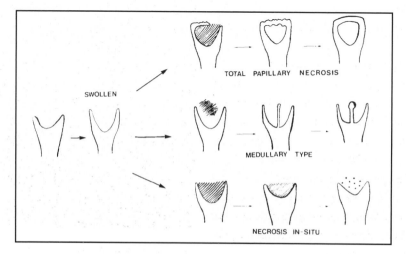

Fig. 11.24   Renal papillary necrosis. Diagram showing the patterns of sloughing which may follow the acute episode of papillary swelling.

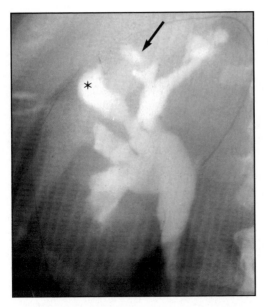

Fig. 11.25 Analgesic papillary necrosis. Total sloughing of a middle calyx (*), partial sloughing in calyx above (arrow) and mixed lesion at upper pole. Necrosis-in-situ of lower calyces. Similar lesions in left kidney.

were diagnosed, with a high incidence in Australia, and this continued until the 1980s when legislation and education concerning analgesics resulted in a dramatic and rapid decline in the incidence.

Causes of RPN

- Diabetes.
- Ureteric obstruction with infection above.
- Analgesics.
- Sickle cell disease (prevalent in the USA).

Radiological appearances

The urographic manifestations of RPN are varied and can be confused with other pathology. The extent of necrosis within a papilla may vary and three degrees are described in order of decreasing severity (Figs 11.24,11.25).

a. Total papillary sloughing

The entire papilla becomes necrotic and sloughs away leaving, at first, an irregular papillary bed which becomes smoother in outline, resulting in a clubbed calyx on urography.

b. Partial papillary sloughing

The necrotic focus involves only the central portion of the papilla. Softening of the lesion leads to a communication with the calyx through a sinus which drains through the papillary tip. On urography, the typical lesion is a single contrast filled cavity placed centrally in the papilla, the so-called 'ball in a cup' appearance.

c. Necrosis in-situ

In the mildest form only very small foci of necrosis occur in the papilla and no communication with the calyx occurs. The necrotic tissue is replaced by connective tissue and calcification may occur in the necrotic papillary focus. The papillary shape is preserved on urography, although the papillae are smaller.

Complications

A totally sloughed papilla may remain in the calyx and it may be difficult to appreciate that it has separated on urography (Fig. 11.26). Papillae may fragment and be passed in the urine to leave an

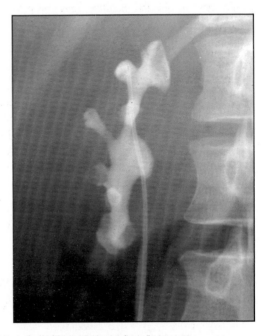

Fig. 11.26 Analgesic papillary necrosis. Poor renal function. Retrograde pyelogram. Sloughed papilla in uppermost calyx of this small kidney. Left kidney similar.

empty clubbed calyx. Papillary fragments may cause ureteric obstruction. Papillary residues may act as a nidus and calcify, behaving as other urinary calculi. The presence of an opaque calculus with a radiolucent centre should always suggest the possibility of RPN.

Transitional cell carcinoma incidence is significantly increased throughout the urinary tract in analgesic nephropathy.

'Clubbed' calyces

Loss of papillae results in calyces having a rounded or clubbed appearance on pyelography rather than the normal conical indentation. Loss of papillary impressions and clubbing occurs in a number of the conditions already described:

- Reflux nephropathy.
- Back pressure atrophy.
- Papillary necrosis.
- Tuberculosis.

11.9 Bladder Neck Obstruction

Interference with bladder emptying, and sometimes the development of acute retention, may occur at any age. Most common is the transient dysfunctional retention which may follow abdominal operations or trauma. Leaving these aside the commonest causes are included in the following list:

a. Mechanical

i. Children and infants

Posterior urethral valves (males).

ii. Adult males

Prostatomegaly – hyperplasia or neoplasia. Acute prostatitis. Urethral stricture.

iii. Adult females

Pregnant uterus at term. Retroverted gravid uterus usually at about five months gestation. Massive uterine fibroids. Uterine prolapse (procidentia).

b. Functional

i. Drugs

Certain drugs may contribute to disturbed bladder emptying:

- Drugs with an anticholinergic effect e.g. tricyclic antidepressants.
- Drugs which stimulate sympathetic receptors in the bladder wall, e.g. ephedrine.
- Diuretics including alcohol.

ii. Neurological abnormalities

Multiple sclerosis. Cauda equina tumours. Elderly males with a neurogenic bladder are frequently misdiagnosed because the altered micturition is attributed to prostatism.

Clinical presentation

Patients with interference of bladder emptying may present with:

- Dysuria.
- Acute retention of urine.
- Chronic retention with overflow.
  These patients present usually with dribbling incontinence.
- Chronic renal failure (the sequel to longstanding obstruction).

Careful clinical history and detailed examination including suprapubic percussion will usually point to the diagnosis in the majority of cases. Radiology may be helpful in confirming the diagnosis and also provides information significant in further management.

Prostatism

In the older population benign prostatic hypertrophy (BPH) and carcinoma of the prostate (CA) are the common causes of bladder neck obstruction (BNO). The severity of the BNO and the level of inconvenience to the patient is very variable. Managing such cases requires careful assessment of the following matters by the clinician, and to some degree by the patient.

1. Are symptoms due to BPH or CA?

Although transrectal US displays the internal architecture of the prostate in some detail, it does not differentiate the nature of nodules, which are usually echolucent (Fig. 11.27). Most clinicians rely on the **prostatic specific antigen (PSA)** test together with the assessment of the prostate digitally per rectum. Should the results be suspicious of CA then transrectal US is performed to demonstrate the anatomy. Nodules detected are then biopsied and several biopsies are taken from the prostate elsewhere. If carcinoma is detected there may be an indication for radical prostatectomy. In making that assessment a radionuclide bone scan is usually indicated to detect distant metastases.

2. What are the effects of BNO?

The following objective tests are frequently used to assess the effects of BNO which include residual urine, bladder trabeculation, diverticulum formation, poor urinary stream and, in time, renal failure.

a. Ultrasound

US allows for approximate assessment of residual urine in the bladder, assuming the bladder to be roughly spherical in shape (Fig. 11.28). Bladder volume is assessed before and after micturition from the dimensions of the bladder displayed in various projections. US also demonstrates dilated ureters and the width of the renal parenchyma.

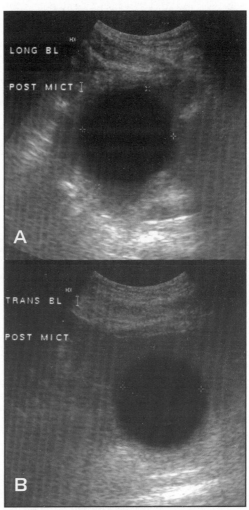

Fig. 11.28 Residual bladder volume measurement. Transabdominal US. (A) Sagittal view shows the bladder depth and length. (B) Transverse view shows the width. Assessed residue was 75 mL.

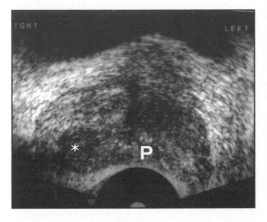

Fig. 11.27 Transrectal prostate US. Non-specific nodular area (*) was carcinoma on biopsy. Note the slightly more echogenic peripheral zone (P).

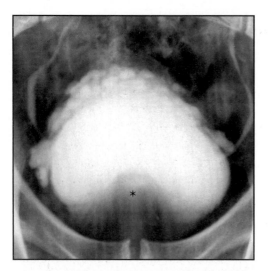

Fig. 11.29 Benign prostatomegaly. IVU. The dense bladder contrast indicates good renal function. The ureters are not dilated but the bladder is heavily trabeculated with a prostatic filling defect (*).

b. Serum creatinine

This provides a further check on the influence of BNO on renal function.

c. Weakness of urinary stream

A flow test is available which allows quantitative assessment of the rate of bladder emptying, which may act as a basis for comparison after surgery.

d. IVU

Patients with BNO complicated by haematuria or symptoms suggesting urinary calculi or severe infection, where an overview of the urinary tract is required, are usually referred for IVU. In the elderly with BNO the urogram should be limited to a plain radiograph, one or two films following contrast injection and an after-micturition film (Fig. 11.29).

3. Management decisions

Carcinoma

Apart from clinical matters, e.g. age and general health, the decision as to whether radical prostatectomy is recommended or conservative management depends on evidence of whether local or distant spread of the tumour has occurred. Local spread may be detected by transrectal US. CT or MRI provides information concerning abdominal metastases particularly to pelvic and para-aortic lymph nodes. Radionuclide bone scan is used to detect skeletal metastases.

Benign prostatic hypertrophy

A decision is required as to whether treatment is necessary, and if so whether it be medical or surgical. Drug treatment of BPH has had limited success but improvements are expected. Transurethral resection (TUR) is the usual operation, but is not without complications. Failure of ejaculation may result and, particularly in large prostates, haemorrhage may require blood transfusion. Urologists carefully assess the situation with their patients prior to recommending therapy. In making the decision the following are significant.

1. *Demonstrable effects of BNO (see above).*

2. *Severity of symptoms*

   Nowadays urologists adopt a more quantitative approach to assessing the symptoms of BNO by scoring such symptoms as sensation of incomplete emptying, frequency, intermittency, urgency, weak stream, straining, and nocturia.

3. *Effect on quality of life*

   Many urologists quantitate the attitude of patients to their problem by the response given to the question 'How would you feel if the urinary symptoms were to continue for the rest of your life?'

11.10 Urethral Obstruction

Ascending retrograde urethrography is the investigation of choice to demonstrate the male urethra. The contrast medium is injected from the external urethral meatus after local anaesthesia (Fig. 11.30A).

Stricture

Strictures in the membranous urethra result from pelvic fractures. Gonococcal strictures and traumatic strictures (Fig. 11.30B) following a fall astride involve the bulbous urethra, whilst strictures resulting from indwelling catheters tend to involve the anterior penile urethra.

Posterior urethral valves

The condition is seen in about 1 in 6,000 male births but is extremely rare in females. More severe cases are detected during antenatal US when distension of the bladder and frequently the pelvicalyceal systems is detected. Because back pressure atrophy of the kidneys may occur during the latter stages of pregnancy interventional methods have been developed to overcome the back pressure until birth. About 50% of patients with the condition present in the first few months of life when transabdominal US can be used to assess the kidneys and upper urinary tract. Transperineal US during micturition sometimes shows the abnormality but MCU is the definitive test demonstrating dilatation of the urethra down to the level of the obstruction (Fig. 11.31). Valves cause a characteristic defect in the contrast column. VUR is a common accompaniment of the condition and is also well seen on the MCU.

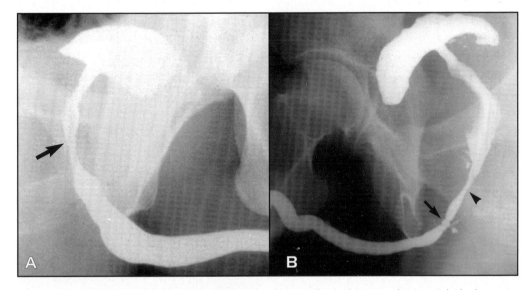

Fig. 11.30 Ascending retrograde urethrography. (A) Normal urethrogram. The membranous urethra (arrow) divides the anterior urethra below from the posterior urethra above. Note the central filling defect in the posterior urethra due to the verumontanum. (B) The posterior urethra above the membranous portion (arrowhead) is elongated and irregular resulting from previous transurethral prostatic resection with regrowth. Severe stricturing (arrow) is seen in the bulbous portion of the anterior urethra as a result of previous gonococcal infection.

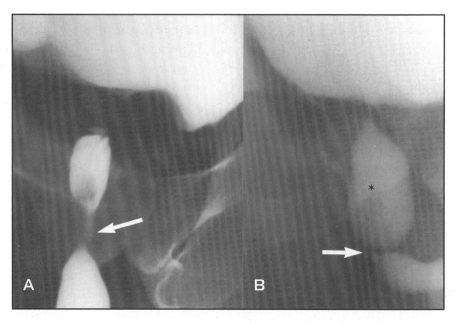

Fig. 11.31 Congenital posterior urethral valves. (A) Retrograde urethrogram showing a narrowing just below the verumontanum (arrow). (B) Micturating urethrogram. The localized narrowing is clearly contrasted with the dilated prostatic urethra (*).

11.11 Scrotum and Penis

Scrotum

Clinical problems in this region which may require diagnostic imaging include:

- Development of an **acute scrotum** associated with pain and swelling.
- A gradually enlarging **scrotal mass,** usually less painful.
- Search for an **occult primary tumour**.
- Search for an **undescended testis**.

Acute scrotum

Epididymitis and epididymo-orchitis and torsion of the testis, the commonest causes, require differentiation as torsion if neglected for more than about six hours results in loss of function, atrophy and in some necrosis. Torsion may occur at any age but the vast majority occur about the time of puberty. Colour Doppler US should be performed when torsion is suspected as it can show the loss of blood supply to the testis, an indication for surgery. Of all young people presenting with an acute scrotum only

less than 30% require open surgery and US is proving of great benefit in reducing unnecessary exploration. Torsion is likely to occur in cases where the attachment of the testis to the soft tissues is not broadly based, but by a pedicle, the so-called 'bell clapper' testis, and US can demonstrate this clearly.

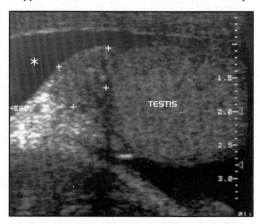

Fig. 11.32 Acute scrotal pain and swelling. US shows an hydrocoele (*) and normal testis. The head of the epididymus (marked) is swollen consistent with epididymitis.

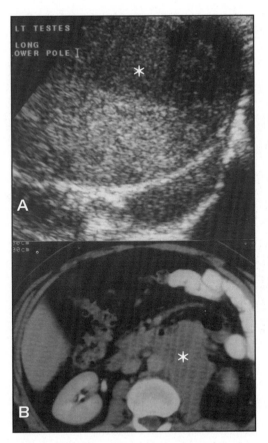

Fig. 11.33 Testicular germ cell tumour. (A) The hypoechoic tumour anteriorly (*) is well demarcated from the normal testicular echo pattern posteriorly. (B) Contrast-enhanced CT shows enlarged matted lymph nodes (*) at the typical drainage site in the para-aortic region.

Scrotal swelling

Ultrasound is the primary investigation and can clearly display hydrocoeles, cysts of epididymis and testis, varicocoeles and tumours. In particular, it can demonstrate the state of the testis hidden by a hydrocoele (Fig. 11.32). The range of germ cell and stromal tumours of the testis and also lymphoma may be shown, but US appearances, in which the abnormal tissues are hypoechoic, are quite nonspecific (Fig. 11.33). CT is used for staging testicular neoplasms, particularly for demonstrating the para-aortic nodes and is approximately 90% accurate.

Searching for an occult primary

Occasionally testicular metastases are much larger than the primary and are the main presenting feature in such cases. Ultrasound may reveal a small primary lesion in the testis.

Undescended testis

Ultrasound is useful in demonstrating an undescended testis in the inguinal canal, but if it lies in the retroperitoneum CT and particularly MRI are more effective. The increased risk of a malignant neoplasm developing in such a testis is well recognized.

Penis

Male impotence has many causes. A vascular cause is suspected when the intracavernous injection of vaso-active drugs fails to induce erection, and US is the initial imaging investigation. Adequate arterial blood supply and effective venous closure are both necessary to sustain erection and US flow tracings of the cavernosal arteries can demonstrate the status of both. In some cases further investigation by selective internal iliac arteriography or by intracavernous venography may be indicated (Fig. 11.34).

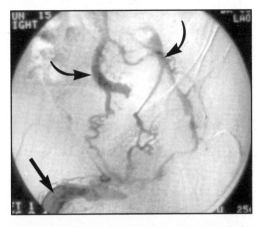

Fig. 11.34 Penile venogram. Contrast injection into a corpus cavernosum (arrow) shows flow via the prostatic plexus to the internal iliac veins (curved arrows) indicating failure of venous closure.

11.12 Urinary Tract Trauma

A degree of haematuria is common following blunt trauma to the trunk or the pelvis. The damage may be to the kidney, bladder or urethra, but rarely the ureter. Other intra-abdominal organs and the diaphragm may be damaged also (see Chapter 12). Clinically, it is usually possible to determine whether the damage is to the upper or lower urinary tract. The presence of pelvic fractures and blood at the external urethral meatus point to damage below, whilst loin tenderness and lower rib fractures suggest the upper tract.

Monitoring the progress

It is useful to keep a sample of each urine specimen passed in a test tube and to place these tubes in a rack. In this way it is possible, over a period of days, to determine easily whether the haematuria is abating or not.

Urinary tract injuries

Kidney

Developmentally fused kidneys, e.g. horseshoe kidney (Fig. 11.35) are more prone to traumatic injury.

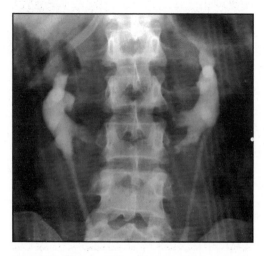

Fig. 11.35 Horseshoe kidney. The lower poles overlap the psoas margins and lower pole calyces are directed medially.

Three main categories of injury are recognized:

1. Contused kidney

In these cases, the renal capsule remains intact. The swelling of the renal parenchyma results in compression of the pelvicalyceal system and slight renal enlargement.

2. Ruptured renal parenchyma

When the capsule is torn, tension in the kidney is reduced and the calyces are no longer compressed. Administered contrast medium may be seen to track out through the rent in the capsule into the perinephric tissue.

3. Avulsed renal pedicle

The kidney becomes non-functioning with no excretion of contrast medium. Surprisingly, there may be very little, if any, retroperitoneal haemorrhage if prompt retraction of the artery occurs.

Ureter

An hydronephrotic renal pelvis may be ruptured from direct injury and very occasionally the ureter may be avulsed at the pelviureteric junction. However, the relatively thick-walled ureter throughout its length is rarely injured.

Bladder

1. Intraperitoneal rupture

Relatively uncommon. This results from blunt trauma to a distended bladder and the patient presents with signs of peritoneal irritation.

2. Extraperitoneal rupture

Because the peritoneum is reflected over the dome of the bladder, rupture, associated with pelvic fractures, is usually into the extraperitoneal space in the pelvis.

Urethra

1. Membranous urethra

Also associated with pelvic fractures complete or partial rupture may occur at the level of the perineal membrane.

2. Bulbous urethra

Classically resulting from a 'fall astride', disruption of the bulbous urethra may occur with the potential for later stricture formation.

Investigation and management

If clinically the damage is likely to be to the upper urinary tract and significant haematuria is present CT is indicated particularly if damage to other organs is likely. With less severe haematuria intravenous urography (IVU) or US may suffice to exclude major renal damage. On IVU a contused kidney retains renal outline but the calyces may be difficult to discern due to compression. On CT and US the perirenal tissues

appear relatively normal. With rupture of the renal capsule contrast may be seen leaking into the perirenal tissue and on CT or US the perirenal space is expanded by haematoma (Fig. 11.36). With avulsion of the renal pedicle non-function of the kidney is seen on IVU and CT and the obstructed renal artery may be seen on dynamic CT or aortography (Fig. 11.37).

Patients with pelvic fractures frequently have acute retention of urine, and in males it is important to differentiate in such cases between **extraperitoneal rupture of the bladder** and **ruptured membranous urethra**. Catheterization to relieve retention in a partially ruptured membranous urethra may convert the damage to complete rupture which is more likely to result in stricture formation later. In such patients an **ascending retrograde urethrogram** should be performed in the emergency department prior to

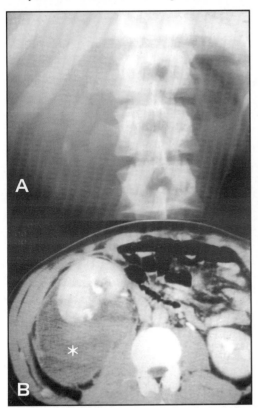

Fig. 11.36 Ruptured kidney. (A) The IVU shows poor excretion on the right with loss of the right psoas margin consistent with a perirenal mass. The details of the kidney damage are uncertain. (B) Contrast-enhanced CT in the same patient shows a very large right perirenal haematoma (*) with the right kidney largely intact. Conservative surgery followed.

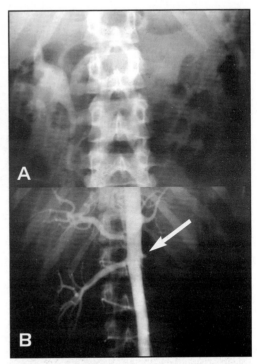

Fig. 11.37 Traumatic avulsion of renal pedicle. (A) IVU following injury shows no excretion on the left. The psoas margin is not clearly seen consistent with perirenal haemorrhage. (B) Aortogram showing occluded left renal artery near the origin (arrow).

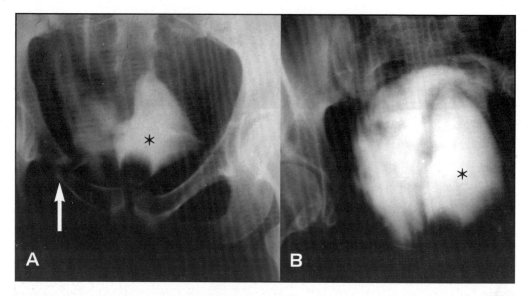

Fig. 11.38 Extraperitoneal rupture of the bladder. (A) Retrograde cystogram shows leakage of contrast from the bladder (*) into extraperitoneal tissue. Note fracture through the right pubic ramus (arrow). (B) With further filling the extraperitoneal fluid surrounds the bladder. Self-retaining balloon catheter in the bladder neck.

urethral catheterization. If patient discomfort due to retention is extreme then suprapubic needling of the bladder for relief should be performed as a preliminary. If the urethrogram, performed by injecting contrast into the external meatus shows a satisfactory passage to the bladder then a soft rubber catheter should be passed and contrast injected (Fig. 11.38). If peri-urethral extra-vasation occurs (Fig. 11.39), catheterization should not be performed and the assistance of a urologist is indicated. **Intraperitoneal rupture** is less common, resulting from direct trauma to a full bladder and the patients present with peritonitis (Fig. 11.40).

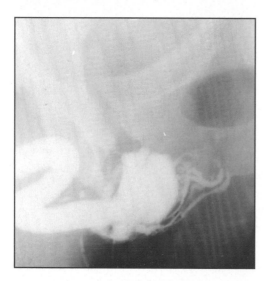

Fig. 11.39 Retrograde urethrogram in patient with pelvic trauma. Rupture of the membranous urethra has allowed extravasation of contrast medium into soft tissue and veins.

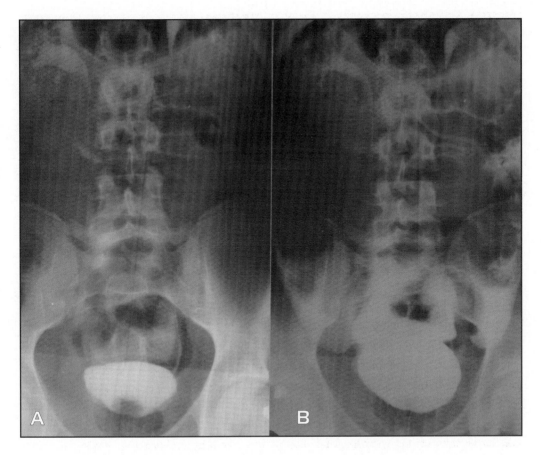

Fig. 11.40 Intraperitoneal rupture of the bladder. (A) IVU shows no leakage of contrast from the bladder, which contains a catheter and is elevated. (B) Cystogram via the catheter shows leakage to the left paracolic gutter.

Reference

Pollack, H. M. (ed.), *Clinical Urography*.
W. B. Saunders Co., Philadelphia, 1990.

Abdominal Emergencies

Acute onset of abdominal symptoms, usually pain, may be due to a wide range of pathological conditions including inflammations, perforations, obstructions, torsions, and haemorrhage. Such patients pose particular diagnostic problems because:

1. Prompt surgical intervention may be required.
2. The patient is often distressed and only limited investigation is warranted before commencing treatment.

Information obtained from the history and careful bedside clinical examination will indicate the probable nature of the intra-abdominal pathology. The decision to further clarify the diagnosis by investigations will depend on the time available, the degree of confidence in the clinical diagnosis, and the imaging resources available. In patients requiring urgent intervention immediate **exploratory laparotomy** may be obligatory. With more time available investigations are warranted to confirm the clinical diagnosis and provide additional detail, or, in some cases, to obtain a diagnosis as a basis for management.

When the diagnosis is obscure

When the nature of acute abdominal pain is uncertain CT scanning is recommended as providing the best overview of both the intraperitoneal and retroperitoneal tissues. Particularly with upper abdominal pain it is important to remember that myocardial infarction may be a cause in adults, whilst lower lobe pneumonia may be the cause in children.

When a confident clinical diagnosis is made

According to the clinical diagnosis specific investigations are recommended to confirm the clinical opinion and to provide further information which may assist in management. These particular investigations are dealt with in the following sections.

12.1 Acute Peritonitis

Peritoneal irritation, manifest clinically by release tenderness and muscle guarding or rigidity, is a common accompaniment of pathology involving abdominal organs. Occasionally peritonitis may be primary, eg. tuberculosis. Frequently, the locality of these signs suggests the underlying diagnosis and determines the appropriate investigations. If the diagnosis remains obscure, and time permits, CT may prove helpful.

A diagnosis of **acute appendicitis,** particularly in the male, generally requires no radiological investigations. In women pelvic inflammatory disease, ovarian pathology, or ruptured ectopic pregnancy may also cause right iliac fossa pain and US is recommended in patients where doubt arises. Evidence of acute appendicitis may be seen on US or CT (Fig. 12.1).

A diagnosis of **acute cholecystitis** (see section 9.3) may be confirmed with US by demonstrating gallstones, which are usually present, thickening of the gall bladder wall, and, in some cases, pericholecystic fluid collections.

When **acute pancreatitis** is suspected clinically, differentiation from a perforated peptic ulcer, which also results in upper abdominal peritonitis, may be difficult. Erect chest radiography is important to demonstrate the presence of free gas following perforation, and if gas is not present CT is indicated (see section 10.11).

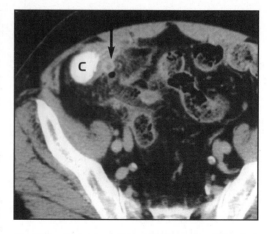

Fig. 12.1 Acute appendicitis. CT shows the thick-walled dilated appendix (arrow) is associated with a small gas collection next to it suggesting local perforation. Caecum (C).

12.2 Free Intraperitoneal Gas

The PA chest film made erect is used to demonstrate quite small amounts of gas beneath the diaphragm (Fig. 12.2). If the patient is unable to sit up, then a left lateral decubitus view using a horizontal x-ray beam is satisfactory. The air is then seen lying between the liver and the right lateral lower chest wall.

Free intraperitoneal gas results from rupture of an intraperitoneal gas-containing structure or is introduced artificially.

Causes:

- Postoperative.
- Perforated peptic ulcer.
- Perforated diverticulitis.
- Via the female genital tract.
- Pneumatosis coli.

Gas introduced at operation absorbs over several days. An increase in the volume of gas in the postoperative period suggests leakage from the gastrointestinal tract. Most patients with perforation of a peptic ulcer present with severe peritoneal irritation. The presence of free gas helps to distinguish the condition from acute pancreatitis and other conditions which might be confusing. The absence of free gas does not exclude an intraperitoneal rupture of a peptic ulcer, as the sign is dependent on the upper gastrointestinal tract containing swallowed air. In older patients, and if symptoms are atypical for ulcer, the possibility of a perforated large bowel

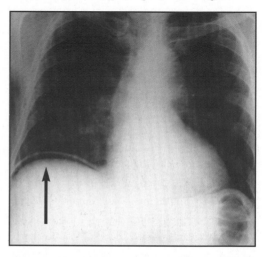

Fig. 12.2 Erect chest film showing a small amount of free intraperitoneal gas beneath the right hemidiaphragm (arrow).

diverticulum should be considered, particularly when planning the site of the operative incision.

Gas introduced via the female genital tract in tests for tubal patency (Rubin's test) may be associated with some degree of peritoneal irritation and shoulder tip pain.

Pneumatosis coli is a most unusual condition in which gas cysts are scattered along the length of the bowel, particularly the large bowel. Occasionally the cysts rupture causing peritoneal irritation and rarely a small amount of free gas is seen beneath the diaphragm. The gas cysts may be seen sometimes on plain films but barium enema or CT is necessary to confirm the diagnosis (Fig. 12.3).

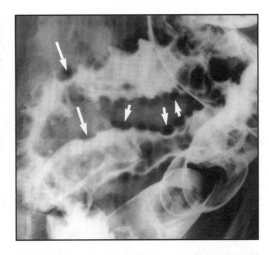

Fig. 12.3 Pneumatosis coli. The gas containing cysts within the bowel wall produce polypoid indentations in the barium and appear radiolucent (arrows).

12.3 Abdominal Abscesses

Although plain radiography may show gas within an abscess, and in a subphrenic abscess show elevation of a hemidiaphragm with, perhaps, a small pleural effusion, CT generally is indicated as the first investigation, particularly when the abscess site is indefinite. Because abscesses containing air can be confused with bowel loops, it is essential that oral contrast medium should be given prior to CT (Fig. 12.4). In specific sites US demonstrates abscesses well, particularly subphrenic, perirenal and deep in the pelvis. Elsewhere, gas-filled bowel causes US interference. Intravenous injection of a sample of the patients leucocytes labelled with Technetium may be used to show the inflammatory nature of an abdominal collection. By 72 hours the patient's labelled white cells can be detected in the abscess (Fig. 12.5). Most abscesses can be drained and treated using interventional radiological methods in conjunction with systemic antibiotic therapy.

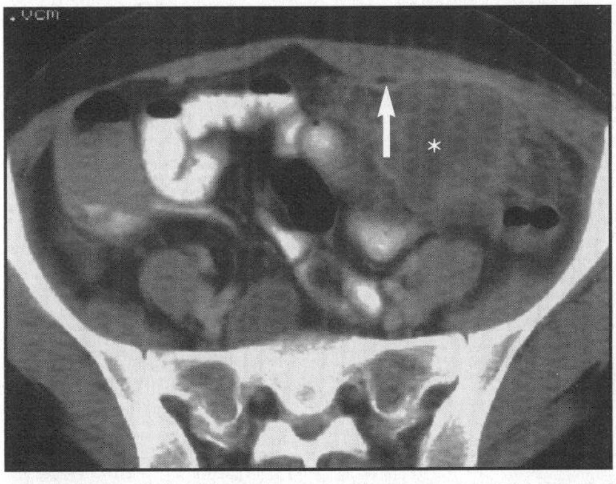

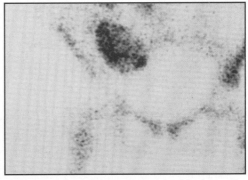

Fig. 12.4 Paracolic abscess. (*) in left iliac fossa. CT shows the loculated collection adherent to the anterior abdominal wall. Note the small gas collection (arrow).

Fig. 12.5 Abdominal abscess in right iliac fossa. The patient's white blood cells were labelled with radionuclide, re-injected and were taken up in the abscess wall.

12.4 Acute Intestinal Obstruction

The presence of intestinal obstruction (Figs 12.6, 12.7) is diagnosed clinically and in many cases the level and degree of obstruction and the cause can be determined satisfactorily. Radiology is used to confirm the clinical findings and establish the level of obstruction, and in some cases the nature of the pathology. From amongst the many possible causes of bowel obstruction this list includes most.

Mechanical

In the lumen

• Foreign bodies, including gallstones.

In the wall

• Carcinoma, diverticulitis, Crohn's disease, lymphoma.

Outside the wall

• Postoperative adhesions, peritoneal metastases, hernia, sigmoid and caecal volvulus.

Functional

• Paralytic ileus.
• Toxic megacolon.

The most common cause by far is postoperative adhesions so the presence of an abdominal scar is highly significant. The absence of an abdominal scar should be recorded in the clinical notes when referring a patient for radiology because it is important information for the radiologist interpreting the films.

Plain radiology should include:

• PA erect chest film.
• AP supine abdomen.
• AP erect abdomen.
• Right and left lateral decubitus views of the abdomen, particularly for those who cannot sit up.

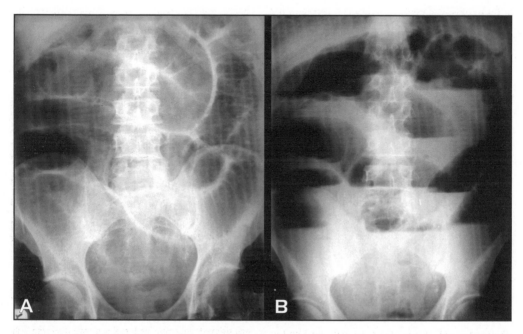

Fig. 12.6 Small bowel obstruction: supine (A) and erect (B) views. Note the absence of large bowel content. The band of soft tissue between adjacent gas-filled loops in the supine view indicates the width of the combined bowel walls; normal in this case.

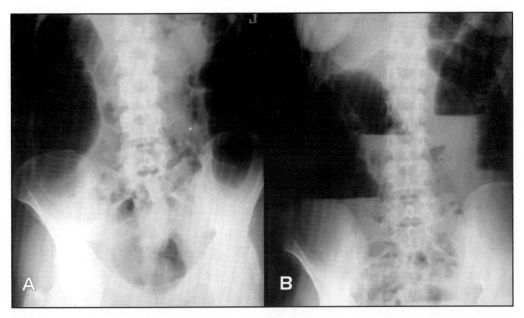

Fig. 12.7 Large bowel obstruction: supine (A) and erect (B) views. Gas-distended colon, but not rectum, with fluid levels consistent with obstruction in the distal descending colon.

Mechanical obstruction

The evidence for mechanical intestinal obstruction can be grouped as follows:

- Accumulation of material proximal to the obstruction.
- Absence of material beyond the obstruction.
- Evidence of the obstructing lesion itself.
- Complications, particularly perforation.

1. Accumulation of materials proximal to the obstruction

Fluid, gas and, in the large bowel, faeces, accumulate proximal to a site of obstruction. The result is distension of bowel loops and this can be assessed if there is sufficient gas within the bowel to demonstrate the luminal width. The upper limits of normal for various levels of bowel is given as:

Jejunum   3 cm

Ileum   2 cm

It is important for students to realize that the presence of air-fluid levels within the small bowel in the erect film is not, per se, a sign of bowel obstruction. Most bowel gas is swallowed and as the small bowel content is normally fluid, there will usually be air-fluid levels in an erect film. In patients with very little bowel gas a clue to the presence of obstruction can be obtained from the supine view in which small ellipses of gas accumulate anteriorly in the bowel, separated by the mucosal folds, giving an appearance sometimes referred to as 'the necklace of death' because of the poor prognosis in what are often very debilitated patients (Fig. 12.8).

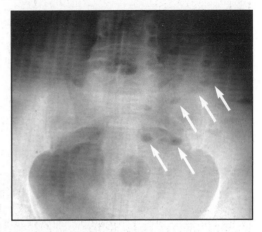

Fig. 12.8 Small bowel obstruction: supine view, in a patient with delayed diagnosis. The bowel is grossly distended with fluid but very little air, which is arranged in rows ('necklace of death') (arrows).

With large bowel obstruction there may be extreme ballooning of the caecum, but in the majority of cases the ileocaecal valve becomes incompetent so that small bowel distension develops secondarily. The degree of tone and peristalsis in small bowel loops may be gauged from the erect abdomen film. With mechanical obstruction, if a moderately large amount of gas is present in a loop it will be noted that the fluid levels in the two limbs of the loop are at slightly different levels. If the tone is lost, as in paralytic ileus, levels tend to equalise and the bowel lumen dilates further.

2. Absence of materials beyond the obstruction

This is equally important in establishing the diagnosis of bowel obstruction. Clinically an empty rectum is a significant finding. The absence of gas, fluid and faeces beyond an obstruction is expected in mechanical obstructions which have persisted for some hours.

3. Evidence of the cause of obstruction

Plain radiography is very limited in providing this information. However, sometimes it can be quite specific.

In gallstone ileus (Chapter 9, Fig. 9.16), as a result of a fistula between the gall bladder and the gut, a gallstone obstructs the small bowel, usually ileum, but it takes quite a large stone to do it, i.e. more than 1.5 cm across. Sometimes the calcified stone itself can be detected, but this is difficult because it usually overlies the pelvic bones. More frequently the clue is given by the presence of gas in the biliary tree.

With sigmoid volvulus (Fig. 12.9) the greatly distended sigmoid loop can usually be identified extending upwards and to the right and containing long fluid levels. The large bowel proximally is usually not distended to anywhere near the same degree as in simple large bowel obstruction, pointing to the closed loop nature of the volvulus.

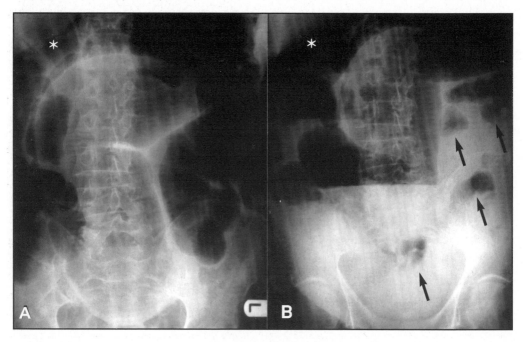

Fig. 12.9 Sigmoid volvulus: supine (A) and erect (B) views. Grossly gas-distended sigmoid loop (*) is displaced upwards and to the right over the liver. Note the absence of gas in the rectum and the only slightly-dilated loops of small bowel (arrows).

Caecal volvulus (Fig. 12.10) is less easily recognized. The gas-distended caecum twists to take up a position in the left upper quadrant of the abdomen, having an appearance very suggestive of a gas-distended stomach. The absence of the caecum from the iliac fossa and its replacement with small bowel loops is a further clue.

4. Complications of bowel obstruction

CT is used frequently to provide additional information concerning the obstructing lesion, particularly to detect neoplastic masses, intussusceptions and bowel wall thickening, e.g. in Crohn's disease (see Chapters 7 and 8).

It is important to inspect the erect chest film for the presence of gas beneath the diaphragm, indicating rupture of the distended bowel. Also, a generalized hazy opacity of the entire abdomen in the supine film with loss of the soft tissue landmarks, i.e. psoas margins, is consistent with the presence of ascites.

Functional obstruction

Differentiating paralytic ileus from mechanical obstruction may be difficult at times radiologically.

Paralytic ileus usually affects the entire bowel so that dilatation extends to the rectum with air fluid levels throughout small and large bowel (Fig. 12.11). Small bowel loops lack tone so that the levels in the two limbs of an individual loop come to the same height in the erect film. Occasionally paralytic ileus may be localized to a segment of small intestine, e.g. if lying in a pelvic abscess, and differentiation from mechanical obstruction is difficult.

Toxic megacolon (Chapter 8, Fig. 8.10), a complication of ulcerative colitis, may present with absolute constipation and unless fulminating ulcerative colitis is suspected clinically the films may be misinterpreted.

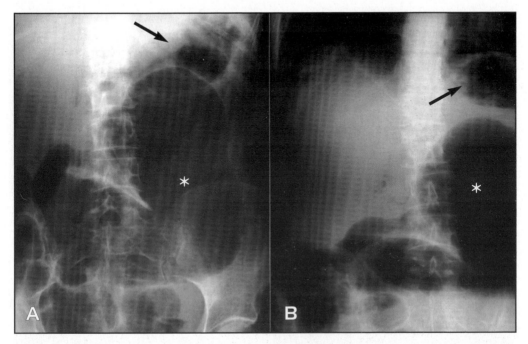

Fig. 12.10 Caecal volvulus: supine (A) and erect (B) views. The twisted gas-distended caecum is displaced towards the left to a position simulating the stomach (*). However, the gastric air bubble (arrow) can be seen above. Small bowel occupies the right iliac fossa.

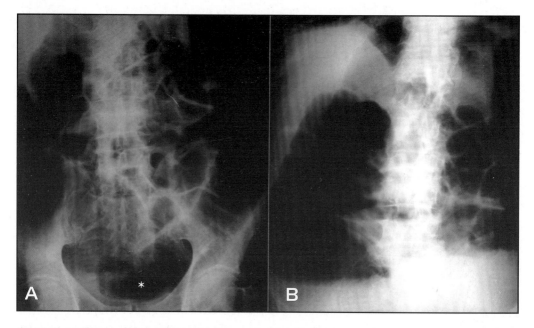

Fig. 12.11 Paralytic ileus following lumbar sympathectomy: supine (A) and erect (B) views. Large and small bowel distended with gas extending to the rectum (asterisk).

Repeat examinations in suspected bowel obstruction —

the value of water soluble contrast medium (Fig. 12.12)

In many cases intestinal obstruction is incomplete and management is conservative with careful monitoring of progress. Often, further plain films of the abdomen are requested after 24 to 48 hours to

show variation in the degree of intestinal distension. However, these follow-up studies are difficult to interpret. Much more information, particularly concerning the obstructing lesion, is obtained if water-soluble contrast medium, Gastrografin, is present in the intestine at the time of the follow-up request when, in addition to further plain films, CT may be performed. It is recommended that in cases of intestinal obstruction in which an operation is not performed immediately, oral Gastrografin be given through the intragastric tube after aspirating the stomach. Further gastric aspiration should be delayed for four hours to allow the Gastrografin to proceed down the small intestine. Management should continue along usual lines but if follow-up views are required, say after 24 hours, then the presence of the positive contrast material provides much more information. Gastrografin has the following advantages:

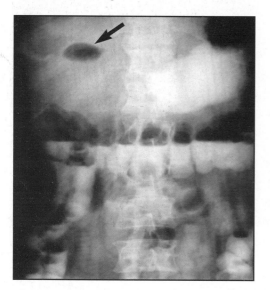

Fig. 12.12 Use of water-soluble contrast (Gastrografin; Schering) in suspected bowel obstruction. Erect view shows contrast in large bowel, excluding obstruction, and an abscess (air-fluid level) in the gall bladder area (arrow).

- It demonstrates the degree of dilatation of the bowel (only shown by gas on plain films).
- It provides more specific information concerning the degree of obstruction and the nature of the lesion.
- It diffuses through segments of paralytic ileus.

- If it enters the peritoneal cavity it causes no reaction (barium produces dense fibrosis).
- It is hypertonic, acting as a mild purgative, which frequently has dramatic therapeutic effects in mild degrees of obstruction!

12.5 Gastro-Intestinal Obstruction in Infants

Radiology may provide helpful supportive evidence in the diagnosis of obstructive lesions occurring in the first two years of life. Plain radiography demonstrates the presence of air in the bowel, which reaches the stomach within 2 hours of birth, the small bowel by 6 hours and the rectum by about 24 hours. Unlike the adult the distinction between small and large bowel is often difficult in this age group.

Hypertrophic pyloric stenosis

Non-bilious vomiting developing in the first two months of life suggests hypertrophy of the pylorus and a mass may be palpable clinically. If so, surgery is often performed without radiology. If confirmation is required US does so by showing the ovoid mass of hypertrophied muscle (Fig. 12.13A). In less definite cases a barium study is indicated to assess the degree of pyloric obstruction (Fig. 12.13B).

Duodenal atresia
Midgut volvulus

These conditions commonly occur in association with polyhydramnois. Duodenal atresia may be associated with Down's syndrome, and on a plain film the gas-distended duodenum and stomach give a 'double-bubble' sign (Fig. 12.14). With volvulus involving the small intestine the plain film shows gas extending further down into the abdomen.

Meconium ileus
Hirschsprung's Disease

If obstruction is suspected in a neonate and the plain film shows gas-filled bowel throughout the abdomen except the rectum these conditions should be considered. Inspissated meconium is common in cystic fibrosis and a barium enema using water-

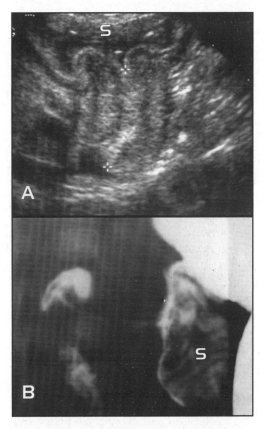

Fig. 12.13 Hypertrophic pyloric stenosis in an infant. (A) US shows the hypertrophied cuff of muscle (between +'s). (B) Barium shows the elongated narrowed segment. Stomach (S).

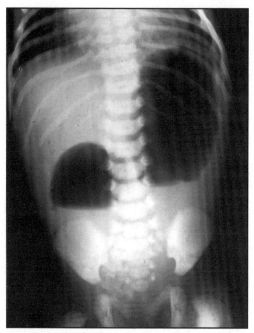

Fig. 12.14 Duodenal atresia in neonate with Down's syndrome. Gasless abdomen apart from the 'double bubble' in stomach and duodenum.

soluble contrast medium demonstrates the **microcolon**, a result of non-function in foetal life. In Hirschsprung's disease, considered due to absent neural cells in a distal colon segment, barium enema may show the narrowed segment with dilated colon proximally.

Intussusception in infants is referred to in section 7.3 and ***tracheo-oesophageal fistula*** in section 6.3.

12.6 Acute Gastro-Intestinal Bleeding

Patients sometimes present with life-threatening acute blood loss from the gastro-intestinal tract. The principles of management are:

- Replacement of blood loss.
- Control of the bleeding point.

It is necessary to diagnose the site of bleeding and this may be difficult. The clinical history is crucial. Bright blood per rectum points to a large bowel or distal small bowel source, whilst haematemesis points to upper tract bleeding. Melaena favours haemorrhage above the level of the mid-small intestine, and is most frequently due to duodenal ulcer.

Upper GI tract bleeding

The commonest causes of bleeding from the oesophagus, stomach, duodenum and proximal small bowel are:

1. Peptic ulceration – acute or chronic.
2. Oesophageal varices.
3. Mallory–Weiss tear of the oesophageal mucosa.
4. Carcinoma of the stomach.

There may be a history of proven peptic ulceration which provides a clue. Remember, however, that patients with oesophageal varices frequently have gastric ulceration which may be the site of bleeding, and not the varices.

The generally accepted protocol for investigation is:

1. Endoscopy

This provides the answer in about 90% of cases and allows for injection sclerotherapy, particularly in varices. Very severe haemorrhages may obscure the endoscopist's view and consideration is given then to performing immediate surgery after resuscitation or performing arteriography with a view to embolisation of the bleeding site.

2. Arteriography

With rapid haemorrhage from the upper gastro-intestinal tract selective coeliac and superior mesenteric arteriography may demonstrate the site of bleeding. Superselective placement of the catheter into the feeding vessel provides the opportunity of injecting vasoconstrictor substances and particulate emboli and this has proven effective in a range of conditions. The method is useful in severely debilitated patients not fit for surgery (Fig. 12.15).

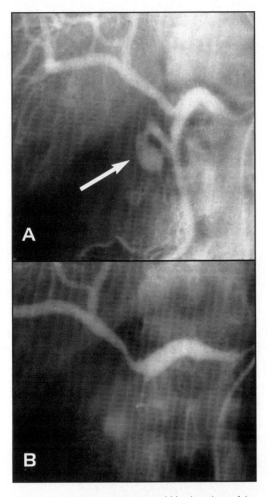

Fig. 12.15 (A) Upper gastro-intestinal bleeding due to false aneurysm (arrow) on gastroduodenal artery following pancreatitis. (B) Aneurysm obliterated with coils and emboli introduced by selective catheterization.

3. Barium meal

Barium studies have limited application in severe acute upper tract bleeding. If endoscopy proves negative and the patient is fit to attend the radiology department then a barium meal should certainly be performed as the bleeding abates.

Lower GI tract bleeding

The commonest causes of bleeding from the distal small bowel and the large intestine are:

1. Haemorrhoids.
2. Diverticular disease.
3. Polyps – benign and malignant.
4. Colitis – ischaemic, ulcerative and occasionally Crohn's disease.
5. Angiodysplasia – this abnormality of blood vessels in the submucosa of the colon, usually right side, has been identified in elderly patients as a source of severe haemorrhage. The cause of the abnormality is unknown. On arteriography abnormal vessels may be seen in the bowel wall.
6. Meckel's diverticulum – said to be the commonest congenital abnormality of the gut. It usually arises within 50 cm of the ileocaecal valve from the antimesenteric border of the ileum. It occurs in about 3% of individuals but is symptomatic in very few, and then usually in childhood. Acid-secreting gastric mucosa within the diverticulum may result in peptic ulceration and bleeding and should be thought of particularly in the younger age groups with rectal bleeding.

Clinically, conditions such as haemorrhoids should be diagnosed without difficulty. The commonest cause of severe bleeding is diverticulosis in the elderly and it may be extremely difficult to determine which of a large number of diverticula is the offending one. The protocol recommended for patients with lower GI tract haemorrhage is:

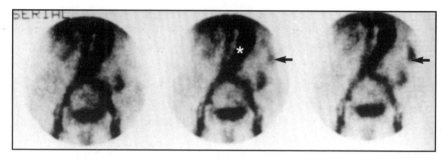

Fig. 12.16 Profuse bleeding from diverticulum in descending colon. Technetium-labelled red cell scans at two-minute intervals show the bleeding site (arrow). Note aneurysmal aorta (*).

1. Plain radiography

Generally plain films do not assist but should be performed. Occasionally toxic megacolon, a manifestation of acute ulcerative colitis, may be associated with severe bleeding and can be recognized on plain films. The mucosal changes of ischaemic colitis may also show up in gas-filled segments of colon.

2. Technetium-labelled red cell scan

The use of serial Technetium-labelled red cell scans (Fig. 12.16) can help in indicating the general region of bleeding. The red cells which pass into the lumen of the gut accumulate and the localized gamma emission can be detected if scans are made over a number of hours. However, because the red cells migrate along the gut the site of maximum intensity does not necessarily coincide with the site of bleeding, particularly in cases where the bleeding is at a slow rate.

3. Arteriography

If bleeding is proceeding at the rate of 2 mL per minute the bleeding site may be detected by selective arterial studies. If the Technetium red cell scan is negative there is little point in performing arteriography. If a bleeding point is found in the small or large bowel by arteriography then a vasoconstrictor drug can be infused in an attempt to control the bleeding (Fig. 12.17).

4. Barium enema

Although previously the main diagnostic investigation for lower tract bleeding, it has many

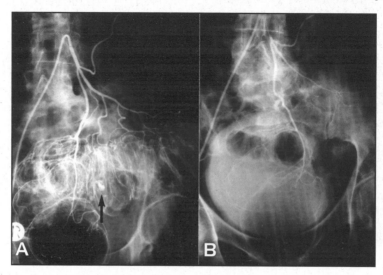

Fig. 12.17 (A) Inferior mesenteric arteriogram in elderly patient with severe bleeding from a diverticulum (arrow). (B) Film after infusing a vasoconstrictor drug shows the bleeding controlled.

disadvantages. First, with multiple foci of disease, e.g. diverticulosis, it provides no information as to which diverticulum is bleeding. Secondly, once barium is filling the colon it obscures the field if arteriography is to be performed. Nowadays, the barium enema in these cases is reserved for patients which remain undiagnosed or to gain further information in patients in whom the bleeding site has been determined by other means.

5. Sodium pertechnetate scan

Sodium pertechnetate is taken up avidly by gastric mucosa and, particularly in young patients, this agent can be used to demonstrate the presence of a Meckel's diverticulum (Chapter 7, Fig. 7.3).

12.7 Blunt Abdominal Trauma

Blunt injury to the abdomen is far more common than penetrating injury and may be due to direct impact, seat belt injury, or rapid deceleration. Localized pain, tenderness and muscle-guarding may indicate the nature of the internal injury but clinical evidence of severe injury may be slight, or absent, if diminished consciousness is present. The liver, spleen, kidneys and the retroperitoneal pancreas and duodenum are most commonly damaged, and diaphragmatic rupture, far more common on the left side than the right, is not uncommon and important to detect. Diaphragmatic rupture is frequently misdiagnosed until herniation of abdominal content into the chest occurs, with catastrophic results. Such herniation is likely to occur at the conclusion of positive pressure respiration, which is frequently employed in the seriously injured, or even days later. The role of radiology depends on the urgency of management and the resources available. Haematuria indicates probable urinary tract damage, a matter discussed in section 11.12.

1. Plain radiography

Films of the chest, preferably erect, and the abdomen can be made at the bedside and may show diaphragmatic irregularity or elevation

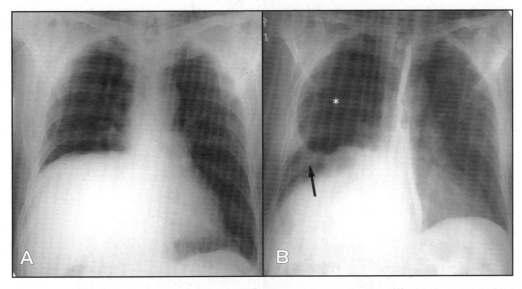

Fig. 12.18 Ruptured right hemidiaphragm. (A) Two weeks following blunt abdominal trauma. Apparent marked elevation of the hemidiaphragm. (B) Five months later, clinically thought to have had a spontaneous pneumothorax. Film shows gas-filled bowel loops at right base (arrow) and probable large gas-distended bowel loop (*) in the chest. At operation, liver, large and small bowel with omentum had passed through the large tear.

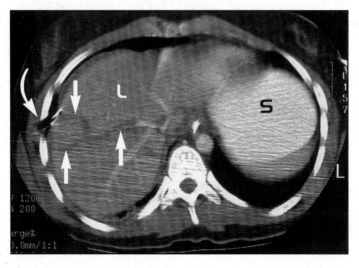

Fig. 12.19 Ruptured liver following blunt trauma. Rent (arrows) extends across right lobe in CT following IV contrast. No contrast leakage from vessels. Note drain tube (curved arrow). Peritoneal fluid around liver (L) and spleen (S).

suggesting rupture (Fig. 12.18) and free gas beneath the diaphragm indicates bowel perforation (Fig. 12.2).

2. Computed Tomography (CT)

If CT is readily available in the emergency department this should be performed as the first investigation following blunt trauma. If obtaining CT involves delays then peritoneal lavage may be preferable. CT demonstrates damage to liver and spleen and kidneys well and can demonstrate intraperitoneal fluid (Fig. 12.19). It is less helpful with retroperitoneal damage to the pancreas and duodenum and the sensitivity of CT for significant abnormalities following blunt trauma is still debated, some reported series putting it at only 65%.

3. Peritoneal lavage

This procedure can be performed at the bedside and if the aspirate is significantly bloodstained or contains bowel content immediate surgery may be indicated. Prior to performing peritoneal lavage plain radiography is recommended to demonstrate free gas, if present, as the lavage procedure itself introduces a small amount of air.

Reference

Harris, J. H., Harris, W. H., & Novelline, R. A.
The Radiology of Emergency Medicine, 3rd edn, Williams and Wilkins, Baltimore, 1993.

Female Reproductive System and Breast

13.1 Imaging the Female Pelvis

A range of radiological methods is available to image the uterus, Fallopian tubes, the ovaries, and the adnexal tissues.

1. Ultrasound (US)

US is the primary imaging modality and generally provides excellent detail of the uterus, in which the echogenic endometrium is clearly distinguished from the surrounding myometrium. The ovaries are clearly demonstrated in most cases and US is particularly sensitive in the detection of cystic lesions. Transabdominal US is performed with a distended bladder which allows excellent sound transmission to the organs of interest. Transvaginal US is being used with increasing frequency in particular clinical situations because it provides far greater detail of ovaries, uterus and adnexae. Colour flow Doppler US is valuable in assessing the vascularity of tissues. Because US is considered to have no harmful effects on the ovaries and developing foetus US is used exclusively in pregnancy except for occasional indications for plain radiography and CT, e.g. to determine pelvic dimensions.

2. Plain radiography

Intrauterine contraceptive devices (IUCD) may be demonstrated and also calcified lesions, such as degenerating fibroids and dermoids which may show calcification, teeth and radiolucency due to fat (Fig. 13.1).

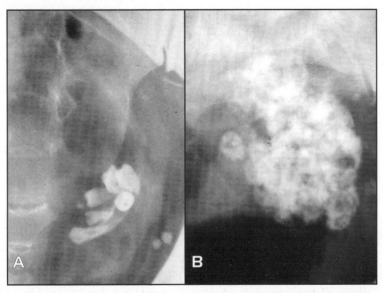

Fig. 13.1 (A) Left ovarian dermoid containing dental elements and translucent fat. (B) Calcification in large degenerate uterine fibroid in postmenopausal patient.

3. Hysterosalpingography

In this technique a viscous iodine containing contrast medium is injected through the cervix to outline the cavity of the uterus and the tubes. Flow of contrast medium into the peritoneum confirms tubal patency. Developmental uterine anomalies may be well shown, e.g. cornuate uterus.

4. Computed Tomography (CT)

Demonstrates the outline of the uterus but provides limited information concerning the uterine wall and pathological processes, eg carcinoma. Enlarged ovaries are evident but normal-sized ovaries may not be displayed. The structures in the pelvic wall, particularly enlarged lymph nodes, may be well seen.

5. Magnetic Resonance Imaging (MRI)

Provides similar information to CT, but demonstrates more detail of the uterine wall and pathological processes.

Interventional radiological techniques have replaced open surgery in some instances and US is used for guidance during many of these therapies.

13.2 Pelvic Radiation

The developing foetus and to a lesser extent the gametes in the ovary are sensitive to the ionizing effects of x-rays and it is important to avoid the possibility of irradiating unsuspected pregnancies. The clinician should consider the menstrual history when referring patients in the reproductive age group for pelvic investigations such as plain radiography, CT, hysterosalpingography, intravenous pyelography and even elective skeletal examinations. The most sensitive period for the developing embryo is about six weeks following conception when organogenesis is progressing rapidly. Irradiation in the early weeks prior to this is now considered to be less significant. For practical purposes when arranging appointments for radiology involving the pelvis in women of reproductive age it is prudent to select a time during the first three weeks following menstruation. Certainly such an examination should not be performed if the patient has missed a regular period. Clinicians should advise patients accordingly and appropriate questions should be asked at reception in the Radiology Clinic. Non-irradiated foetuses have a 2–4% possibility of a congenital abnormality. This risk is not increased by an x-ray examination of the pelvis during the sensitive period. Debate continues as to whether there is a slightly increased risk of childhood malignancy developing.

13.3 Pregnancy

In known pregnancy and particularly in the first trimester pelvic x-rays should be avoided. In later pregnancy, when necessary for patient management, the number of films should be reduced, e.g. limited IVP for suspected calculus obstruction.

Because US is considered to have minimal biological effects there should be no hesitation in using it to assist diagnosis in complications throughout pregnancy. It is recommended that all pregnancies should have an US scan between 18 to 20 weeks of gestation.

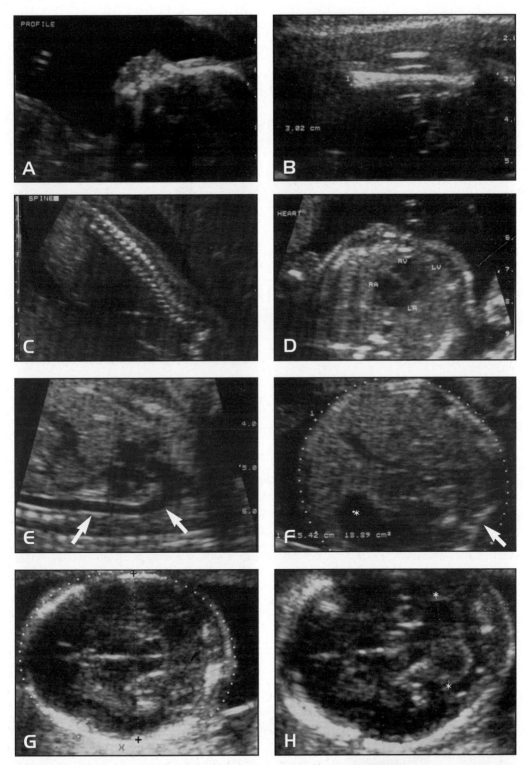

Fig. 13.2 Antenated US – 18 weeks gestation. Normal. (A) Face. (B) Femoral shaft (3.22 cm normal). (C) Thoraco-lumbo-sacral spine. (D) Four chamber heart view. (E) Thoracic aorta (arrows). (F) Abdominal circumference (15.42 cm normal). Spine (arrow). Stomach (*). (G) Skull. Biparietal diameter (between +'s) and circumference (marked). (H) Skull. Posterior fossa. Cerebellar hemispheres (between *'s)

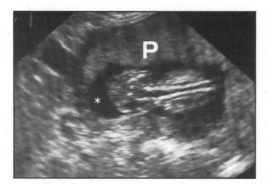

Fig. 13.3 Anencephaly. Typical US appearance at 18 weeks. Absent skull vault (*). Placenta (P).

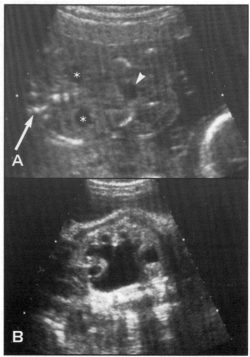

Fig. 13.4 (right) (A) Foetal urinary tract dilatation at five months. Both renal pelves (*) are moderately dilated and the bladder filled (arrowhead). Spine (arrow). (B) US at 37 weeks shows persisting moderate pelvic dilatation. Note the normal echogenic cortex at this age. Micturating cystourethrogram after birth showed posterior urethral valves in this male child.

US pregnancy scan at 18 to 20 weeks

US at this stage (Fig. 13.2) is the most cost-effective pregnancy investigation. It provides assessment of gestational age, which is more accurate than the clinical information; it allows diagnosis of multiple pregnancies and will detect a low–lying placenta. US at this time will also detect many serious foetal anomalies (Figs 13.3,13.4). Gestational age is assessed from measurements of the biparietal diameter and femoral length and is accurate to plus or minus one week. In checking the foetal anatomy particular attention is paid to the head, face, diaphragm, heart, abdomen, spine, extremities and the umbilical cord and placental site. Major congenital malformations occur in approximately 2% of pregnancies. Up to 50% of these may be detected by a well-performed US at 18–20 weeks gestational age. At 18 to 20 weeks should an abnormality be detected there is still sufficient time to undertake further investigation and to make decisions about the future of the pregnancy.

A normal US at this time does not guarantee a perfectly healthy baby. Cardiac abnormalities and some gastrointestinal anomalies may not be apparent at this stage and the final site of the placenta may be indefinite because of the later elongation of the lower uterine segment.

US in the first trimester

US is recommended if there is clinical concern in the early months of pregnancy or in patients assessed at high risk of maternal or foetal complications. US may provide the following information:

- Evidence of an intrauterine pregnancy, particularly if ectopic pregnancy is suspected. Pregnancy should be diagnosed by blood test but may be confirmed by the presence of a gestational sac within the uterus and later a developing embryo. Ruptured ectopic pregnancy may present as an acute abdomen. US may sometimes demonstrate the ectopic in the adnexal tissues; the uterus is empty and there may be fluid, consistent with blood, in the pouch of Douglas (Fig. 13.9).

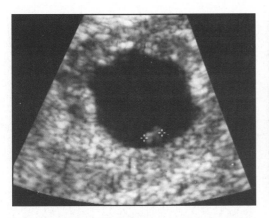

Fig. 13.5 Missed abortion. Last menstrual period 12 weeks ago. Transvaginal scan. The gestational sac is irregular measuring 19 mm across (equivalent to 7 weeks gestation). The foetal pole (marked) measures 3.3 mm (equivalent to 6 weeks gestation). No foetal heart movement detected. Falling B-human chorionic gonadotropin level.

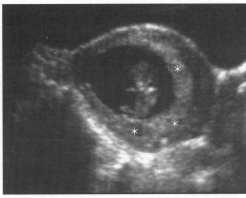

Fig. 13.6 US of normal eight week pregnancy. The embryo has several echogenic foci consistent with the developing skeleton. The choriodecidual reaction (*) is slightly more echogenic than the myometrium external to it.

- Evidence of an early complication. 20–50% of pregnant women experience bleeding ('spotting') in the first few weeks, which is insignificant, but 20–30% of these will proceed to a threatened abortion (Fig. 13.5). US may show the site and extent of retrochorionic bleeding.

- Evidence of viability. By five weeks following menstruation (i.e. five and one half weeks gestational age or three weeks postconception) a gestational sac should be visible within the uterus using transvaginal US. By seven to eight weeks postmenstrual age US should depict a gestational sac, a developing embryo with its heartbeat, together with the surrounding membranes and choriodecidual reaction (Fig. 13.6). Absence of an embryo within the sac, the so-called 'blighted ovum' or anembryonic pregnancy is usually a reflection of a chromosomally aberrant pregnancy. During the first trimester growth is monitored by measuring the crown-rump length.

- Evidence of an IUCD associated with pregnancy, an occasional occurrence.

US in the third trimester

If the 18 to 20 week routine antenatal US scan reveals no abnormality the majority of pregnancies require no further imaging. Further monitoring by US may be indicated in the following circumstances in the later stages of pregnancy.

- If an abnormality is suspected at 18 to 20 weeks.

- If the clinical assessment of progress, based mainly on the height of the uterine fundus

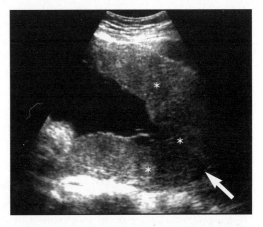

Fig. 13.7 Central placenta praevia. The placenta (*) extends from the anterior to the posterior walls across the position of the internal cervical os (arrow).

clinically is out of step with the earlier US assessment. This may indicate **intrauterine growth retardation**, or if the uterus is larger than expected the possibility of **polyhydramnios** may require clarification.

- Multiple pregnancy because clinical monitoring is inadequate. Identification of a monochorionic twin pregnancy increases the risk of twin to twin transfusion. US may display discordant growth between twins and provides important information concerning the placenta and membranes.
- Maternal insulin dependent diabetes because of the increased frequency of malformations and complications in this group.

- Bleeding. Assessment of the final placental site may be inaccurate at 18 to 20 weeks and US is required later if bleeding occurs to determine whether placenta praevia is present and whether it is marginal or central (Fig. 13.7). Patients with placental abruption need review for signs of foetal compromise.

US at time of presentation

At this stage of pregnancy US is of value in specific clinical situations, particularly for patients with antepartum bleeding in the second and third trimester. US may be diagnostic in suspected premature rupture of membranes or suspected foetal death.

13.4 Gynaecology

Gynaecological pathology involving the internal reproductive organs may present acutely suggesting conditions such as complicated cyst, ruptured ectopic pregnancy, acute pelvic inflammatory disease, or ovarian torsion; or the onset may be gradual when the symptoms may include amenorrhoea, abnormal bleeding, lower abdominal pain, dyspareunia or a discharge. Infertility may be the indication for investigation.

In women presenting with acute abdominal symptoms and signs pointing to the pelvis and particularly with women in the reproductive age group pelvic US is advisable and may avoid exploratory laparotomy by providing the diagnosis and, in some cases, indicating conservative management. For example, physiological follicular or corpus lutein cysts may be larger than the usual 5 cm, due to haemorrhage which may resolve in subsequent cycles and can be monitored by US (Fig. 13.8). Ovarian torsion is usually associated with a cyst in the ovary and Doppler US may indicate impaired blood supply.

Acute pelvic inflammatory disease may not be evident on US unless a hydrosalpinx or tubo-

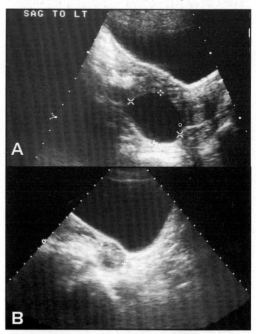

Fig. 13.8 Left ovarian follicular cyst. (A) The unilocular cyst measures 6 cm across. (B) 14 months later the cyst has regressed and the ovary appears normal.

ovarian abscess has developed. A ruptured ectopic pregnancy should be considered in any woman of child-bearing age with a positive pregnancy test and pelvic pain. The US signs are an empty uterus, fluid in the pouch of Douglas and an adnexal mass (Fig. 13.9).

With non-acute presentations digital vaginal examination is performed routinely in adults and if a pelvic mass is detected US is indicated. However, increasingly, the use of pelvic US is being used routinely by gynaecologists as an extension of the digital examination. In prepubertal females transabdominal US replaces the vaginal digital examination in most cases (Fig. 13.10).

Pelvic masses

Gynaecological causes of pelvic masses, excluding pregnancy include:

Uterus

*   Developmental – haematometrocolpos.
*   Tumours – fibroids – carcinoma.

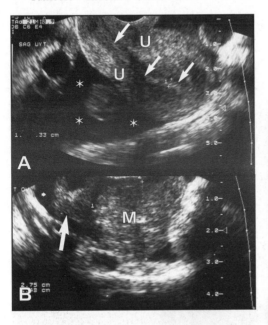

Ovary

*   Cysts – follicular or luteal.
*   Tumours – germinal cell, eg dermoid cyst.
    *   – cystadenoma or carcinoma.
    *   – metastasis.

Tubes and associated tissues

*   Hydrosalpinx.
*   Endometrial cysts.

If a pelvic mass is suspected clinically US is the initial diagnostic investigation, and shows:

*   Whether a mass is present or not.
*   The size and location of a mass and in most instances its site of origin.
*   The internal structure and walls of the mass.
*   The presence of hydronephrosis, ascites or other masses suggesting metastases.
*   Vascularity using Colour Doppler.

If a malignant neoplasm is suspected on US, CT or MRI provides more detail concerning the retroperitoneal structures and pelvic walls, particularly lymph nodes, and the adnexal tissues. However, these methods have been disappointing in determining the extent of the primary tumour, particularly in the body of the uterus.

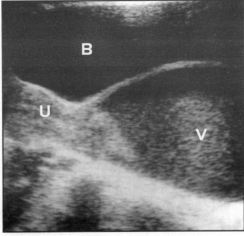

Fig. 13.9 Ectopic pregnancy. Transvaginal US. (A) Slightly enlarged empty uterus (U) with echogenic endometrium (arrows). Echolucent blood in pouch of Douglas (*). (B) Round echogenic mass (M) in the right adnexal region consistent with ectopic pregnancy and separate from R ovary (arrow). Pregnancy test positive.

Fig. 13.10 Haematocolpos in 12 year old. The vagina (V) is markedly distended with blood retained behind an intact hymen. The uterus (U) appears normal and the bladder (B) is distended.

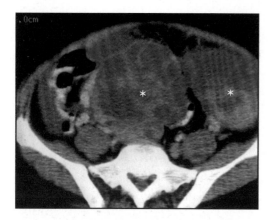

Fig. 13.11 Bilateral cystic ovarian tumours (*). Numerous denser soft-tissue areas suggest the tumours may be malignant.

Ovary

The commonest mass is a physiological ovarian follicular or lutein cyst. A normal follicle generally does not exceed 2.5 cm in size but follicular cysts may be as large as 8 cm across and may spontaneously regress. Ovarian tumours may be entirely cystic, partly cystic or solid (Fig. 13.11). In general the likelihood of malignancy increases according to the amount of solid tissue within the ovarian mass. Ovarian carcinoma accounts for 25% of gynaecological cancer and is usually 'silent'. Staging is made at operation using biopsies.

On presentation CT shows 75% have extended beyond the ovarian capsule. Ovarian carcinoma is most common in the postmenopausal period and in this age group even a purely cystic ovarian mass, discovered incidentally, of more than 5 cm in diameter is removed surgically because of the inherent risk. Metastases to the ovary are relatively common and may be the presenting sign of an occult primary, e.g. Krukenberg tumour from the stomach or more often from large bowel.

Uterus

Uterine **fibroids** are extremely common. Usually hypoechoic, they lie most commonly within the myometrium (Fig. 13.12) but may be subserosal or submucosal, where they may simulate a pregnancy or hydatidiform mole. In the elderly degeneration leads to calcification with acoustic shadowing on US and the calcification may be seen on plain radiography (Fig. 13.1). The diagnosis and staging of **cervical carcinoma** is generally clinical and CT or MRI is used mainly for follow-up. Parametrial invasion of cervical carcinoma usually contra-indicates surgery. If the ring of cervical stroma surrounding the tumour is intact on MRI parametrial extension is usually not

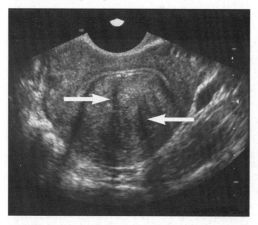

Fig. 13.12 Uterine fibroid, 8 cm across, causing arc-shaped displacement of the echogenic endometrium on transvaginal US. Acoustic shadows within the mass (arrows) caused by calcified foci.

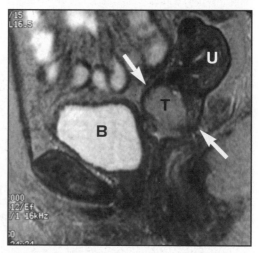

Fig. 13.13 Cervical carcinoma on T_2 weighted MRI. The tumour (T) is well defined within the cone of cervical muscle (arrows). The high signal of bladder urine (B) is seen on T_2 imaging. Uterine body (U).

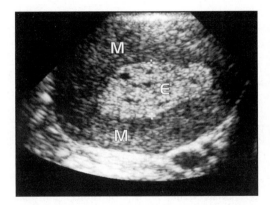

Fig. 13.14 Endometrial hyperplasia (E) following tamoxifen therapy. Such an appearance is seen in endometrial carcinoma. Myometrium (M).

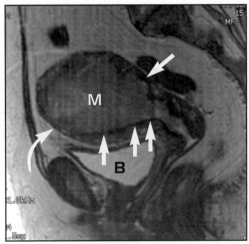

Fig. 13.15 Endometrial carcinoma on T$_2$ weighted MRI. Inferiorly the darker line of the junctional zone (arrows) is well seen. Superiorly the line is lost (curved arrow) indicating myometrial invasion by the tumour (M) which has expanded the uterus. Bladder (B).

present (Fig. 13.13). **Endometrial carcinoma** of the body of the uterus frequently presents as postmenopausal bleeding. US demonstrates the width of the endometrium, which appears hyperechoic and normally should not exceed 4 mm in width. In the postmenopausal period, particularly if associated with bleeding, an endometrial width greater than 5 mm is usually an indication for diagnostic curettage (Fig. 13.14). Occasionally endometrial hyperplasia may result from drug therapy, i.e. tamoxifen. On normal T$_2$ weighted MRI images a lower signal (greyer) 'junctional zone' is seen beneath the endometrium corresponding to the inner myometrium. The

depth of myometrial penetration of endometrial carcinoma may be assessed (Fig. 13.15).

Tubes and associated tissues

Pelvic inflammatory disease resulting in closure of the fimbriated end of a Fallopian tube resulting in an hydro or pyosalpinx may be seen on US as a cystic tortuous structure and confirmed by hysterosalpingogram (Fig. 13.16). A tubo-ovarian abscess is usually less well defined. Cysts of endometriosis are often multiple, implanting in

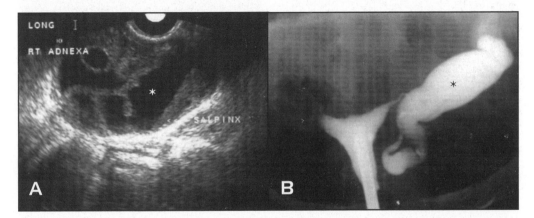

Fig. 13.16 Hydrosalpinx (*). (A) Transvaginal US. (B) Hysterosalpingogram. Injected contrast medium has not entered the peritoneal cavity indicating obstructed fimbriated end of the left Fallopian tube. Right tube blocked at isthmus.

the peritoneum and adjacent tissues, and these 'chocolate' cysts have a typical US appearance of low level echoes, posterior wall enhancement and no blood flow on Doppler US.

Infertility

Infertility, generally defined as inability to conceive after one year, affects between 10 to 15% of couples and in about 60 to 70% the disorder is with the female partner. Very approximately about 40% are due to occlusive tubal disease or endometriosis; in 30% ovarian disorders, and in 10% uterine abnormalities are the cause. In about 5 to 10% the cause of infertility remains unexplained.

In the management of infertility patients, US has an important role which can be divided into:

- Performing a baseline scan.
- Assessing the ovulatory cycle.
- Monitoring induction of ovulation.
- Monitoring for complications of assisted pregnancy.

1. Baseline ultrasound scan

Polycystic ovaries are diagnosed on the basis of numerous follicles which generally lie peripherally in the ovaries which have increased stroma (Fig. 13.17). More than 15 follicles in each ovary is consistent with the diagnosis. Ovarian cysts may be detected and dermoids suspected on the detection of hyperechoic fat, evidence of hair

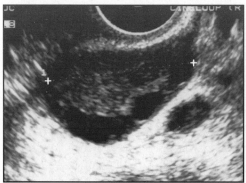

Fig. 13.17 Polycystic ovaries. US of right ovary which is slightly enlarged (+'s) with many peripherally placed follicles.

and calcification (Fig. 13.18). The tortuous cystic nature of an hydrosalpinx is characteristic (Fig. 13.16) and abnormalities within the uterine cavity such as polyps, submucous fibroids or adhesions following curettage may be demonstrated. Saline installation into the uterine cavity may be used to assist the demonstration of such intrauterine lesions with US.

Hysterosalpingography is used to demonstrate obstructed Fallopian tubes, which may be corrected nonsurgically by a technique of balloon dilatation similar to that employed for stenosed arteries.

2. Assessment of the ovulatory cycle

US is valuable for studying the cycle in infertility patients. Normally, one or two follicles mature up

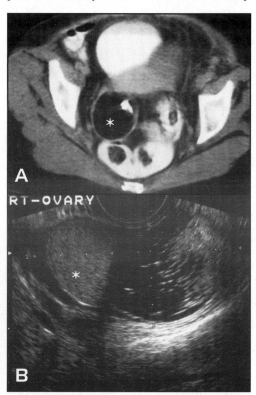

Fig. 13.18 Ovarian dermoid cysts. (A) CT showing lucent fat (*) and a dental type calcification. (B) Transvaginal US showing an homogenous echogenic area (*) consistent with fat. Linear appearance adjacent suggests hair within the cyst.

to the time of rupture, when the follicle measures between 17 to 25 mm. The presence of a corpus luteum is readily detected using Doppler US because of the increased surrounding vascularity. Non-ovulatory cycles may be associated with reduced maximum follicle size and the absence of a corpus luteum.

3. Monitoring following induction of ovulation

Transvaginal ultrasound is used to monitor the development of follicles up to a size of about 15 to 18 mm when, for in vitro fertilisation (IVF), the follicles are aspirated under US control.

4. Monitoring for complications of assisted pregnancy

Multiple pregnancies are common following ovarian stimulation with a high loss rate. Ectopic pregnancies also are more frequent. US is helpful in monitoring for evidence of **ovarian hyperstimulation disorder** (OHSS) in patients undergoing ovulation induction. OHSS is associated with persisting large follicles and stromal oedema of the ovaries leading to considerable enlargement greater than 10 cm, the development of ascites, and in its severest form to maternal respiratory and circulatory compromise and electrolyte imbalance.

13.5 Breast Cancer

Carcinoma of the breast affects 1 in 16 Australian women and together with carcinoma of the cervix is one of the two main causes of cancer deaths amongst women. Patients present clinically usually because of a palpable lump or occasionally because of a serous or bloody discharge from the nipple or because of metastases. With a view to earlier diagnosis a number of nations have established screening programs based on self-examination or particularly mammography and the Swedish Mammography Screening Programme has reported a 31% decrease in mortality amongst the screened population. The anatomy of the breast is suitable for soft tissue radiography and the breast is so shaped that various views may be obtained to assist detection and localization of abnormalities. Mammography can be divided into **diagnostic mammography** in which a patient with symptoms is investigated and a report given to the referring doctor and **screening mammography** in which asymptomatic non-referred patients are examined and any abnormality detected is investigated further, usually in a screening assessment centre. US is a valuable supplement to mammography and MRI also has a role in certain cases.

13.6 Mammographic Anatomy

The breast contains a large amount of radiolucent fat so that the glandular tissue and ducts of the breast are displayed in contrast, much as the air in the lungs allows the pulmonary blood vessels to be outlined. The proportions of fat and parenchymal tissue vary from person to person and change gradually throughout life with a relative increase in fat occurring after the menopause. Normally the pattern in the two breasts is remarkably symmetrical and this is a great help in detecting focal abnormalities, by comparison.

Mammography is performed using special equipment to compress the breast. The images are recorded on fine grain film which requires particular processing. Routinely two views are made of each breast, a **cranio-caudal** and an **oblique view** on each side to allow for accurate localization within the breasts. The oblique view shows the axillary tail of breast parenchyma and some of the axillary lymph nodes. If a focal abnormality is suspected greater detail is obtained by performing a further view with localized compression and magnification. In patients with a nipple discharge, suggesting a duct papilloma, the duct can be injected with contrast medium at the nipple, a technique known as **galactography**. Following breast implantation mammography technique has been modified to show the breast tissue and also the status of the implant, and whether rupture is present (Fig. 13.19).

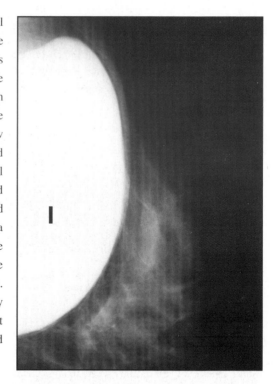

Fig. 13.19 Mammogram in patient with silicone implant (1).

13.7 Mammographic Appearance of Breast Cancer

The radiologist must try to distinguished breast cancer from a number of other conditions including cyst, fibroadenoma, lobular hyperplasia, fat necrosis and haematoma. In a significant number of cases this distinction cannot be made with sufficient confidence and biopsy is required. The presence of a cancer may be evident as a circumscribed mass, a stellate lesion, or by a focus of calcification.

Circumscribed lesion
(Fig. 13.20)

A rounded discrete soft tissue mass in the breast may be due to several pathologies including cancer. If the mass is sharply defined on all borders and has a surrounding halo of radiolucency it is more likely to be benign. If solid on US, with features of cancer (Fig. 13.23), virtually all such masses require biopsy.

Stellate lesion
(Fig. 13.21)

Invasive breast cancer, such as scirrhus carcinoma, induces a fibrotic reaction and distorts the surrounding stroma producing a radiating stellate appearance with often only a very small soft tissue mass at the centre.

Calcification
(Fig. 13.22)

Many breast lesions may contain calcification but cancers frequently contain tiny foci less than 1 mm, referred to as **microcalcifications,** and these have been reported in as high as 40% of breast carcinomas. Microcalcifications are commonly seen in non-invasive **carcinoma in-situ**. Breast cancer usually commences in the ducts and ductal carcinoma in-situ (DCIS) has a characteristic

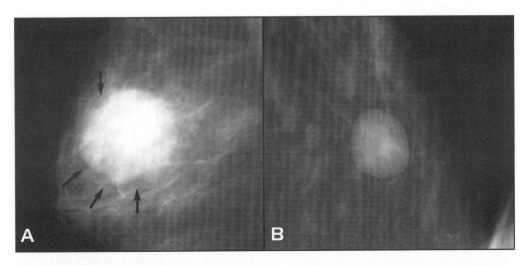

Fig. 13.20 Circumscribed breast lesions. (A) Carcinoma. The rather dense mass is well-defined posteriorly but irregular anteriorly (arrows). (B) Cyst. The lump is less dense than carcinoma (A) but very well-defined and has a radiolucent rim ('halo' sign) commonly seen in benign lesions.

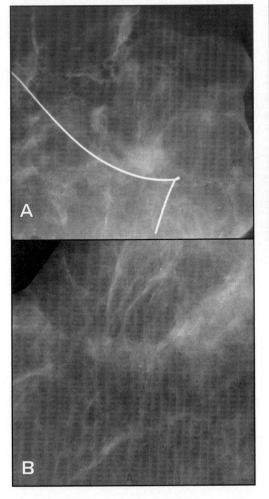

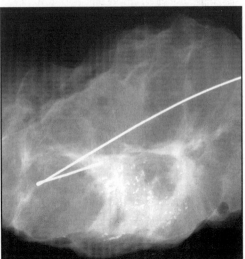

Fig. 13.22 (above) Malignant microcalcifications in excised carcinoma. The fine J-wire was inserted prior to surgical biopsy as a guide.

Fig. 13.21 (left) Stellate carcinoma. (A) Oblique view shows the lesion with a fine biopsy guide wire prior to surgical biopsy. (B) Compression magnification view of the lesion shows irregular strands radiating from the central mass.

appearance with granular microcalcifications. Because of the invasive potential it is usual to excise areas of DCIS, which may be quite extensive, leaving a clear zone of tissue around.

13.8 Breast Ultrasound and MRI

Although US is inadequate as a primary investigation for suspected breast cancer it is an important supplement to mammography. On US the fibroglandular tissue and the stroma of the breast appear hyperechoic in contrast to the fatty background, which appears hypoechoic. The fasciae and retromammary tissues are well demonstrated. As in other areas US clearly demonstrates cysts which are relatively echo-free and show posterior enhancement (Fig. 13.23A). Occasionally US will show a mural tumour within a cyst. Carcinoma usually appears ill-defined and hypoechoic compared with the surrounding tissues, and acoustic shadowing is usually, but not always, present deep to the tumour (Fig. 13.23C). Doppler US allows assessment of vascularity within a focal lesion.

Contrast medium-enhanced MRI mammography is reported to have an excellent sensitivity in detecting cancer and may allow the distinction between benign and malignant tumours, but further evaluation is required. It does appear that MRI has a role in differentiating postoperative scar tissue from recurrent tumour. Also, it may be valuable for cancer detection following breast implantation.

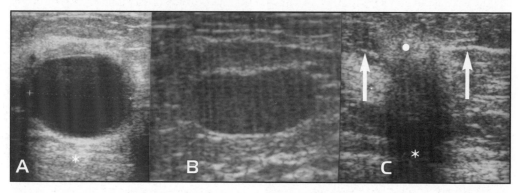

Fig. 13.23 US of breast lumps. (A) Cyst. Well-defined and with posterior wall enhancement (*) consistent with fluid content. (B) Fibroadenoma. Well-defined, elliptical and containing low level echoes. (C) Carcinoma (•). Ill-defined, interrupted fascial line (arrows) and acoustic shadowing (*).

13.9 Breast Biopsy

Because of the high sensitivity of mammography and US in detecting focal breast lesions, and the relative nonspecificity in many instances, biopsy is frequently required to establish the diagnosis and is performed in many, if not most, patients prior to definitive surgery. Breast screening results in more women requiring further investigations of suspicious areas on mammography and this usually means biopsy. In the Swedish program 50 women in every 1000 screened have an abnormality detected requiring further investigation, and only 7 turn out to have cancer, a positive predictive value of about 14%. Biopsy is performed in various ways. Open surgical **excisional biopsy** is assisted by the radiologist placing a fine wire as an indicator with its tip in the lesion (Fig. 13.22). **Fine needle aspiration** (FNA) may be performed under US or mammographic control if the lesion is impalpable but the diagnosis depends on cell cytology. Stereotactic needle **core biopsy** is performed using special radiological equipment which provides very accurate localization. The core of tissue obtained allows conventional pathological sections to be examined. Following open surgical or core biopsy it is helpful to x-ray the specimen to be sure that the biopsy has been successful. If a suspicious lesion on mammography turns out to be normal it may be wise to perform a further mammogram to be sure that the lesion was sampled.

13.10 Role of Breast Imaging

A number of significant issues should be considered by a clinician referring patients for mammography and breast ultrasound.

- Mammography and US are no substitute for clinical examination of the breast. Because of a significant false negative rate of diagnosis of these techniques clinical judgement is required when advising a patient with a palpable lump in the breast and a negative result from these tests. Based on clinical signs, age and family history, open surgical biopsy may be wise.
- Mammography may fail to demonstrate a focal mass in the breast, even, on occasions, a palpable mass. In those instances US may demonstrate the mass. When referring a patient with a palpable mass for mammography it is helpful to request that US be performed if required, in this way saving the patient a delay. Negative imaging of a suspected lump means clinical assessment must be relied upon and FNA is usually indicated
- Regular two-yearly mammography is recommended for all over the age of 50 years. The progressive atrophy of glandular tissue within the breast in the older age groups assists cancer detection and screening in this age group is of proven value. The menopausal breast remains relatively dense and cancers are harder to detect. However, the trend is to reduce the age of regular breast screening to 40 years.
- Mammography is not recommended for young women, say less than 30 years of age. The breasts are usually very dense, with little fat making detection of focal lesions difficult. Cancer is very unusual in this age group. If imaging is thought to be indicated US should be used initially.
- Availability of previous mammograms for comparison is important in breast cancer detection and it is wise for women to retain previous mammograms and present them for comparison whenever mammography is performed.
- Modern mammography equipment delivers a very low dose of radiation to the breast, but there is a hypothetical risk of contributing to the development of cancer. This risk is minimal compared with the benefits of mammography and has been compared with the risk involved in travelling 200 miles in a plane, or 30 miles by car!

Reference

Rumack, C. M., Wilson, S. R. & Charboneau, J. W.
Diagnostic Ultrasound (vol. 2), Mosby, 1998.

Tabar, L. and Dean, P. B.
Teaching Atlas of Mammography, 2nd edn.
George Thieme Verlag, 1985.

Musculo-Skeletal System

Plain radiography demonstrates bones extremely well because of their high calcium content, bearing in mind that absorption of x-rays is dependent on the fourth power of the atomic number, which for calcium is moderately high. For the same reason CT demonstrates bone and in addition provides greater detail of surrounding soft tissues. MRI, which depends on the distribution and environment of hydrogen protons displays the soft tissues, particularly the bone marrow, but because bone is relatively devoid of hydrogen atoms it emits a very low signal, appearing black on MRI images. Radionuclide imaging using a complex phosphate molecule, labelled with Technetium, which is taken up by the bones, is useful in particular cases. Focal increase in bone metabolism results in increased radionuclide uptake and a 'hot spot' on the image. US is also of help in certain cases, particularly for demonstrating tendon sheaths and soft tissues.

14.1 Indications for Musculo-Skeletal Imaging

- Following trauma.
- Symptoms of a bone lesion, e.g. pain, usually of a boring unrelenting nature.
- Clinical signs of a bone lesion, e.g. a lump or local tenderness.
- To demonstrate spread of an established primary condition, e.g. metastases.
- To demonstrate evidence of metabolic bone disease.

  Occasionally, unsuspected bone lesions are demonstrated when diagnostic imaging is performed for an unrelated reason.

14.2 Imaging Role in Fracture Management

Blunt trauma to the bony skeleton may result in fractures and dislocations and also damage to the soft tissues particularly ligaments, tendons and cartilage. In general, following musculo-skeletal injury it is relevant to perform plain radiography. It is important to appreciate certain general principles concerning the use of radiology during the various stages of managing fractures.

1. In diagnosis of fractures

a. Precise clinical localization improves the yield from radiology

The more confined the area examined by x-ray the better the quality of the image and the lower the likelihood of missing a fracture line. The clinical signs of fracture should be well known to students, allowing the suspicious area to be carefully localized. Referred pain may be misleading, e.g. knee pain following hip injury.

b. Request x-ray examination
   of a specific region

Radiology departments use examination protocols for specific regions. For example, ankle, foot, wrist, hand, are all separate examinations. If clinically the injury is specifically in the wrist then to obtain optimal definition the request should be for 'wrist' and not 'hand'. For rib fracture specify the particular ribs where maximal tenderness is experienced, again allowing the radiographer to obtain maximal definition in the suspicious area. With long bones do not request examination of 'femur' or 'humerus', but rather specify the portion of those bones under suspicion, e.g. hip, knee or femoral shaft, or shoulder, elbow or humeral shaft. It is better to request examination of a particular bone rather than a region. The 'arm' extends from the shoulder to the elbow and the 'forearm' from elbow to wrist. Using bone names overcomes the occasional misinterpretation that 'arm' implies the entire upper limb.

c. X-raying regions with two long bones

When a fracture is suspected in one of paired long bones it is important that the x-ray covers the full length of both bones. Not infrequently a fracture of one long bone is associated with a dislocation or injury to the joint above or below, e.g. fractured ulnar shaft with dislocated head of radius. There are reasonable exceptions to the rule, e.g. Colles and Pott's fractures are virtually always local.

d. Demonstrating epiphyseal fractures

Juxta-epiphyseal fractures (Fig. 14.2) may be difficult to demonstrate and the appearances seen may be difficult to interpret because of normal variations in appearance. When in doubt the corresponding normal region on the other side of the body should be examined to allow comparison. Appearances in the contralateral limb usually are similar.

e. Clinical assessment is paramount

A normal x-ray report in the presence of a strong clinical suspicion of fracture should be queried, particularly in areas such as the scaphoid, hip, cervical spine and supracondylar region of the elbow in children. In these regions fine fracture lines are notoriously missed and have been the basis of litigation. When a significant discrepancy exists between the clinical findings and the x-ray report then the radiologist should be consulted. Further views may be required or CT or radionuclide bone scan recommended. Radionuclide uptake is apparent in a recent fracture site two days following injury.

f. Damage to adjacent and
   passing structures

It is a basic principle that careful clinical examination is required to assess the integrity of blood vessels and nerves passing a region of injury. They may be damaged directly by bone fragments, or indirectly by swelling within closed fascial compartments, e.g. tibia and fibula, when surgery and relieving incisions may be necessary. Occasionally, arteriography is required to demonstrate trauma to the arterial system.

2. In the reduction of fractures

The standard method of checking the adequacy of reduction in most fractures is by the use of plain radiography with two views obtained at right angles. Often mobile X-ray units are used for this purpose in wards, clinics and operating theatres. In certain circumstances fluoroscopy is of advantage in checking for adequate reduction. Fluoroscopy is also used for the introduction of intramedullary nails which are passed across the fracture site. However, it is important to appreciate that the potential radiation dose to patient and physician using fluoroscopy is significantly greater than for plain radiography.

3. In maintaining reduction

Malposition is likely to develop soon after adequate reduction of many fractures, particularly if a padded plaster is used. For this reason an early check x-ray in the days after the initial treatment is wise. Remanipulation may be required to correct malalignment, e.g. Colles' fracture. Again the checking of the position is done by obtaining two views at right angles for most fractures.

4. In assessment of union

It is important to realize that the radiological signs of union are dependent on demonstrating calcifying or ossifying callus and lags far behind the clinical evidence of union. To avoid unnecessary radiation it is important to appreciate the time required for the common fractures to heal and to time the radiography accordingly. With oblique fractures of long bones the views obtained from standard radiology may not display developing callus optimally. For example, in a spiral fracture of the tibia it is usual to follow progress using an AP and lateral view. Neither of these views clearly demonstrates the line of the fracture and in such cases the radiological evidence of bridging 'callus' may be considerably delayed. Again clinical examination and assessment should be stressed in estimating union. Radiology may demonstrate the presence of established non-union, e.g. in the scaphoid. The bony margins adjacent to the fracture line become slightly sclerotic and the fracture line itself remains clearly evident in such cases.

It is important for students to be familiar with the radiology of commonly encountered injuries because, on graduation, in an emergency, they may be required to not only treat the condition but make the initial radiographic diagnosis.

14.3 Types of Fracture

Avulsion

A bony fragment is torn away at the attachment of a tendon or ligament.

Compound

Associated with an open wound as a result of penetration from within by bone fragments, or from without at the time of injury, when the risk of infection is greater.

Complicated

Associated with damage to vital structures, i.e. nerves, arteries, viscera.

Comminuted

A fracture with more than two fragments.

Compression

Occurs in cancellous bone, e.g. vertebral body, calcaneus, tibial plateau.

Green stick

An undisplaced fracture in children often seen as a buckling of the cortex opposite to the deforming force. The periosteum remains intact (Fig. 14.1).

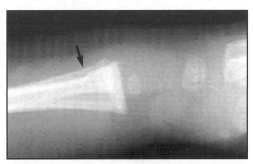

Fig. 14.1 Green stick fracture. Buckling of the dorsal radial cortex (arrow).

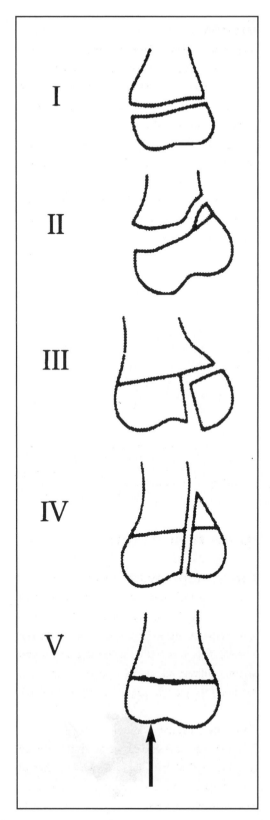

Growth plate

Salter and Harris classified epiphyseal fractures (Fig. 14.2).

Type I

Transverse fracture across the growth plate. May be difficult to see on X-ray.

Type II

Transverse fracture across the growth plate but including a triangular portion of the margin of the metaphysis. The commonest type.

Type III

Involves a fracture line extending from the growth plate into the joint and separating a portion of the epiphysis.

Type IV

Similar to Type III but extending proximally across the growth plate to separate a portion of metaphysis.

Type V

A crushing injury of the growth plate which is difficult to diagnose on x-ray.

Types V and IV have the worst prognosis as regards arrest of growth whilst Types I and II have the best prognosis.

Osteochondral

A fragment consisting of a thin layer of bone attached to overlying articular cartilage is sheered off. It may form a loose body.

Pathological

Occurs through an area of previously diseased bone and may occur spontaneously. Tumours, cysts, chronic osteomyelitis, and generalized bone diseases such as osteoporosis, osteogenesis imperfecta, and Paget's disease are prone to fracture. The fractures in Paget's disease in the long bones tend to be transverse, but they heal readily.

Fig. 14.2 Salter–Harris classification of epiphyseal injuries (see text).

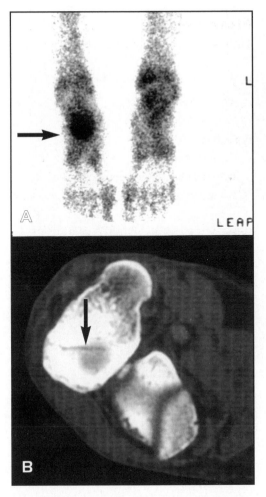

Stress

Sometimes called **fatigue fractures**, these occur in regions subjected to excessive persistent stress. If the underlying bone is abnormal, e.g. osteomalacia, the term **insufficiency fracture** is sometimes used. Often difficult to see on plain radiography, particularly in the tarsus, they may be detected by radionuclide scan, revealing a 'hot-spot', or by CT (Fig. 14.3). The best known is the March fracture of the neck of the second metatarsal, which may be difficult to see on X-ray until callus develops.

Fig. 14.3 Stress fracture of the right navicular in an athlete. (A) Radionuclide bone scan showing increased uptake in the right navicular (arrow). (B) CT scan reveals linear fracture (arrow) in the bone. Plain films were normal.

14.4 Injuries to the Skull, Spine and Pelvis

Skull

In general, linear fractures of the skull vault are not of themselves particularly significant following head injury; it is the damage to the underlying brain and blood vessels which determines management and these abnormalities are best demonstrated by CT. If there is a clinical indication for radiology CT is indicated and plain radiography is no longer used, unless CT is unavailable. Depressed skull fractures and fractures involving the air-containing sinuses are of more significance in management but these also are best shown by CT. Facial fractures are discussed in section 4.9.

The unconscious patient

Occult injuries may be present in patients unconscious following a head injury. It is wise to obtain at least a lateral view of the cervical spine in such patients and this can be made as a lateral digital radiograph (scout view) during CT. Alternatively, plain radiographs may be obtained.

Cervical spine

The cervical spinal cord is at risk when an unstable cervical spine injury is present. Careful assessment of a lateral radiograph should detect most unstable injuries, which are commonest in

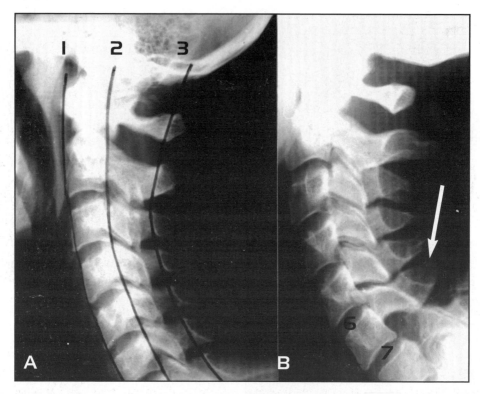

Fig. 14.4 (A) Contour lines in cervical spine. 1 – The anterior vertebral line. 2 – Posterior vertebral line. 3 – Spinolaminar line extending up to the posterior margin of the foramen magnum. (B) Dislocation at the C6–7 level. Note the forward displacement of the lateral masses of C6 on C7, the disturbed spinolaminar line, and the fracture of C6 spinous process (arrow).

the upper cervical region. It is essential to assess the three contour lines of the cervical spine when assessing stability (Fig. 14.4A). The anterior line is formed by the anterior margins of the vertebral bodies. The second line along the posterior margins of the vertebral bodies outlines the anterior margin of the spinal canal. The third line, known as the spinolaminar line, is drawn along the anterior margins of the bases of the spinous processes and indicates the posterior margin of the spinal canal. The spinolaminar line should extend upwards in a gentle curve to the posterior margin of the foramen magnum. In addition the width of the retropharyngeal soft tissues anterior to the upper cervical vertebral bodies should be measured, and if it exceeds one half the width of the mid-portion of C4 vertebral body it suggests bleeding into that space. Also important in the lateral view is the relationship of the anterior arch

of the atlas to the odontoid process. In adults the distance between the anterior surface of the odontoid and the posterior edge of the arch should not exceed 3 mm, but in children it may be normal up to about 5 mm.

Any bone in the cervical spine may fracture and it may be difficult to display. Persisting symptoms after adequate plain radiography should lead to CT which provides more detail.

Odontoid fracture

The fracture line usually passes across the very base of the process, resulting in instability (Fig. 14.5). The skull, atlas and odontoid may be displaced anteriorly or posteriorly on the cervical column.

Hangman's fracture

Bilateral fractures across the pedicles of the second cervical vertebra (the axis) is an injury which is frequently seen after road trauma

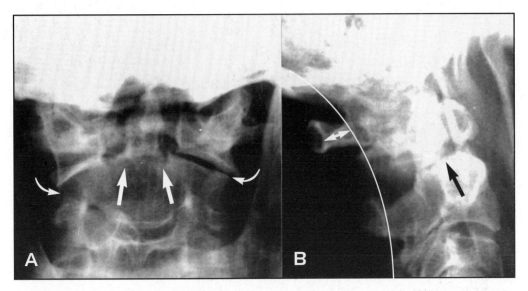

Fig. 14.5 Fractured odontoid process at the base (arrows). (A) View through the open mouth shows subluxation of the atlas with asymmetry of the atlanto-axial joints (curved arrows). (B) Lateral showing slight posterior displacement of the odontoid and atlas (double arrowhead) with interruption of the spinolaminar line (curved white line).

(Fig. 14.6). It is the lesion produced in judicial hanging. The spinal cord is not always damaged because of the relatively capacious spinal canal at that level.

Jefferson fracture

This occurs when a direct blow is received to the vertex of the head, such as in diving into shallow water. The arches of the atlas are fractured in several places and if the transverse ligament is ruptured the atlas may subluxate on the axis with a risk of spinal cord compression. CT demonstrates the lesion best (Fig. 14.7).

Hyperextension injuries

Acute hyperextension, sometimes called 'whiplash', may result in complete rupture through an intervertebral disc, usually in the mid-

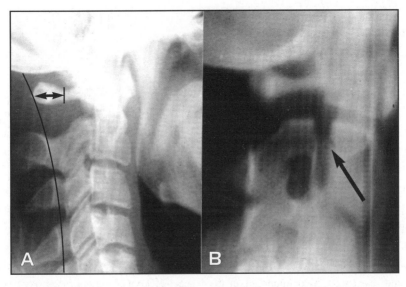

Fig. 14.6 Hangman's fracture. (A) Interruption of the spinolaminar line (double arrowhead) indicates forward displacement of the atlas on the axis. The fracture lines are not clearly shown. (B) Linear tomography shows the fractures across the pedicles of the axis (arrow).

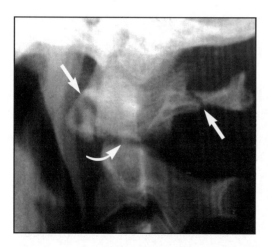

Fig. 14.7 Jefferson fracture following a dive into shallow water. Fractures in the arch of the atlas (arrows) were better shown on CT. Note also a fracture across the base of the odontoid (curved arrow).

cervical region, and may be unstable. Such an abnormality may not be seen on the lateral radiograph, although there may be some retropharyngeal swelling. Occasionally a small bony fragment is avulsed from the antero-inferior aspect of a vertebral body, providing a clue to the nature of the injury. Initially the disc space is not narrowed. It is wise in such cases, particularly for medico-legal reasons, that a further radiograph be made two or three months later when in many instances the disc space will be seen to have reduced considerably, consistent with a previous disc rupture (Fig. 14.8).

Apophyseal joint dislocation

The synovial joints in the lateral masses between vertebrae, sometimes called facet joints, may dislocate and if bilateral the injury is unstable (Fig. 14.4B).

Thoracic spine and ribs

Compression fractures of the vertebral bodies with wedging is the predominant injury at this level, usually affecting the mid and lower thoracic regions. Pain is frequently referred to the rib cage suggesting rib fracture.

Multiple rib fractures are best shown by chest radiography. More localized injuries in which rib fracture is suspected may not require investigation. If views of the ribs are requested it is important that the sites of maximum tenderness are determined clinically so that the radiography can be localized to the area, with a greater chance of demonstrating fracture lines if present. They may be difficult to show initially but with the development of callus are readily detected.

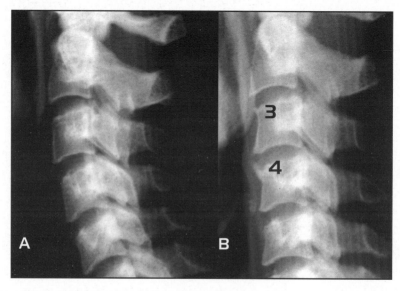

Fig. 14.8 Extension ('whiplash') injury. (A) No abnormality soon after the car accident. (B) One year later. The C3–4 disc is slightly narrowed with adjacent vertebral osteophytes.

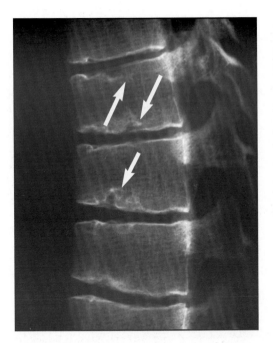

Wedged dorsal vertebrae and Scheuermann's disease

Medico-legally a problem sometimes arises as to whether wedged lower dorsal vertebrae are the result of trauma or not. Scheuermann's disease, or juvenile kyphosis, is a relatively common condition in which the vertebral body end-plate epiphyses are fragile and easily damaged during teenage development (Fig. 14.9). The end plates appear irregular and small herniations of the nucleus pulposis (Schmorl's nodes) may occur into the vertebral bodies. With maturity wedging persists, the fused end-plates appear slightly irregular and the presence of Schmorl's nodes may indicate the nature of the abnormality.

Fig. 14.9 Scheuermann's disease (autopsy specimen). Multiple Schmorl's nodes (arrows) indent the vertebral bodies and result from herniations of the nucleus pulposus through fragile epiphyseal end-plates during development. Note associated vertebral wedging.

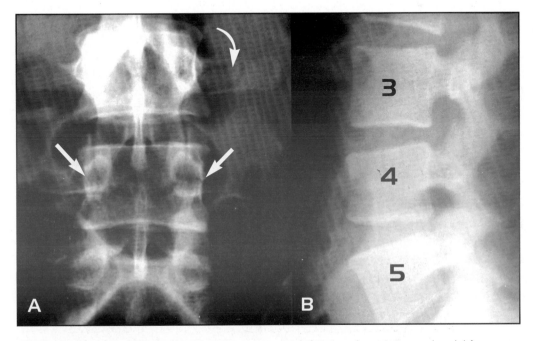

Fig. 14.10 Chance fracture of L4. (A) Fracture in transverse process of L3 (curved arrow). Fracture through left transverse process of L4 and the pedicles of L4 (arrows). (B) Lateral view shows slight wedging of L4 vertebral body.

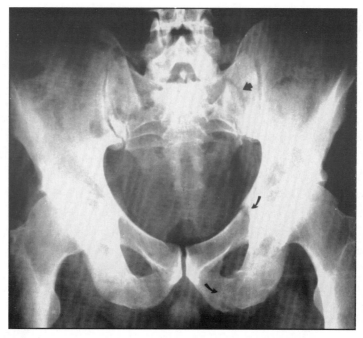

Fig. 14.11 Fractures through the left ischio-pubic rami (curved arrows), and through the left side of the sacrum (arrow). Note the slight upward subluxation of the left hip bone with the left acetabulum lying slightly higher than the right.

Lumbar spine

Flexion injuries predominate with wedging of vertebral bodies. In the elderly senile, osteoporosis, myeloma, or metastases may predispose to compression fracture and the nature of the underlying condition may be difficult to determine in some patients, short of percutaneous biopsy. Fractures of transverse processes are relatively common and retroperitoneal haemorrhage may result in obliteration of the psoas outlines.

Chance fracture

A Dr Chance described a lumbar extension injury with a characteristic appearance usually related to wearing a seat belt. A horizontal fracture across the vertebral body passes posteriorly through the body and pedicles and sometimes the transverse processes. It may be difficult to diagnose if unaware of the condition (Fig. 14.10).

Pelvis

Fractures most commonly involve the ischio-pubic rami, but may occur through the acetabula, the iliac wings, the sacroiliac joints, and the symphysis pubis (Fig. 14.11). It is important to note that if a single fracture is detected and the pelvic ring is deformed there is likely to be a second injury, particularly in the sacroiliac region, and CT may be indicated for detailed assessment.

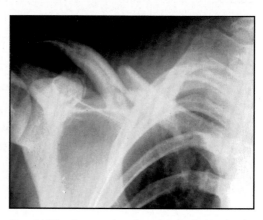

Fig. 14.12 Fracture through mid-shaft of the clavicle.

14.5 Upper Extremity Injuries

Shoulder and shoulder girdle
Clavicle

The commonest injury is a fracture of the mid-shaft, usually resulting from a fall on the outstretched hand, and responding well to conservative management (Fig. 14.12). Fractures through the outer end are usually stable, but in some the coracoclavicular ligament is ruptured allowing considerable distraction of fragments and indicating the need for surgery in most cases. The sternoclavicular joint may be dislocated anteriorly by a fall on the shoulder region and less commonly direct trauma may result in posterior dislocation of the clavicular head, which may damage upper mediastinal structures. Ligamentous damage to the acromio-clavicular joint results in subluxation, but complete dislocation usually indicates associated rupture of the coracoclavicular ligament. Persisting laxity of acromio-clavicular ligaments may be demonstrated radiographically by examining the patient erect holding weights in both hands, and with a film positioned to include both shoulder regions.

Anterior gleno-humeral dislocation

Usually results from a fall on the outstretched hand. The humeral head is displaced medially anterior to the neck of the scapula below the coracoid process. Fracture across the greater tuberosity is a common accompaniment and occasionally axillary nerve palsy may occur with loss of deltoid muscle contraction (Fig. 14.13). In patients with recurrent dislocation plain radiography may demonstrate a groove on the humeral articular surface (Hill–Sachs lesion) and, in some, an avulsion fracture of the anterior glenoid rim (Bankhart lesion), but both are better shown on CT.

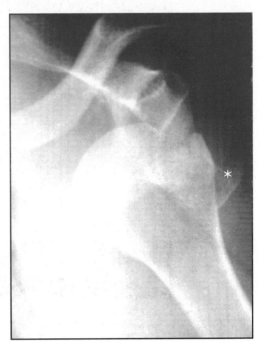

Fig. 14.13   Anterior subcoracoid dislocation of the left humeral head with fracture of the greater tuberosity and displacement of a bony fragment (*).

Posterior gleno-humeral dislocation

Relatively uncommon, the diagnosis of posterior dislocation is missed in at least 50% of patients at initial presentation. Resulting from the forced internal rotation of the humerus the condition is likely to occur during an epileptic fit. Doctors should be familiar with the normal antero-posterior view of the shoulder, which is made with the arm externally rotated (Fig. 14.14A). Clinically, inability to externally rotate the arm should raise suspicion. The x-ray shows no obvious dislocation of the humeral head but the internally rotated position is a strong indicator (Fig. 14.14B), which may be confirmed by an infero-superior view of the shoulder through the axilla, which may be difficult to obtain under the circumstances.

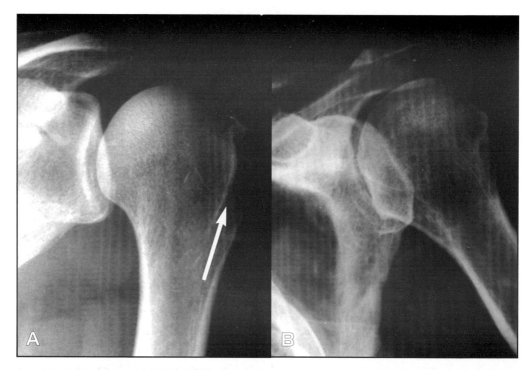

Fig. 14.14 (A) Normal antero-posterior view of the shoulder shows the bicipital groove clearly (arrow). (B) Posterior dislocation shows the internally rotated position of the humeral head, i.e. the so-called 'ice cream cone' appearance.

Fractures

Direct injury may fracture the greater tuberosity. Fracture across the surgical neck of the humerus is commonly seen in the elderly following a fall on the outstretched arm. Most are impacted but some are displaced and in those the axillary nerve may be damaged. In young children, minimally displaced fractures of the growth plate at the upper end of the humerus are common and respond to conservative treatment.

Rotator cuff syndrome

The combined tendinous insertions of the supraspinatus, infraspinatus and teres minor muscles blend with the capsule and insert into the

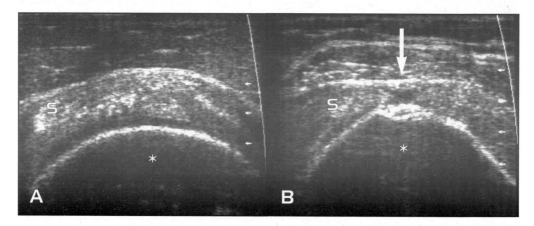

Fig. 14.15 (A) US of normal rotator cuff showing supraspinatus tendon (S) and humeral head (*). (B) Ruptured supraspinatus tendon (arrow).

greater tuberosity of the humerus. This cuff is commonly injured producing a characteristic syndrome with pain in the middle range of abducting the arm from the side. In longer standing injuries plain radiography may show calcification in the line of the tendons. Ultrasound can image the rotator cuff and adjacent muscles, the bursae and tendon of the long head of the biceps muscle, and can view these structures during movement. It is reliable in detecting complete tendon rupture but less reliable in cases

of partial damage (Fig. 14.15). MRI provides more detail.

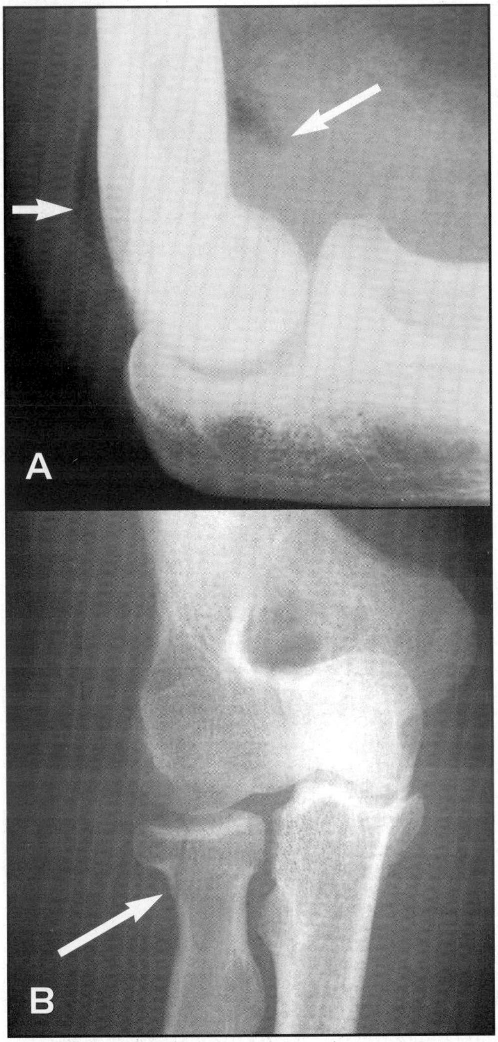

Elbow and forearm

Fractures may occur following a fall on the outstretched hand and more severe injuries, including dislocations, may result from more direct trauma.

Fat pad sign

Some fractures involving the joint may be difficult to detect but are usually accompanied by a joint effusion. The small fat pad which nestles in the coronoid fossa on the anterior aspect of the lower humerus is not normally seen in a lateral view of the elbow, but is displaced forwards in the presence of a joint effusion and should be looked for on a lateral view following injury (Fig. 14.16A). This sign should prompt a further look at the film to detect a fracture line.

Fracture of the radial head

Commonly in adults a fall on the outstretched hand results in a longitudinal fracture through the radial head towards the lateral aspect. If the lateral fragment involves less than 1/3 of the articular surface usually conservative management is used (Fig. 14.16B). If there is a significant step in the articular surface or if more than 1/3 of the articular surface is damaged or loose fragments are present in the joint then surgery and resection of the radial head is the usual treatment. In some cases the capitellum is fractured. In children fracture is usually across the radial neck just below the head and is managed conservatively, because the radial head is an important growth centre.

Supracondylar fractures

Whilst in adults a more severe injury may result in T-shaped fractures of the lower end of the humerus, involving the elbow joint, in children, after a fall on the outstretched hand, the lower humeral growth centre may be fractured transversely. If the lower humeral fragment is considerably displaced the diagnosis is not

Fig. 14.16 (A) Both anterior and posterior fat pads (arrows) are clearly visible, indicating an elbow joint effusion. (B) Vertical fracture through the radial head with insignificant displacement (arrow).

difficult, but the only evidence may be slight rotation either anteriorly or posteriorly of the distal humeral fragment, and this is best detected by comparison with a lateral of the other elbow. The fat pad sign is often positive with these fractures.

Postero-lateral dislocation of the elbow

This is the usual type of dislocation and is associated with disruption of the medial ligament and sometimes avulsion of the medial epicondyle to which it is attached. Occasionally the epicondylar fragment becomes trapped within the joint.

Forearm bones

Injuries resulting in fracture of radial and ulnar shafts are easily diagnosed. When fracture of only one forearm bone is demonstrated it is essential to include views of the elbow and wrist joints. Fracture of the ulna may be associated with a dislocated radial head (Monteggia fracture) and fracture of the radial shaft with dislocation of the inferior radio-ulnar joint (Galleazzi fracture).

Wrist joint

Normal anatomy

To detect and manage fractures and dislocations certain normal features should be understood. In the lateral view the distal articular surface of the radius should be angulated about 10–15 degrees in the volar direction from the longitudinal axis of the radius (Fig. 14.17A). Also, in the lateral view the lunate, the head of the capitate, and the longitudinal axis of the third metacarpal should be in correct alignment. In the postero-anterior view of the wrist it is important to note that the tip of the radial styloid extends about 1 cm more distally than the tip of the ulnar styloid. The scaphoid bone bridges between the proximal and distal rows of carpal bones. In injuries to the carpal bones fractures may result and these tend to be along a curved stress line which passes through the waist of the scaphoid, the body of the capitate, and the body of the triquetrum (Fig. 14.17B).

Colles' fracture

Colles described this fracture of the distal radius in 1786 (Fig. 14.18). The typical 'dinner fork' deformity seen clinically results from the posterior and lateral rotation with impaction of the distal radial fragment. A fractured ulnar styloid process is frequently associated. Several important aspects of the fracture should be appreciated.

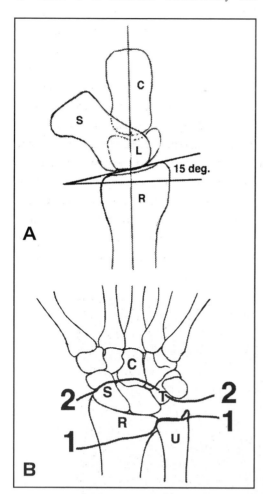

Fig. 14.17 (A) Showing that normally the distal radial articular surface is angled forwards by about 15 degrees on the long axis of the shaft. (B) Showing the lines along which fractures mostly occur. The proximal line (1) passes through the distal radius (R) and the base of the ulnar styloid (U). The distal line (2) passes through the scaphoid waist (S), the capitate (C) and triquetrum (T).

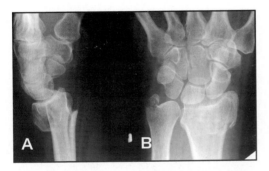

Fig. 14.18 Left-comminuted Colles' fracture. (A) Lateral view shows posterior rotation of the distal radial fragments. (B) Postero-anterior view showing marked lateral impaction of radial fragments with the radial styloid tip level with the ulnar styloid, which is also fractured.

- Non-union does not occur, but because the region consists of mainly cancellous bone there is a tendency for the bone to collapse and union to occur with some deformity.
- The prognosis with comminuted fractures, particularly if a fracture line extends into the wrist joint is less favourable as regards developing future osteoarthritis.
- It is important to maintain the reduced position. Nowadays management responsibility may be fragmented. Initial reduction made in an emergency department

requires checking by x-ray one week later when swelling has subsided. This may fall to the local practitioner and it is important, particularly with younger adults, that remanipulation be carried out if adequate reduction is not maintained.

Smith's fracture is far less common and results in the distal radial fragment being displaced anteriorly. Maintenance of adequate reduction is more difficult.

Scaphoid fracture

Most commonly the fracture line is across the waist, although fractures may occur distally or proximally in the bone (Fig. 14.19A). The blood supply to the proximal portion comes from a nutrient artery which enters the bone distally and which may be damaged by a fracture across the waist resulting in avascular necrosis of the proximal fragment. The fracture in the bone may be difficult to detect initially. Patients with classical tenderness over the bone but with no definite fracture on x-ray should have a radionuclide bone scan which will be positive about two to three days following the injury. Alternatively a plaster can be applied for about ten days, following which x-ray

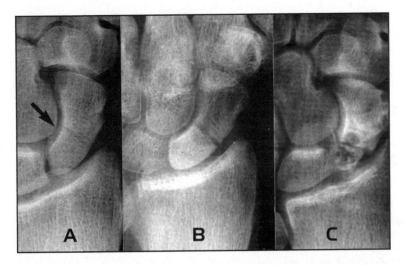

Fig. 14.19 Scaphoid fractures. (A) Recent fracture line (arrow). (B) Non-union indicated by increased density of the relatively avascular proximal fragment with a wide fracture line. (C) Late stage non-union with avascular necrosis of the shrunken proximal fragment.

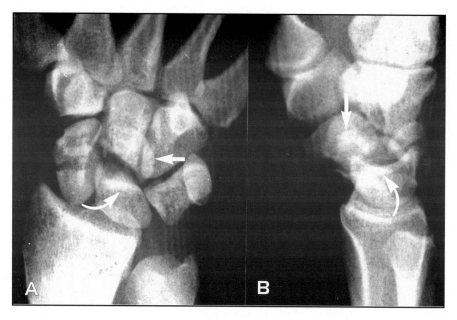

Fig. 14.20 Right wrist. Transcapho-perilunar fracture dislocation with fractures also in the capitate and the triquetrum. Postero-anterior (A) and lateral (B) show absence of the head of the capitate from the distal lunar articular surface (curved arrows) and the dislocated proximal capitate fragment (arrow). The triquetral fracture was seen in an oblique view.

will most likely demonstrate the fracture line (Fig. 14.19B). Prolonged immobilisation is usually required and non-union may result. Established non-union is manifest radiologically by widening of the fracture line and the development of sclerosis along the margins. Also the proximal fragment, with the poorer blood supply, may appear relatively dense (Fig. 14.19C).

Fracture dislocations of the carpus

These serious injuries may require open reduction. The most common dislocation is a displacement of the distal carpal bones from the proximal row and this is usually associated with a fracture through the scaphoid (Fig. 14.20). Careful study of the lateral view will show a disturbance of the alignment of the third metacarpal, the capitate, and the lunate. Fractures may also be present in the capitate and triquetrum.

Bennett's fracture dislocation of the first metacarpal

The proximal articular surface of the first metacarpal is saddle-shaped and a fall on the outstretched thumb may result in an oblique fracture into the first metacarpo-carpal joint. Because of the shape of the articulation the fracture is unstable, with subluxation of the end of the first metacarpal proximally (Fig. 14.21B).

Fractured neck of 5th metacarpal

Second to Bennett's fracture as the most common metacarpal fracture, this usually results from punching with a clenched fist (Fig. 14.21A).

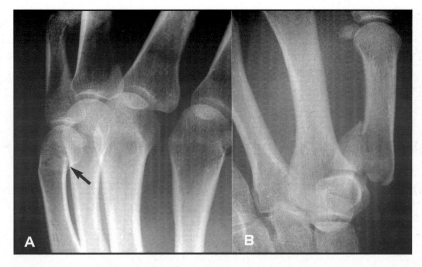

Fig. 14.21 (A) Fracture across the neck of the fifth left metacarpal (arrow) with slight forward rotation of the head. (B) Bennett's fracture dislocation of the first metacarpal.

14.6 Lower Extremity Injuries

Hip joint

Fracture of the femoral neck

Although various names are used to describe the anatomical sites of these fractures, for practical purposes they are of two types, subcapital and basal.

Subcapital

The fracture line may occur anywhere along the length of the neck, but usually in the mid-cervical region or towards the head of the femur. Very commonly seen in the elderly and osteoporotic, these fractures are likely to damage the arterial blood supply which runs in the retinacula on the surface of the bone towards the head, resulting in avascular necrosis. Sometimes the fracture is undisplaced, but more often displacement occurs with external rotation of the lower limb.

Displaced subcapital fractures are usually diagnosed clinically. Radiologically these fractures are clearly seen (Fig. 14.22), particularly on a lateral view, but in the acutely injured patients it may not be possible to obtain a lateral. In the AP view the fracture line may be seen but the external rotation and angulation of the neck may not be appreciated. With external rotation of the femoral shaft the lesser trochanter becomes more obvious in the AP view when compared with the normal side.

Undisplaced subcapital fractures may be very difficult to detect on the plain radiograph. If an undisplaced subcapital fracture is suspected because of continuing pain in the elderly, detailed films confined to the femoral neck should be obtained and CT may be helpful. It is reasonable in such patients to rest them in bed for two days and to perform a radionuclide scan. The prognosis is considerably better when treating an undisplaced fracture and it is important that displacement should not occur following injury and prior to therapy. Femoral neck fractures, particularly undisplaced fractures, may be immobilised using a trifin nail introduced percutaneously under fluoroscopic control, but the risks of non-union and avascular necrosis have made excision of the head fragment and replacement with a prosthesis a feasible option in many elderly patients but requires an open operation. Radiology has a role in monitoring for complications of hip joint

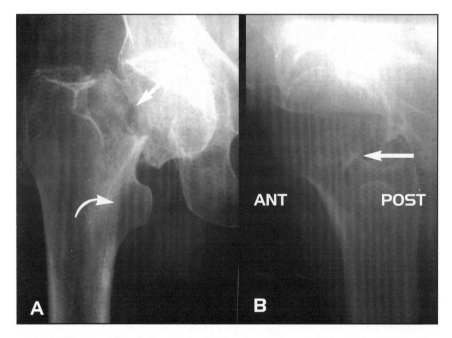

Fig. 14.22 Subcapital fracture of the right femur. (A) Antero-posterior view showing the fracture line (arrow) and a prominent lesser trochanter (curved arrow) indicating external rotation of the femoral shaft. (B) Lateral view showing anterior angulation of the femoral neck at the fracture site.

prostheses. The radiolucency which may develop around the metal stem in the femoral shaft may, or may not, be due to chronic infection. Infection is confirmed if the site is 'hot' on scanning following injection of radionuclide-labelled white cells (see section 12.3).

Basal

The fracture line passes through cancellous bone at the base of the femoral neck and the fracture is often described as pertrochanteric or intertrochanteric (Fig. 14.23). The blood supply to the upper end of the femur is not in jeopardy and these fractures unite well. On x-ray the fracture line is usually clearly seen and the external rotation of the femoral shaft results in a prominent lesser trochanter. Occasionally these fractures are comminuted. The usual treatment is with a trifin nail in the femoral neck coupled to a plate and screws along the femoral shaft.

Dislocation of the hip

Most commonly the head of the femur dislocates posteriorly and in some cases the posterior rim of

the acetabulum is fractured. The injury often results from a motor vehicle accident and the force is transmitted through the femur of a person

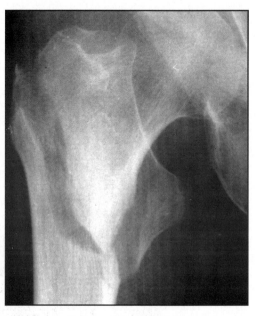

Fig. 14.23 Basal fracture of the right femur. The fracture line extends from the greater to the lesser trochanter, i.e. intertrochanteric.

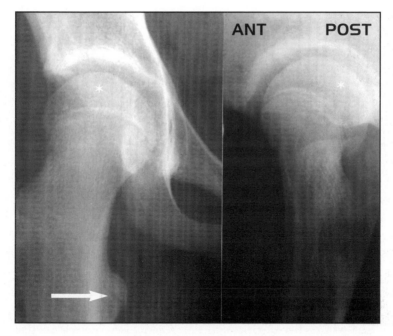

Fig. 14.24 Slipped femoral epiphysis. (A) Antero-posterior view shows the epiphysis (*) lying slightly laterally on the neck. The prominent lesser trochanter (arrow) indicates external rotation of the shaft. (B) The lateral view shows the epiphysis to have slipped posteriorly also causing anterior angulation with the shaft.

seated. In contrast to femoral neck fractures the lower limb is internally rotated, adducted and flexed. This injury is frequently seen in younger people and avascular necrosis of the femoral head may occur through damage to the blood supply at the time of injury or during reduction, which often requires open surgery. Usually the dislocation is obvious radiologically, the main purpose of which is to detect associated fractures.

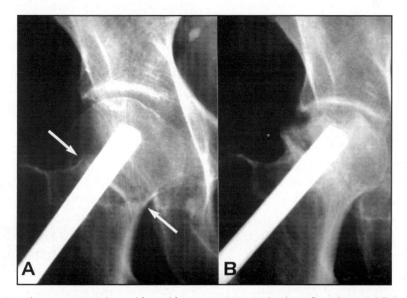

Fig. 14.25 Avascular necrosis. (A) Subcapital femoral fracture (arrows) treated with a tri-flanged intramedullary nail. (B) Five years later. The fracture site is well healed but irregularity, collapse and sclerosis have developed in the necrotic femoral head.

Slipped upper femoral epiphysis

This condition of childhood usually presents with a history of hip pain and limp but occasionally the slipping may be acute following injury when the patient presents with external rotation of the lower limb. In some children only referred knee pain is present. Radiologically the slipping may be subtle and it is necessary to compare the positions of the femoral epiphyses on the two sides (Fig. 14.24). The epiphysis tends to slip posteriorly and laterally in respect to the femoral neck.

Avascular necrosis of the femoral head

This may not be apparent for several years after femoral neck fracture or dislocation. Radiologically, irregularity of the articular surface of the femoral head with associated sclerosis is seen (Fig. 14.25). The condition is painful. MRI provides evidence of the condition well before changes are visible on the plain radiograph. Avascular necrosis of the femoral head is seen also after steroid administration, Cushing's syndrome, Legg–Perthes disease of childhood, barotrauma of deep sea divers and sometimes in alcoholics.

Knee and leg

In this complex joint damage may occur to bones, ligaments, cartilage and the quadriceps mechanism. Severe injury may produce gross fractures but more frequently indirect and minor injury affects the knee, often during sports. Soft

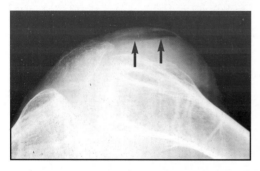

Fig. 14.26 Lipohaemarthrosis of the knee. Lateral view made with an horizontal beam shows the fluid - fluid (arrows) level consistent with an underlying fracture.

tissue damage, particularly to ligaments and menisci, predominates in this type of injury.

Acute knee injury

Plain radiography is indicated to detect fractures, particularly of the patella, the tibial plateau and avulsion fractures. An avulsed fracture of the tibial spine is consistent with anterior cruciate ligament injury and bony avulsion from the posterior margin of the tibial plateau is consistent with posterior cruciate damage. More often cruciate injuries are not associated with avulsions. A depressed fracture of the tibial plateau may indicate rupture of a collateral ligament, particularly rupture of the medial ligament in association with depression of the lateral aspect of the tibial plateau due to impaction of the lateral femoral condyle.

A lateral view of the knee using a horizontal beam may show evidence of **lipohaemarthrosis**, which results from osteochondral damage and seepage of bone marrow into the joint space (Fig. 14.26). A fluid-fluid level is seen due to the less dense lucent fatty fluid rising to the highest point. Such a finding should encourage a further search for a fracture and this may require CT.

In some acute knee injuries general anaesthesia is performed to aspirate a tense effusion and perhaps perform arthroscopy. In these circumstances a stress X-ray may show abnormal mobility consistent with ligamentous rupture. In adolescence a stress view may reveal a fracture across the lower femoral epiphyseal plate.

Fractured patella

The patella is the largest sesamoid bone and lies in the tendinous extension of the quadriceps muscle. It may be fractured indirectly by muscle pull, producing usually a transverse fracture line. If separation of the patellar fragments is present it indicates some damage to the surrounding tendon and surgical correction, usually with wiring, is indicated (Fig. 14.27B). If no distraction is present conservative management is appropriate (Fig. 14.27A). Direct violence may result in

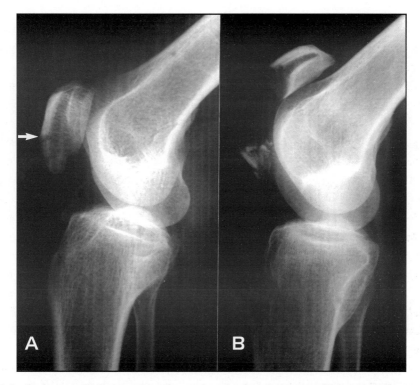

Fig. 14.27 Patellar fractures. (A) Transverse linear fracture (arrow) without displacement. (B) Comminuted fracture with wide separation indicating rupture of the quadriceps tendon.

comminution of the patella with disturbance to the patello-femoral articular surface. This usually requires patellectomy and tendon repair. A developmentally bi-partite patella may be confused with a fracture (Fig. 14.28). A separate ossification centre develops at the upper lateral aspect of the patella and may remain separate. The lucent line between the centre and the body of the patella is usually wider than a fracture, but if doubt exists comparison with the opposite knee may show a similar centre.

Internal derangement of the knee

Severe soft tissue injuries may be present with a normal plain radiograph. Arthroscopy provides diagnosis and allows treatment of certain abnormalities and is now well established. MRI is capable of demonstrating many of the common abnormalities, particularly cruciate ligament damage (Fig. 14.29) and meniscal injuries, such

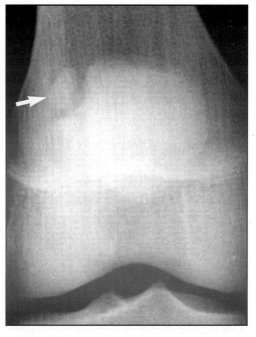

Fig. 14.28 Bi-partite patella. The separate ossicle at the usual superolateral site (arrow) is smaller than the gap in the patella.

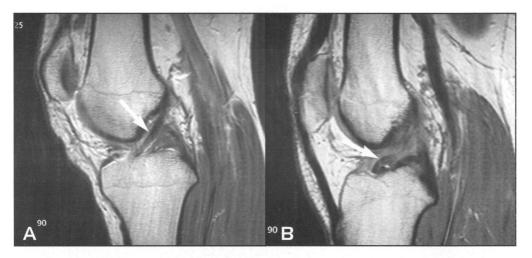

Fig. 14.29 Sagittal MRI of the knee. The T$_2$ weighted scans show (A) a normal anterior cruciate ligament (arrow) and (B) a ruptured anterior cruciate (arrow).

as 'bucket-handle' tears. When available MRI is recommended, following plain radiography, as the next investigation, with the more invasive arthroscopy reserved for those cases in which endoscopic therapy may be necessary.

Tibia and fibula

The fibula may be fractured by direct trauma. More commonly, fractures of the tibia and fibula occur and usually at the junction of the middle and lower thirds of the shafts. Occasionally, swelling in the deep fascial compartments of the leg embarrass nerves and vascular structures to the foot and requires urgent surgical decompression.

Ankle joint and foot

Ankle

In normal radiographs the articular surface of the talus is seen to fit accurately into the mortice made up of the lower tibial articular surface, including the medial malleolus, and the articular surface on the medial aspect of the external malleolus of the fibula. The lower ends of the tibia and fibula are held closely together by interosseous ligaments. On the posterior margin of the lower tibial articular surface a bony prominence, usually called the posterior malleolus, gives rise to the posterior tibio-fibular

ligament. It is important to detect disturbances in this normal arrangement and to restore normality when treating such injuries.

Ankle injuries vary in severity. When viewing the films it is important to determine the likely extent of ligamentous damage as well as detecting fractures, often referred to as Pott's fractures, because stability of the joint is the main concern. The following points are relevant.

- Serious ligamentous injury may result without any x-ray evidence. Dislocation of the talus may occur and the talus return to its normal position without radiological evidence of the happening. When suspected the presence of such an injury may be determined by performing a stress radiograph by abducting or adducting the foot and demonstrating on the radiograph the displacement of the talus. The person applying the stress should wear lead gloves and an apron and anaesthesia may be necessary.

- Injuries result from forces causing mainly inversion or eversion of the talus. On the side of the initial force, ligament damage with or without avulsion of a bone fragment from the adjacent malleolus occurs, e.g. with eversion the medial collateral ligament (deltoid) may tear or a medial malleolar avulsion may occur,

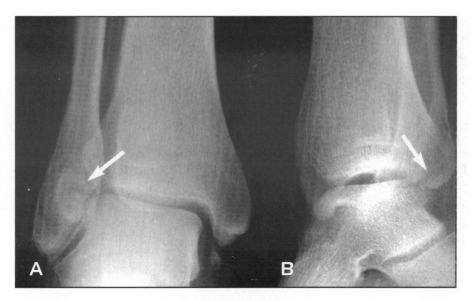

Fig. 14.30 Tri-malleolar Pott's fracture. Eversion injury. (A) The AP view shows avulsion of a fragment from the medial malleolus with slight lateral displacement of the talus and a fracture in the lateral malleolus (arrow) at the level of the talo-tibial joint line. (B) Oblique. A posterior malleolar fracture of the tibia (arrow) is seen. The lateral displacement of the talus indicates that this Weber B injury is unstable and after reduction requires surgical internal fixation of the lateral malleolar fragment.

usually, below or at the level of the talo-tibial joint line (Fig. 14.30A).

- On the side of secondary impact of the talus a fracture is seen at or extending above the talo-tibial joint line, e.g. with eversion the oblique fracture occurs in the fibula (Fig. 14.30B) and with inversion the oblique fracture extends obliquely above the talo-tibial joint line separating the medial malleolus. Thus an oblique fibular fracture indicates significant damage to the medial ligament even if an avulsion fracture is not seen in the medial malleolus.

- With eversion injuries damage to the interosseous membrane and tibio-fibular ligaments may result in separation of the two bones (**diastasis**) with instability, and this can be predicted from the level of the oblique fibular fracture, using the Weber classification of 1972 (Fig. 14.31). Weber A with the fracture below the transverse talo-tibial joint line is stable (Fig. 14.31A), Weber B at the joint line has a 50% chance of instability (Figs 14.30, 14.31B) and Weber C above the line even up to the fibular neck, has extensive

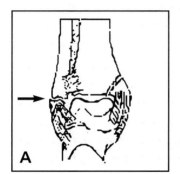
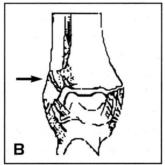
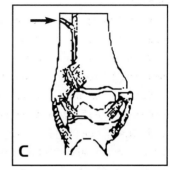

Fig. 14.31 Weber classification of fibular fractures. Fracture (arrow) below the talo-tibial joint line (A), at the line (B) and above (C). Rupture of interosseous and tibio-fibular ligaments causing instability (diastasis) occurs in (C), in about 50% of (B) and not in (A) fractures.

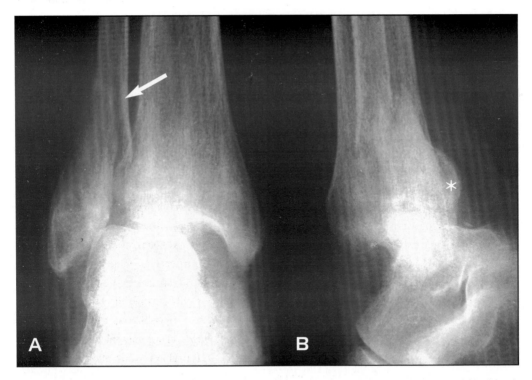

Fig. 14.32 Bi-malleolar Pott's fracture dislocation. Eversion injury. (A) AP showing marked lateral displacement of the talus with a fracture through the fibula (arrow) above the talo-tibial joint line. Rupture of medial ligament. (B) The talus is markedly displaced posteriorly. This Weber C injury requires internal fixation of the lateral malleolus after reduction and probably the posterior malleolus (*) also.

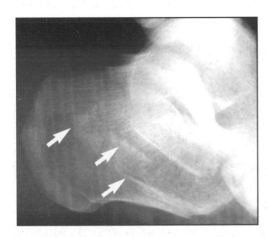

Fig. 14.33 Fractured calcaneus. The dense bands in the lateral view (arrows) indicate compressed cancellous bone. The patient jumped from a height.

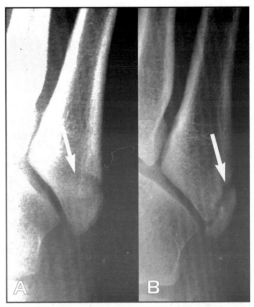

Fig. 14.34 (A) Transverse avulsion fracture at base of fifth metatarsal (arrow). (B) Developmentally separate ossicle at base of fifth metatarsal. Note the longitudinal direction of the lucent line (arrow) compared with fracture (A).

interosseous ligament damage requiring internal fixation (Figs 14.31C,14.32).

- With posterior displacement of the talus, the posterior tibial malleolus may be separated and, if the fragment is large, it may require internal fixation (Fig. 14.32).

Calcaneus

Those who 'fall on their feet' may be less fortunate than the idiom suggests as they may sustain a compression fracture of a vertebral body, a fracture dislocation of the ankle or a compression injury of the calcaneus. Many calcaneal fractures are easily diagnosed from the x-ray but in some the cancellous bone compacts producing only a fine sclerotic band seen best in the lateral view (Fig. 14.33).

Fifth metatarsal

A fracture across the base of the fifth metatarsal is common and results from avulsion by the tendon of peroneus brevis. Confusion may arise with a separate bony ossicle which may develop at the base of this metatarsal. However, the fracture line is always transverse whilst the line of separation of the ossicle runs longitudinally (Fig. 14.34).

Forefoot

Multiple fracture dislocations at the metatarso-tarsal level may result from a wheel crushing the foot. This fracture, named after Lisfranc, was described at the time of the French Revolution when it is said spectators watching the guillotine ran the risk of a tumbrel squashing their feet! It is of importance because of the likelihood of damage to blood vessels resulting in gangrene of toes, requiring amputation.

Stress fractures

These commonly involve the bones of the foot and may not be visible on plain radiography. Radionuclide scanning may show a 'hot-spot' and in many CT is able to show the occult fracture line. (Fig. 14.3).

14.7 Osteochondroses

This group of conditions, often called osteochondritis, includes growth centre abnormalities at various sites throughout the body. Best known is Legg-Perthes disease of the femoral head epiphysis. Much more common in boys, the condition affects children aged three to twelve years and the epiphysis undergoes a series of changes over several years. Patients present

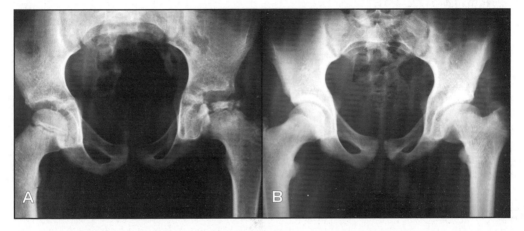

Fig. 14.35 Legg-Perthes osteochondrosis of left hip. (A) Ten year old boy. Fragmentation of capital epiphysis. (B) Eight years later. Flattened left femoral head.

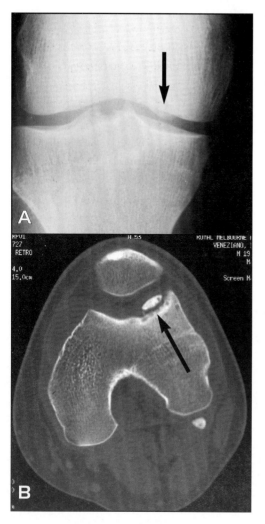

with a limp and the initial film may show minor fracturing of the epiphysis, which over time leads to necrosis followed by a healing phase sometime later (Fig. 14.35). The cartilage over the head is usually preserved. Radionuclide scanning initially shows deficient uptake suggesting ischaemia and the radiological changes are consistent with ischaemic necrosis. Eponyms abound to describe similar changes at other sites and the best known are Osgood–Schlatter's disease of the tibial tubercle, Kienbock's for the lunate and Freiberg's for the head of a metatarsal. In later life these epiphyses appear fused but deformed and sometimes dense.

Osteochondritis dissecans is somewhat different and is considered to be due to a localized fracture of subchondral bone on the margin of an epiphysis. Typically the lesion is seen on the anterolateral aspect of the medial femoral condyle in the knee. A separate piece of bone lies surrounded by a radiolucent rim (Fig. 14.36). The bone fragment may break through the cartilage to become a loose body within the joint.

Fig. 14.36 Osteochondritis dissecans. (A) Plain film. A bony fragment (arrow) separated from the lateral aspect of the medial condyle: a common site. (B) CT showing a similar lesion on the lateral condyle.

14.8 Bone metastases

Radionuclide bone scanning is more sensitive than plain radiography in demonstrating carcinomatous bone metastases and should be used as the first investigation. The radionuclide employed is a phosphate compound labelled with **technetium 99m.** The phosphate compound is taken up in the region of most metastatic lesions. Suspicious areas are detected by the whole body scanner as 'hot spots' due to increased gamma emission (Fig. 14.37). However, the test is nonspecific and 'hot spots' are seen around osteoarthritic joints and inflammatory foci. For this reason, plain radiography should be performed of suspicious areas on the radionuclide bone scan. Also, because metastases can be present occasionally without increased radionuclide uptake it is important to perform plain radiography of regions of persistent pain despite a negative bone scan. Multiple myeloma does not take up the radionuclide well. On plain radiography most carcinomatous metastases are purely lytic, particularly from lung, kidney, adrenal and thyroid (Fig. 14.38). They are frequently very small and widespread throughout

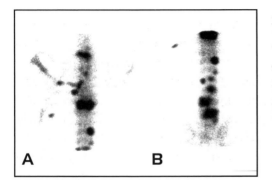

Fig. 14.37 Radionuclide bone scan of thorax (A) and abdomen (B). Multiple rounded foci of increased uptake consistent with carcinomatous metastases.

many bones but occasionally may be larger, measuring several centimetres across, when the diagnosis may be uncertain. An isolated rounded purely lytic lesion in bone may be due to:

- Metastatic carcinoma. Typically from kidney, thyroid, adrenal or lung.
- Multiple myeloma, e.g. plasmacytoma.
- Bone cyst, e.g. hyperparathyroidism.
- Benign tumour, e.g. chondroma, histiocytosis.
- Bone abscess (Brodie's abscess).

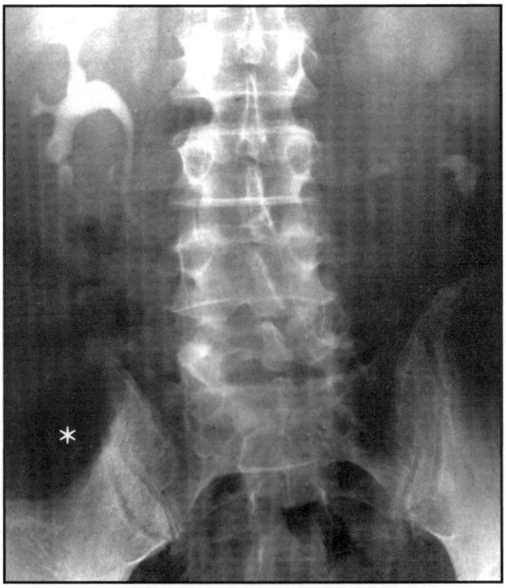

Metastases do not grow across joint cartilage and in the spine the intervertebral disc spaces are preserved. The widespread lytic lesions of multiple myeloma can frequently be distinguished from carcinoma by the characteristic punched-out circular appearance of the myeloma deposits, especially in the skull (Fig. 14.45). Myeloma patients usually do not develop focal lung opacities and in confusing cases this may help differentiation from carcinomatosis in which lung metastases frequently occur.

Some bone metastases evoke an osteoblastic reaction seen as dense areas of bone sclerosis and some metastases show a mixed lytic and sclerotic pattern. When widespread sclerotic bony opacities are present, diagnosis may be difficult and the following possibilities should be considered.

- Sclerotic carcinomatous metastases. Typically from prostate, breast and occasionally stomach or bladder (Fig. 14.39).
- Sclerotic form of Paget's disease (Fig. 14.42).
- Lymphoma (usually some lytic areas present also).
- Myelosclerosis.

Clinical features and further tests, e.g. prostate-specific antigen, usually clarify the diagnosis.

Fig. 14.38 Renal cell carcinoma of left kidney distorting the pyelogram. Large lytic metastasis in right ilium (*).

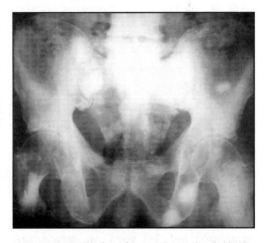

Fig. 14.39 Multiple foci of bone sclerosis due to bladder carcinoma metastases.

14.9 Paget's Disease

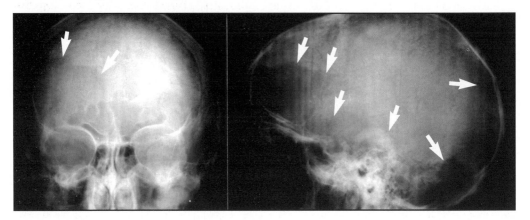

Fig. 14.40 Paget's disease. Osteoporosis circumscripta. A large area of lysis with a well-defined margin (arrows) involves the right side of the calvarium, including the base.

Paget's disease is common and has various manifestations. It is a disease of individual bones but multiple bones may be involved. It is unusual in the hands and feet. Paget's disease is a disturbance of the balance between bone deposition and resorption with an increased rate of bone turnover. Oriental races are rarely affected. Three stages of the condition are recognized.

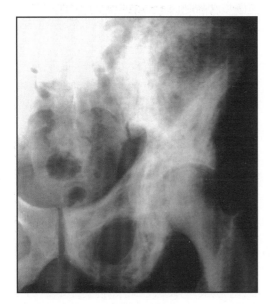

Fig. 14.41 Paget's disease. Fibrillary pattern involving the left hip bone.

1. Osteoporosis circumscripta (Fig. 14.40)

The earliest change is a loss of density and this is seen best in the skull where a large area of demineralised bone with an ill-defined wavy margin is seen in the vault. The tibial shaft also may show this early change. Loss of cortico-medullary differentiation occurs in the area which, in the tibia, has a V-shaped lower edge, well demonstrated in the lateral view.

2. Fibrillary form (Fig. 14.41)

This common form of Paget's disease is usually easily recognized from the following radiographic features.

- Altered architecture of the bone. The trabecular pattern of the bone is altered with the development of an open coarse-stranded or fibrillary appearance. The coarsened trabeculae are most prominent in the direction of the lines of weight bearing.
- Loss of cortico-medullary differentiation.
- Slight increase in size of the bone. A valuable diagnostic point is the abnormal remodelling of bone in Paget's disease, resulting in a slight increase in bulk of the bone and a loss of some

normal contours. Thus, an affected vertebral body is not only slightly enlarged but the slight concavity on the anterior aspect normally seen in the lateral view may be lost.

3. Sclerotic form (Fig. 14.42)

Very occasionally, established Paget's disease may be seen as a uniform sclerosis of an entire bone and this may give rise to confusion in diagnosis, e.g. with prostatic metastases. Careful observation may show subtle features which aid in differentiation, e.g. increase in bulk of the bone indicating Paget's disease, or some isolated rounded nodular opacities suggesting prostatic cancer.

Complications

Paget's disease is frequently a chance finding on radiography or as a 'hot spot' in a radionuclide bone scan. Occasionally, complications occur.

1. Fracture (Fig. 14.43)

The shaft of a Paget's disease long bone snaps like a carrot with a transverse fracture line compared with the oblique fracture seen in normal long bones. These fractures heal quite well.

2. Nerve compression

In severe disease of the skull, the skull base flattens (platybasia) and, together with the narrowing of foramina, the deformity can interfere with cranial nerves and occasionally the brain stem. Deafness is common.

3. Cardiovascular effects

Widespread Paget's disease is associated with high cardiac output. It is only very occasionally that cardiac failure with cardiomegaly occurs.

4. Sarcoma

Primary osteogenic sarcoma usually occurs in young people, but may complicate Paget's disease in the elderly. The radiograph shows an area of lysis within the Paget's bone and an associated soft tissue mass. The prognosis is very poor.

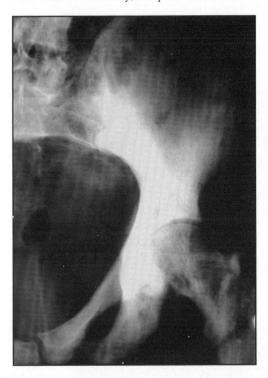

Fig. 14.42 Paget's disease. Sclerotic pattern involving large areas of the left hip bone. Fibrillary pattern in the upper left femur.

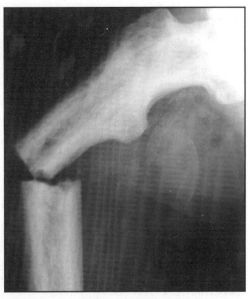

Fig. 14.43 Paget's disease. Typical transverse fracture in the femoral shaft.

14.10 Bone Changes in Blood Diseases

Bony abnormalities may result from diseases affecting the contained bone marrow, particularly in the central skeleton. In congenital haemolytic anaemias such as **thalassaemia** and **sickle cell anaemia**, the increased volume of red marrow alters bony development. The bones have a coarse trabecular pattern and may be expanded and malformed (Fig. 14.44). **Extramedullary haemopoietic tissue** may be seen as extrapleural masses on chest x-ray or may cause spinal cord compression on occasions. In **multiple myeloma**, generalized osteoporosis of the central skeleton may be the only bony manifestation but in some patients focal rounded lytic lesions, particularly in the skull, have a characteristic appearance (Fig. 14.45). Occasionally, a solitary lytic **plasmacytoma** is the first manifestation. Leukaemia may cause widespread ill-defined osteolysis, but lymphoma is usually more localized, causing mixed lytic and sclerotic changes. When the red bone marrow atrophies, e.g. myelosclerosis, the central skeleton responds by becoming slightly denser.

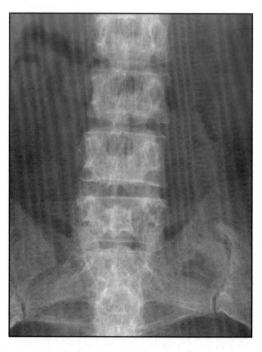

Fig. 14.44 Thalassaemia major. Coarse trabecular pattern due to hyperplastic bone marrow.

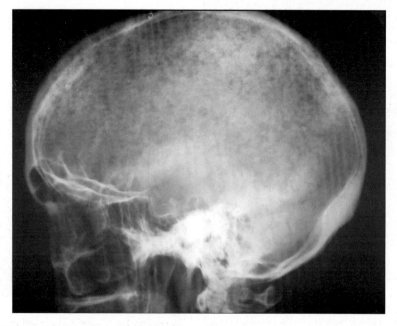

Fig. 14.45 Multiple myeloma. Typical small round lucent foci in the skull vault.

14.11 Generalized Loss of Bone Density

Differentiating osteoporosis, osteomalacia, and hyperparathyroidism may be difficult radiologically, but there are features of these conditions which may be indicative.

1. Osteoporosis

Not only is mineral lost in this condition but also bone matrix. The softening is seen best in lateral views of the spine (Fig. 14.46) which show:

- Altered trabecular pattern. With resorption the remaining trabeculae are arranged in a vertical fashion, giving a striated appearance.
- Reduced cortical width.
- Bulging of intervertebral discs. With softening of the vertebral bodies, the intervertebral discs bulge into the adjacent bones.

Additional features are the tendency for osteoporotic bone to fracture, particularly the femoral neck and compression fractures of vertebral bodies.

The causes of osteoporosis most commonly seen are senile and post-menopausal osteoporosis, prolonged steroid therapy and Cushing's syndrome.

The fractures of Cushing's syndrome are characterized by the development of exuberant callus and, on occasions, multiple rib fractures with callus have been mistaken for multiple pulmonary metastases on a chest film!

2. Osteomalacia

In this condition, there is loss of minerals from the bones but the matrix is relatively unaffected, so that softening is not a major feature. Considerable calcium loss is necessary before changes are apparent radiographically.

In chronic osteomalacia in adults the changes are similar to those in osteoporosis except for

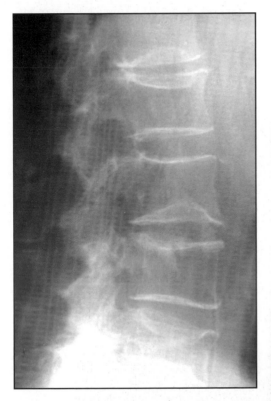

Fig. 14.46 Senile osteoporosis. The softened bone allows expansion of the intervertebral discs into the vertebral bodies, which appear relatively radiolucent with prominent vertical trabeculae.

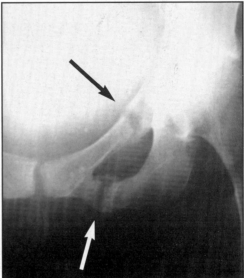

Fig. 14.47 Osteomalacia. Pseudofractures (Looser zones). The relatively broad lucent lines are well seen in the ischio-pubic rami (arrows).

softening. In more acute forms of osteomalacia the diagnosis may be suggested by the presence of **pseudofractures** or **Looser's zones.** These are bands of relatively demineralised bone, looking like fractures, which are seen in the pubic rami, the lateral scapular margins and sometimes in the cortex of long bones (Fig. 14.47).

Demineralisation of bone due to lack of calcium or Vitamin D may be due to:

- Deficient intake – nutritional.
- Deficient absorption – malabsorption syndrome.
- Deficient utilization – hypophosphatasia.
- Deficient tubular reabsorption – chronic renal failure; Fanconi syndrome.

3. Hyperparathyroidism

See section 5.4.

14.12 Focal Destructive Lesions

Practitioners should realize that when confronted with a radiograph which shows a single destructive lesion in a bone the diagnosis can be extremely difficult. The first thing is to exclude other lesions in the skeleton which would widen the field of diagnostic possibilities to include such conditions as metastases, myeloma, lymphoma, or histiocytosis.

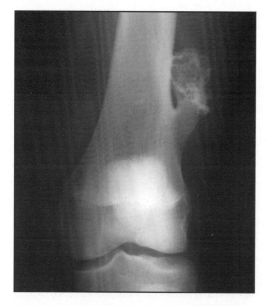

Fig. 14.48 Osteochondroma. Typically directed away from the growing end of the bone. The exostosis has a cartilage cap. Malignant change is very uncommon.

Causes of a focal destructive bone lesion

1. Neoplasms

a. Secondary

Note: Remember the commonest bone lesion in adults is a metastasis, even when apparently solitary (see section 14.8).

b. Primary

- Benign, e.g. enchondroma, contained within a bone; osteochondroma or exostosis seen as a bony spur with a cartilage cap (Fig. 14.48).
- Malignant, e.g. osteogenic sarcoma.

2. Osteomyelitis (including bone abscess and osteoid osteoma).

3. Cysts, e.g. simple bone cyst or cysts of hyperparathyroidism.

4. Fibrous dysplasia

This developmental disturbance may give rise to a local lesion in bone, sometimes solitary, and the appearance can be confused with more sinister conditions. The lesion may be discovered when a complication such as fracture occurs and may give rise to diagnostic difficulty.

5. Histiocytosis, e.g. eosinophil granuloma.

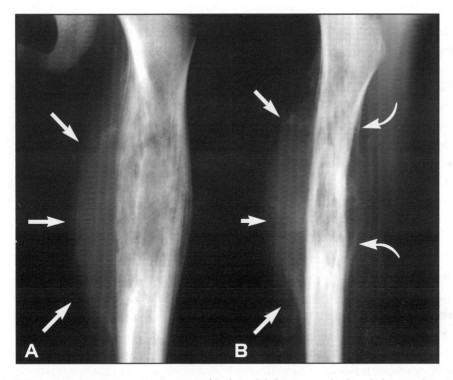

Fig. 14.49 Osteogenic sarcoma. Permeative destruction of the femoral shaft is associated with marked periosteal reaction and a surrounding soft tissue mass (straight arrows). In the lateral view (B) the tumour has grown through the periosteal reaction resulting in Codman's triangles (curved arrows).

Skeletal survey

To detect other bone lesions a radionuclide scan should be performed followed by radiographs of any 'hot spot' areas. Also, because conditions which affect many bones tend to favour the central skeleton a series of radiographs can be selected to provide a reasonable coverage. If adequate clinical notes are provided the radiologist will select a suitable series without the clinician specifying the views. Such a survey would include:

- Lateral skull.
- PA chest.
- Lateral dorsal spine.
- Lateral lumbar spine.
- AP pelvis.
- PA of one hand.
- Lateral of one tibia.

Having excluded, as far as possible, other bone lesions, the focal lesion is then analysed in more detail.

The tissue diagnosis of a solitary destructive lesion of bone may be very difficult in certain cases, even after biopsy. The clinical information from the history and examination of the patient may be helpful. Also, a careful assessment of the radiological changes helps in developing a concept of the type of pathology present and reduces the number of possible diagnoses. However, the radiological features are nonspecific and it is important to realize this. Percutaneous or open biopsy of the lesion provides the pathologist with tissue to study and radiography is helpful in deciding the best site to make the biopsy. However, not uncommonly, pathologists experience difficulty in reaching an exclusive diagnosis and occasionally serious misdiagnoses have occurred and amputations for benign conditions have resulted. In particular, using all diagnostic means available, it may even be difficult to decide whether a lesion is inflammatory, neoplastic, or due to a developmental aberration, such as fibrous dysplasia of bone.

Before considering the radiological features of focal bone lesions, it is important to appreciate that symptoms may be present in advance of a demonstrable lesion on radiography. In acute osteomyelitis, bone changes are not expected until between 7 and 14 days after the onset of symptoms in children. In adults, it may be 3 weeks before changes are detected. In suspicious cases, a radionuclide bone scan will demonstrate a 'hot spot' long before changes are seen radiologically.

Features of localized bone lesions

Careful assessment of these features will be helpful in developing a concept of the underlying pathology.

1. Margin of the lesion

Rapidly spreading processes have an ill-defined margin with a broad zone of transition before normal bone is reached (Fig. 14.49). On the other hand, slowly developing destructive processes are associated with a bone reaction which is seen as a well-defined sclerotic margin (Fig. 14.50). A lobulated edge to the area of destruction suggests that the expansive process is multicentric such as in cartilage tumours.

2. Expansion of the bone

If the lesion causes expansion of the bone and has a well-developed margin it is slow-growing with an increased likelihood that it is benign (Fig. 14.51).

3. The matrix

The matrix is the material within the lesion. In most cases, the appearance is of a loss of bone tissue with no characteristic features. However, degenerating cartilage tumours have a

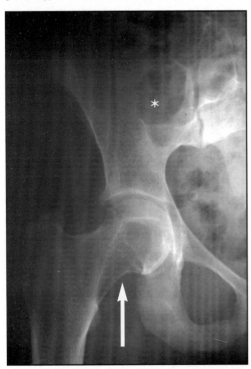

Fig. 14.50 Hyperparathyroidism. Brown tumours in femoral neck (arrow) and ilium (*). Sclerotic rim indicates slow growth and suggests benignity.

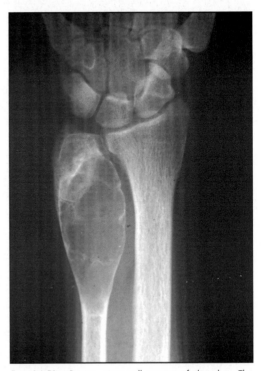

Fig. 14.51 Benign giant cell tumour of the ulna. The symmetrical expansion of the bone with contained bony septa and a clear demarcation from the normal bone are signs of benignity. This tumour typically extends to the end of the bone.

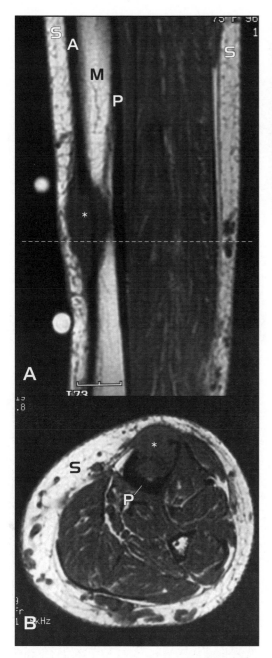

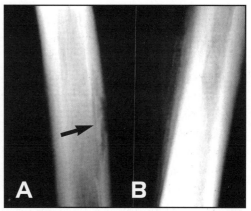

Fig. 14.53 Osteomyelitis. (A) Lateral view showing a dense sequestrum with surrounding cortical lucency (arrow). (B) AP view showing associated periosteal reaction.

characteristic punctate amorphous calcification in the matrix which is easily recognized. Some primary bone tumours retain a trabecular pattern within the matrix. CT is valuable in showing whether the matrix is fluid or solid. MRI is most helpful in demonstrating the extent of tumour tissue, particularly along the marrow cavity, a common route of metastasis in long bones (Fig. 14.52). In osteomyelitis the presence of a sliver of dense bone in the area of destruction, consistent with a **sequestrum**, may be diagnostic (Fig. 14.53). A localized bone abscess known as Brodie's abscess may result from infection and has a cystic appearance with usually some sclerosis of the wall.

4. Overlying cortex

Rapidly enlarging and invasive lesions tend to infiltrate and destroy the overlying cortex, whilst slower processes tend to erode it.

5. Periosteal reaction

The laying down of periosteal new bone locally may be the only radiological feature of a localized bone lesion, and although it is a feature of many malignant neoplasms of bone it is important that the nonspecific nature of the finding be appreciated. In particular it is important to remember that such a reaction may be the only sign of **stress fracture** (Fig. 14.54). Also,

Fig. 14.52 Tibial metastasis from cervical carcinoma (most unusual). T₁ weighted MRI. (A) Sagittal and (B) Axial at level of dotted white line. The tumour (*) has destroyed the anterior cortex (A) and involves the bone marrow (M) locally. (P) = posterior cortex. (S) = Subcutaneous fatty tissue.

periosteal new bone frequently results from **osteomyelitis** (Fig. 14.53). Benign tumours and bone cysts do not develop periosteal reaction unless a fracture or infection is superadded. Small cell sarcoma (Ewing's tumour) is characteristically associated with multilayered periosteal new bone formation **(onion skin layering)**. In osteogenic sarcoma (Fig. 14.49), the initial periosteal reaction is similar but as the tumour breaks through the surface of the bone this parallel periosteal new bone is destroyed and tumour bone is laid down at right angles to the bone in characteristic fashion **(sunray spiculation)**. The remaining cuff of periosteal new bone at the margin of the lesion is also rather characteristic in appearance **(Codman's triangle)**. **Osteoid osteoma** occurs in the cortex, usually of a long bone, and intense periosteal reaction results in localized cortical thickening which is rather characteristic. Within the thickened cortex a small radiolucency or nidus may be seen on plain radiography, and better by CT. Occasionally, **myositis ossificans** resulting from muscle trauma close to a bone can be mistaken for a true periosteal reaction.

Periosteal reaction affecting many bones may be the result of systemic disease. These conditions include:

- Hypertrophic pulmonary osteoarthropathy (see section 15.3).
- Pachydermoperiostitis.
- Scurvy.
- Thyroid acropachy (rare).

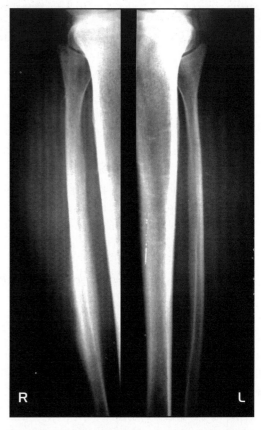

Fig. 14.54 Stress fracture of the right fibula. In this slender basketballer the midshaft of the right fibula shows marked periosteal thickening compared with the left.

6. Soft tissue mass

The presence of a mass in the surrounding soft tissue continuous with the bone lesion strongly suggests a malignant neoplasm or abscess.

Reference

Resnick, D. and Niwayama, G.
Diagnosis of Bone and Joint Disorders, 2nd edn,
W. B. Saunders Co., 1988.

Joints may be involved secondarily from bone disease or trauma (see Chapter 14) or may be the site of a primary process broadly referred to as **arthritis.**

Arthritis has come to mean any disorder of joints, particularly synovial joints. In establishing a diagnosis it is important to realize that clinical manifestations usually precede the radiological evidence by a considerable period. In arriving at a provisional diagnosis, it is important to appreciate the wide range of conditions which may give rise to arthritis.

15.1 Classification of Arthritis

1. Developmental

Congenital hip dysplasia; osteochondroses (see section 14.7).

2. Degenerative

Osteoarthritis; avascular necrosis.

3. Rheumatoid group

Rheumatoid arthritis (including juvenile rheumatoid or Still's disease), and the Spondylarthropathies (including ankylosing spondylitis, psoriatic arthritis, Reiter's syndrome and enteropathic arthritis).

4. Suppurative arthritis

Staphylococcal, tuberculous, gonococcal.

5. Metabolic

Gout, pseudogout, haemochromatosis.

6. Neuropathic

Diabetes, syringomyelia, congenital absence of pain, leprosy, syphilis.

7. Haemorrhagic

Haemophilia.

8. Osteoarthropathies

Hypertrophic pulmonary osteoarthropathy.

15.2 Imaging Modalities

Clinically, following a detailed history and clinical examination, most patients presenting with arthritis can be diagnosed and confirmation established, if necessary, with non-radiological tests. Radiology may be helpful in confirming the diagnosis, staging the disease process, and detecting relevant complications. To this end plain radiography has been the major investigation for many years. Ultrasound is useful in detecting joint effusions, swollen bursae, and Baker's cyst. CT supplements the information from plain radiography, but MRI has particular advantages which will ensure its place in diagnosis of arthritis when the technology is more available. MRI can demonstrate loss of cartilage, and small bony erosions which are not seen on plain x-ray. The extent of vascular pannus, hypertrophy of synovial membrane and subchondral cysts are seen as well as small effusions into joints and synovial sheaths.

On plain radiography only the bony articular surfaces can be seen and the condition of the soft tissues, which are poorly seen, if at all, is inferred. In synovial joints the integrity of the cartilage is assessed from the width of the radiolucent space between the bony articular surfaces. Joint effusions and distended bursae may be seen as slight disturbances in soft tissue density and calcifications can be seen.

Clinically, it is important to determine whether the arthritis is generalized or monarticular. With multiple joint involvement the initial radiological assessment should include the affected joints but also the hands because relatively early changes, particularly in rheumatoid disease, are well shown there.

15.3 Radiological Patterns of Arthritis

1. Developmental joint disease

Developmental abnormalities of the bone ends comprising a joint may lead to dislocation and degenerative arthritis. Congenital dislocation of the hip, better known as **hip dysplasia**, is tested for during neonatal clinical examination by applying the Ortolani or similar manoeuvre. It is important to detect the condition as soon as possible when therapy is most effective. When the Ortolani 'click' test is positive US is used to confirm the diagnosis. US demonstrates the relationship of the femoral head to the bony and fibrocartilaginous acetabulum and the acetabular shape (Fig. 15.1). Plain radiography is no longer used routinely for diagnosis except in patients presenting later (Fig. 15.2). The femoral head epiphysis is not calcified until one year of age.

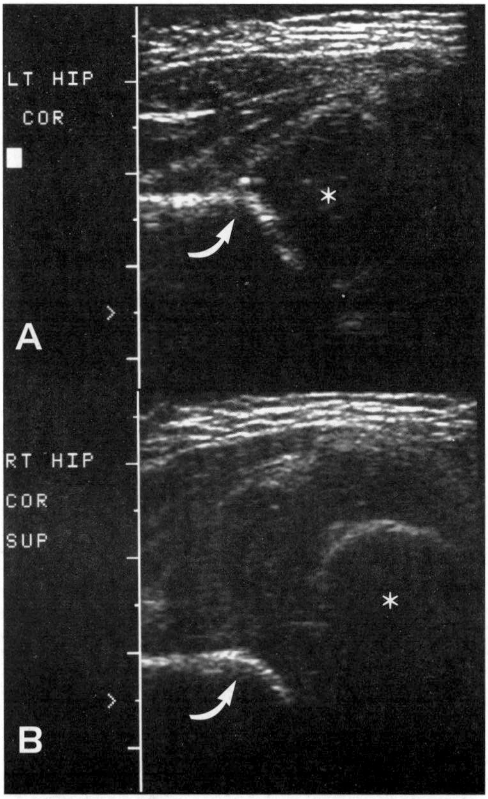

Fig. 15.1 Congenital hip dysplasia. US in neonate. (A) Normal left hip. The cartilaginous femoral head (*) lies in the acetabulum. Note the normal angulation (curved arrow) between ilium and acetabulum. (B) Dislocated right hip. Note the dysplastic curve between ilium and acetabulum (curved arrow) and dislocated femoral head (*).

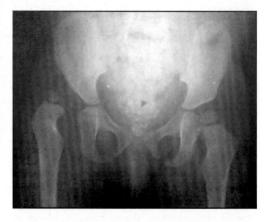

Fig. 15.2 Congenital hip dysplasia. Dislocated right hip. Note the shallow acetabulum compared with the left.

2. Degenerative osteoarthritis (Fig. 15.3)

Weight-bearing joints are often affected, and also joints frequently used, e.g. first metacarpophalangeal joint of the thumb.

- The first change is destruction of joint cartilage with narrowing of the joint space, i.e. the radiolucent area between the bone ends.
- Bony spurs (osteophytes) develop at chondro-osseous junctions.
- Bone density is not significantly altered but with total loss of cartilage the bone ends become sclerotic or 'eburnated'.
- Sub-articular cysts develop. They contain synovial fluid and communicate with the joint.
- Subluxation and false joint formation may eventuate.

Avascular necrosis of bone (see section 14.6) frequently leads to osteoarthritis in the adjacent synovial joint. Avascular bone fragments appear denser and reduced in size.

3. Rheumatoid group

Rheumatoid arthritis and the spondyl-arthropathies, i.e. inflammatory arthritis seronegative to rheumatoid factor, have generally similar radiological appearances, with some variations which may aid diagnosis. Joint cartilage is relatively resistant to pannus, i.e. granulation tissue, and initially it is the intra-articular bone not covered with cartilage which becomes eroded (Fig. 15.4).

The early radiological changes in rheumatoid arthritis are:

- Small erosions seen best at the sides of metacarpal and metatarsal heads and bases of phalanges. Erosive changes may be asymptomatic but indicate the aggressiveness of the disease. If erosions are to appear, 90% will be present within two years of the onset of the disease.
- Joint swellings, particularly proximal interphalangeal joints.
- Juxta-articular osteoporosis.

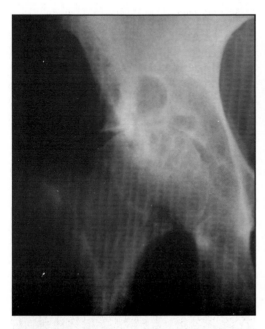

Fig. 15.3 Osteoarthritis of the right hip. Total loss of cartilage centrally with sclerosis of adjacent bone and subarticular synovial cyst formation.

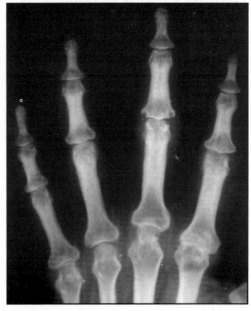

Fig. 15.4 Moderately advanced rheumatoid arthritis. Erosions in the metacarpal heads and, particularly in the base of the middle phalanx of the middle finger. Peri-articular osteopaenia.

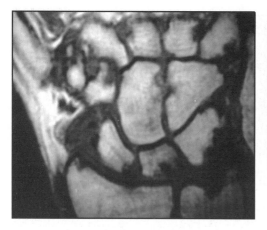

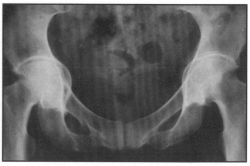

Fig. 15.6   Bilateral protrusio acetabuli. A common manifestation of rheumatoid arthritis.

Fig. 15.5   Rheumatoid arthritis. T_1 weighted MRI shows numerous erosions of carpal bones. With MRI, bone marrow gives a high signal (white) and cortical bone low (black).

- Occasionally, periosteal reaction on adjacent bones.

MRI can show the extent of pannus and the presence of small erosions much earlier than plain radiography, and it is hoped that earlier demonstration and appropriate therapy may limit the destructive process, particularly in juvenile rheumatoid disease (Still's disease) (Fig. 15.5).

In longstanding, advanced rheumatoid arthritis the main features seen in the hands are:

- Gross erosions, often involving the carpus and ulnar styloid ('the rheumatoid lighthouse').
- Ulnar deviation of fingers.
- Subluxation at affected joints.
- Sclerosis of affected bone-ends in some.

In the upper cervical spine, laxity of the transverse ligament may allow forward dislocation of the atlas on the axis with potential cord compression.

In the hip joint there may be no erosions to see in the films, but softening of bone results in **protrusio acetabuli,** i.e. bulging of the acetabulum into the pelvis (Fig. 15.6). In the spondylarthropathies the early joint erosions are similar in nature to rheumatoid. In psoriatic arthritis erosions are seen in the interphalangeal joints with sparing of the metacarpophalangeal joints. In ankylosing spondylitis the initial erosive changes are best seen

in the sacro-iliac joints. In these conditions inflammatory reactions at the site of insertion of ligaments, tendons and muscles into bone may result in bony spur formation (enthesopathy), frequently seen in the pelvis. In Reiter's syndrome these changes may occur on the calcanei. In ankylosing spondylitis complete ankylosis of sacro-iliac joints may occur and ossification may bridge the intervertebral discs, resulting in an appearance referred to as 'bamboo spine' on plain radiography (Fig. 15.7).

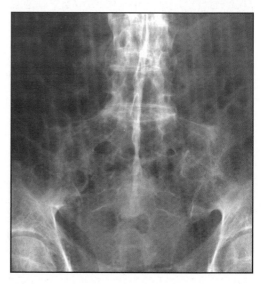

Fig. 15.7 Advanced ankylosing spondylitis. Bony ankylosis of sacro-iliac joints and spinal ligaments.

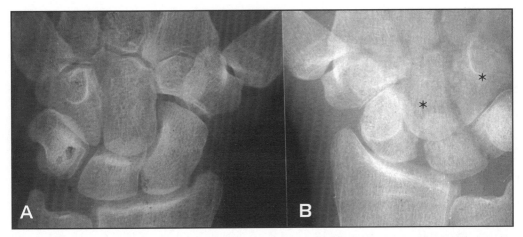

Fig. 15.8 Gonococcal arthritis. (A) Normal left wrist. (B) Generalized loss of density due to soft tissue swelling and osteopenia of the capitate and hamate (*) with loss of cortical outlines. The infection involved the midcarpal joint.

4. Suppurative arthritis

Pyogenic organisms cause acute joint pain, marked osteoporosis and destruction in the affected joint. In tuberculous arthritis the process is more chronic, as is the case with other less virulent organisms (Fig. 15.8).

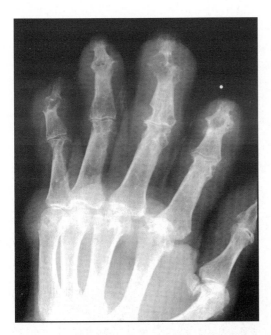

Fig. 15.9   Gout. Large well-defined periarticular bone erosions associated with soft tissue swellings (tophi) but with normal bone density (cf. rheumatoid).

5. Metabolic

Frequently a confident diagnosis of gout (Fig. 15.9) can be made from the radiographs. The following changes are best seen in hands and feet.

- Well-defined arc-shaped erosions, sometimes with a sclerotic margin, seen laterally at the bone ends. Occasionally the process may be more destructive leaving only a bony shell in the affected region.
- Joint swellings.
- Rounded soft tissue opacities due to tophi, i.e, subcutaneous nodules of sodium bi-urate.
- Normal bone density in the region.

Pseudo-gout in which calcium pyrophosphate crystals are found in the joint fluid may be associated with calcification of articular cartilages **(chondrocalcinosis)** particularly the menisci of the knee joints. Cartilage calcification also occurs in the arthritis associated with haemochromatosis.

6. Neuropathic joints

These may occur in patients with diabetes, syphilis, or syringomyelia and in younger patients with congenital absence of pain.

It is frequently stated that neuropathic arthritis is totally painless, but in adults this is not true. Patients usually complain of some pain but this is far less than expected from the degree of damage

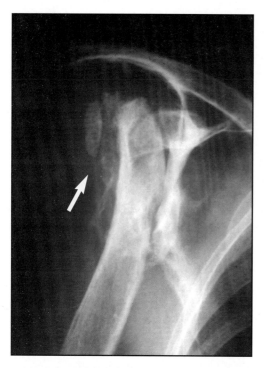

Fig. 15.10 Syringomyelia. Gross destruction of adjacent bones in the shoulder joint with residual bone debris (arrow) and preservation of bone density.

present. In syringomyelia only upper limb joints tend to be affected (Fig. 15.10). The radiological features are:

- Gross bony destruction leading to disorganization of the joint.
- Bone debris in surrounding tissues.
- Joint swelling.
- Normal or increased density of adjacent bones.

7. Haemorrhagic arthritis

Classically, the condition is seen in haemophiliacs. Repeated haemorrhages into a joint from an early age disturbs development. The epiphyses appear relatively enlarged and fuse prematurely. The expanded bone-ends may persist into adult life (Fig. 15.11). In addition, changes similar to osteoarthritis develop, often with large sub-articular cystic spaces.

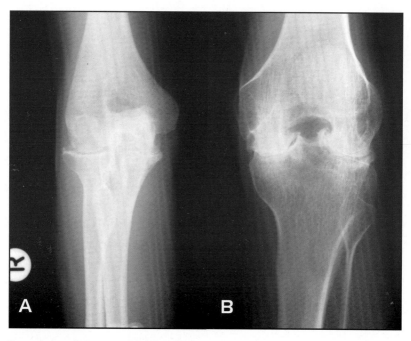

Fig. 15.11 Haemorrhagic arthritis. Gross osteoarthritic changes in elbow (A) and knee joints (B). The relatively expanded bone ends are characteristic. Diagnosis: Haemophilia.

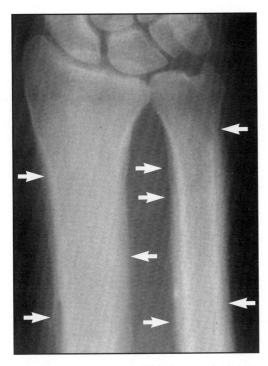

8. Hypertrophic pulmonary osteoarthropathy

Patients with lung pathology, particularly bronchial carcinoma, may first present with aches and pains suggesting polyarthritis. Plain radiography of the lower forearms and hands and distal tibiae, fibulae and feet may reveal periosteal reactions which are bilateral, symmetrical, and often associated with intra-articular effusions (Fig. 15.12). Finger clubbing is another feature of the condition.

Fig. 15.12 Hypertrophic pulmonary osteoarthropathy. Note the ill-defined periosteal reaction involving the distal forearm bones (arrows). Chest x-ray revealed bronchogenic carcinoma.

Reference

See Chapter 14.

A

Abscess
   abdominal, 205
   Brodie's, 267
   cerebral, 79
   lung, 17, 19
   perinephric, 186
   subphrenic, 205
Achalasia, 120
Acoustic neuroma, 83
Acromegaly, 102
Acute abdomen, 203
Addison's disease, 104
Adrenal glands, 104
Adrenogenital syndrome, 106
AIDS, 65
Air bronchogram, 20
Alveolar lung opacities, 33
Alzheimer's disease, 87
Aneurysm
   abdominal aorta, 59
   atheromatous, 57
   dissecting aortic, 57
   traumatic aortic, 58
Angioplasty, 55, 61
Angiography
   coronary, 55
   digital subtraction, 4, 6
   in GI bleeding, 213, 214
   lower limb, 61
   renal, 67
   subarachnoid haemorrhage, 75
Ankle injury, 254
Ankylosing spondylitis, 272
Antegrade pyelography, 183
Aorta
   abdominal, 59
   thoracic, 57

Appendicitis, 203
Arteriovenous malformation
   in brain, 75, 88
   in spinal cord, 91
Arthritis
   classification, 269
   haemorrhagic, 274
   in gout, 273
   in lung disease, 275
   neuropathic, 273
   osteo, 271
   rheumatoid, 271
Asbestosis, 35
Ascites, 165
Aseptic necrosis, 252
Asthma, 36
Astrocytoma, 79
Atalectasis, lung, 23
Atrial septal defect, 49

B

Barium
   enema, 135
   in GI bleeding, 214
   meal, 116
Bennett's fracture, 248
Biliary tract, 147
Biparietal diameter, of foetal head, 219
Bladder, urinary
   diverticulum, 193
   neck obstruction, 192
   neurogenic, 192
   trauma, 199
   tumours, 185
Blebs, 27
Blow-out fracture, orbit, 90
Bone
   fibrous dysplasia, 264